Reconstructive Transplantation and Regenerative Medicine

Gene and Cell Therapy Series

Series Editors: Anthony Atala & M. Graça Almeida-Porada

Published Titles:

Placenta: The Tree of Life
Edited by Ornella Parolini

Cellular Therapy for Neurological Injury
Edited by Charles S. Cox, Jr

Regenerative Medicine Technology: On-a-Chip Applications for Disease Modeling, Drug Discovery and Personalized Medicine
Edited by Sean V. Murphy and Anthony Atala

Therapeutic Applications of Adenoviruses
Edited by Philip Ng and Nicola Brunetti-Pierri

Gene and Cell Delivery for Invertebral Disk Degeneration
Edited by Raquel Madeira Gonçalves and Mario Adolfo Barbosa

Bioreactors for Stem Cell Expansion and Differentiation
Edited by Joaquim M. S. Cabral and Cláudia Lobato de Silva

Biomaterials for Cell Delivery: Vehicles in Regenerative Medicine
Edited by Aaron S. Goldstein

Reconstructive Transplantation and Regenerative Medicine: The Emerging Interface
Edited by Vijay Gorantla, Fatih Zor, and Jelena M. Janjic

For more information about this series, please visit:

https://www.crcpress.com/Gene-and-Cell-Therapy/book-series/CRCGENCELTHE

Reconstructive Transplantation and Regenerative Medicine

The Emerging Interface

Edited by

Vijay Gorantla, Fatih Zor, and Jelena M. Janjic

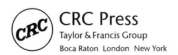

CRC Press
Taylor & Francis Group
Boca Raton London New York

CRC Press is an imprint of the
Taylor & Francis Group, an **informa** business

First edition published 2022
by CRC Press
6000 Broken Sound Parkway NW, Suite 300, Boca Raton, FL 33487-2742

and by CRC Press
2 Park Square, Milton Park, Abingdon, Oxon, OX14 4RN

© 2022 selection and editorial matter, Vijay Gorantla, Fatih Zor, and Jelena M. Janjic; individual chapters, the contributors

CRC Press is an imprint of Taylor & Francis Group, LLC

ISBN: 9780367202088 (hbk)
ISBN: 9781032116761 (pbk)
ISBN: 9780429260179 (ebk)

DOI: 10.1201/9780429260179

Typeset in Times
by KnowledgeWorks Global Ltd.

Contents

Contributors vii

SECTION I   Cellular Therapies in Reconstructive Transplantation

Chapter 1   Cell Therapies in Reconstructive Transplantation 3

   *Curtis L. Cetrulo, Jr., Amalya S. Wilson, Abraham Matar,
   Radbeh Torabi, Mohammadreza S. Pakyari, Elise Lupon,
   Marion Goutard, and Alexandre G. Lellouch*

Chapter 2   Novel T-Regulatory Cell-Based Therapies in Vascularized
   Composite Allotransplantation: Translational Implications 27

   *Yalcin Kulahci, Hulya Kapucu, James D. Fisher,
   and Steven R. Little*

SECTION II   Unique Considerations and Emerging Indications in Reconstructive Transplantation

Chapter 3   Invasive and Non-Invasive Surrogates for Chronic
   Rejection in Vascularized Composite Allotransplantation:
   Claims and Controversies..47

   Nicholas L. Robbins and Warren C. Breidenbach

Chapter 4   Reperfusion Injury in Vascularized Composite
   Tissue Allografts: Impact on Graft Outcomes and
   Preventive Strategies 61

   Kagan Ozer

Chapter 5   Pediatric Upper Extremity Vascularized Composite
   Allotransplantation: Progress and Insights 75

   *Kevin J. Zuo, Anna Gold, Randi Zlotnik Shaul,
   Emily S. Ho, Gregory H. Borschel, and Ronald M. Zuker*

SECTION III Graft Monitoring in Reconstructive Transplantation

Chapter 6   Targeted Imaging and Therapeutic Technologies
in Neuroregeneration 101

*Jelena M. Janjic, Mihály Balogh, Sandeep Kumar Reddy
Adena, Amanda Fitzpatrick, John A. Pollock,
Vijay Gorantla, and Andrew J. Shepherd*

Chapter 7   Biomarkers and Surrogates of Acute Rejection in
Vascularized Composite Allograft Transplantation 121

*Calum Honeyman, Helen Stark, Hayson Chenyu Wang,
Joanna Hester, Henk Giele, and Fadi Issa*

SECTION IV Composite Tissue Graft Manipulation and Engineering

Chapter 8   Bioengineering Composite Tissue Constructs:
Concepts and Challenges 149

*Kavit Amin, David Leonard, Li Yenn Yong, Ralph Murphy,
Roxana Moscalu, Kirsten Liggat, and Jason Wong*

Chapter 9   Advances in Biomaterials for Reconstructive Transplantation 171

Ashish Dhayani and Praveen Kumar Vemula

Chapter 10 Gene Editing Strategies for Immunomodulation:
Translation from Cells to Vascularized Tissues 195

Fatih Zor, Esra Goktas, and Vijay Gorantla

Index 207

Contributors

Sandeep Kumar Reddy Adena
Graduate School of Pharmaceutical
Sciences
Duquesne University
Pittsburgh, Pennsylvania
and
Department of Pharmaceutical
Engineering & Technology
Indian Institute of Technology
(Banaras Hindu University)
Varanasi, India

Kavit Amin
Department of Plastic & Reconstructive
Surgery
Manchester University NHS Foundation
Trust
and
Division of Infection, Immunity
& Respiratory Medicine
University of Manchester
Manchester, United Kingdom

Mihály Balogh
Department of Symptom Research
MD Anderson Cancer Center
The University of Texas
Houston, Texas

Gregory H. Borschel
Division of Plastic & Reconstructive
Surgery
Department of Surgery
Hospital for Sick Children
University of Toronto
Toronto, Canada

Warren C. Breidenbach
AIRMED Program
59th Medical Wing, JBSA Lackland
AFB
San Antonio, Texas

Curtis L. Cetrulo, Jr.
Reconstructive Transplantation Laboratory
Massachusetts General Hospital and
Massachusetts General Hospital for
Children
Harvard Medical School
and
Laboratory for Cellular Immunotherapy
Shriners Hospital for Children
Boston, Massachusetts

Ashish Dhayani
Institute for Stem Cell Science and
Regenerative Medicine (inStem)
Bengaluru, India
and
School of Chemical and Biotechnology
SASTRA University
Thanjavur, India

James D. Fisher
Department of Plastic Surgery
University of Pittsburgh
Pittsburgh, Pennsylvania

Amanda Fitzpatrick
Washington and Jefferson College
Washington, Pennsylvania

Henk Giele
Department of Plastic, Reconstructive
and Hand Surgery
Oxford University Hospitals NHS
Foundation Trust
John Radcliffe Hospital
Oxford, United Kingdom

Esra Goktas
Wake Forest University Health Sciences
Wake Forest Institute for Regenerative
Medicine
Winston Salem, North Carolina

Anna Gold
Department of Psychology
Transplant and Regenerative Medicine
    Centre
Hospital for Sick Children
University of Toronto
Toronto, Canada

Vijay Gorantla
Department of Surgery
Wake Forest University Health Sciences
Wake Forest Institute for Regenerative
    Medicine
Winston Salem, North Carolina

Marion Goutard
Division of Plastic Surgery
Vascularized Composite
    Allotransplantation Laboratory
Massachusetts General Hospital
Harvard Medical School and Shriners
    Hospitals for Children
Boston, Massachusetts

Joanna Hester
Transplantation Research &
    Immunology Group
Nuffield Department of Surgical
    Sciences
University of Oxford
Oxford, United Kingdom

Emily S. Ho
Division of Plastic & Reconstructive
    Surgery
Department of Occupational Science &
    Occupational Therapy
Hospital for Sick Children
University of Toronto
Toronto, Canada

Calum Honeyman
Canniesburn Plastic Surgery and Burns
    Unit
Glasgow Royal Infirmary
Scotland, United Kingdom

Fadi Issa
Medical Sciences Division
Nuffield Department of Surgical Sciences
University of Oxford
Oxford, United Kingdom
and
Department of Plastic Surgery and Burns
Buckinghamshire Healthcare NHS Trust
Aylesbury, United Kingdom

Jelena M. Janjic
Graduate School of Pharmaceutical
    Sciences
Duquesne University
Pittsburgh, Pennsylvania

Hulya Kapucu
Wake Forest Institute for Regenerative
    Medicine
Vascularized Composite
    Allotransplantation Laboratory
Winston-Salem, North Carolina

Yalcin Kulahci
Wake Forest Institute for Regenerative
    Medicine
Vascularized Composite
    Allotransplantation Laboratory
Winston-Salem, North Carolina

Alexandre G. Lellouch
European Georges Pompidou Hospital
    (AP-HP)
Paris, France
and
Vascularized Composite
    Allotransplantation Laboratory
Massachusetts General Hospital
Harvard Medical School
Boston, Massachusetts
and
CEA (French Alternative Energies and
    Atomic Energy Commission)
University of Paris
University Grenoble Alpes
Grenoble, France

David Leonard
Canniesburn Plastic Surgery Unit
Glasgow Royal Infirmary
Glasgow, United Kingdom

Kirsten Liggat
Division of Cell Matrix Biology &
    Regenerative Medicine
University of Manchester
Manchester, United Kingdom

Steven R. Little
Departments of Bioengineering,
    Chemical Engineering, and
    Immunology
McGowan Institute for Regenerative
    Medicine
Departments of Ophthalmology and
    Pharmaceutical Sciences
University of Pittsburgh
Pittsburgh, Pennsylvania

Elise Lupon
Department of Plastic Surgery
University Toulouse III Paul Sabatier
Hôpital Rangueil
Toulouse, France
and
Vascularized Composite
    Allotransplantation
    Laboratory
Center for Transplantation Sciences
Massachusetts General Hospital
Harvard Medical School
Boston, Massachusetts

Abraham Matar
Department of Surgery
Emory University
Atlanta, Georgia

Roxana Moscalu
Division of Cell Matrix Biology
    & Regenerative Medicine
University of Manchester
Manchester, United Kingdom

Ralph Murphy
Department of Plastic & Reconstructive
    Surgery
Manchester University NHS Foundation
    Trust
and
Division of Cell Matrix Biology
    & Regenerative Medicine
University of Manchester
Manchester, United Kingdom

Mohammadreza S. Pakyari
Massachusetts General Hospital and
    Brigham and Women's Hospital
Harvard Medical School
Boston, Massachusetts

John A. Pollock
Bayer School of Natural &
    Environmental Sciences
Duquesne University
Pittsburgh, Pennsylvania

Kagan Ozer
Department of Orthopedic and Plastic
    Surgery
University of Michigan
Ann Arbor, Michigan

Nicholas L. Robbins
AIRMED Program
59th Medical Wing
JBSA Lackland AFB
San Antonio, Texas
and
Department of Orthopedics
School of Medicine
University of Colorado
Aurora, Colorado

Randi Zlotnik Shaul
Department of Bioethics
Hospital for Sick Children
Department of Pediatrics
University of Toronto
Toronto, Canada

Andrew J. Shepherd
Department of Symptom Research
MD Anderson Cancer Center
The University of Texas
Houston, Texas

Helen Stark
Nuffield Department of Surgical Sciences
University of Oxford
John Radcliffe Hospital
Oxford, United Kingdom

Radbeh Torabi
Elite Plastic Surgery Arizona
Phoenix, Arizona

Praveen Kumar Vemula
Institute for Stem Cell Science and
    Regenerative Medicine (inStem)
Bengaluru, India

Hayson Chenyu Wang
Department of Plastic Surgery
Peking Union Medical College Hospital
Chinese Academy of Medical Sciences
    and Peking Union Medical College
Beijing, China

Amalya S. Wilson
Reconstructive Transplantation Laboratory
Massachusetts General Hospital
Boston, Massachusetts

Jason Wong
Department of Plastic & Reconstructive
    Surgery
Manchester University NHS Foundation
    Trust
and
Division of Cell Matrix Biology
    & Regenerative Medicine
University of Manchester
Manchester, United Kingdom

Li Yenn Yong
Department of Plastic & Reconstructive
    Surgery
Whiston Hospital
Liverpool, United Kingdom
and
Division of Cell Matrix Biology
    & Regenerative Medicine
University of Manchester
Manchester, United Kingdom

Fatih Zor
Department of Surgery
Wake Forest University Health
    Sciences
Wake Forest Institute for Regenerative
    Medicine
Winston Salem, North Carolina

Ronald M. Zuker
Division of Plastic & Reconstructive
    Surgery
Department of Surgery
Hospital for Sick Children
University of Toronto
Toronto, Canada

Kevin J. Zuo
Division of Plastic & Reconstructive
    Surgery
Hospital for Sick Children
Department of Surgery
University of Toronto
Toronto, Canada

Section I

Cellular Therapies in
Reconstructive Transplantation

1 Cell Therapies in Reconstructive Transplantation

Curtis L. Cetrulo, Jr., Amalya S. Wilson,
Abraham Matar, Radbeh Torabi,
Mohammadreza S. Pakyari, Elise Lupon,
Marion Goutard, and Alexandre G. Lellouch

CONTENTS

Introduction 4
Hematopoietic Cell Transplantation for Mixed Chimerism
and Tolerance Induction 5
   Preclinical Work 5
   Delayed Tolerance Induction 7
   Clinical Tolerance Studies..8
   Co-Stimulatory Blockade and Local Immunosuppression
   Technologies 8
   Mesenchymal Stem Cells and Regulatory Dendritic Cells 9
T Cells in Reconstructive Transplantation 9
   Regulatory T Cells 9
   Antigen-Specific Regulatory T Cells 10
   Chimeric Antigen Receptor T Cells 11
Decellularization and Recellularization of Composite Tissue
Allografts 14
   The Aim of Decellularization/Recellularization Technology............. 14
   Methods of Decellularization 14
   Approaches to Recellularization 15
   Decellularized Scaffolds Currently in Clinical Use and under
   Investigation... 16
   Vascularized Composite Allograft Decellularization 17
References 19

DOI: 10.1201/9780429260179-2

ABBREVIATIONS

Ag-specific	Antigen-specific
APC	Antigen-presenting cell
ATG	Anti-thymocyte globulin
BM	Bone marrow
BMT	Bone marrow transplant
CAR	Chimeric antigen receptor
CAR-T cell	CAR-modified T cell
CoB	Costimulation blockade
DBM	Donor bone marrow
DCregs	Regulatory dendritic cells
DE/RE	Decellularization/recellularization
DLA	Dog leukocyte antigen
DSA	Donor specific antibody
ECM	Extracellular matrix
ESC	Embryonic stem cell
ESRD	End-stage renal disease
FDA	Food and Drug Administration
GVHD	Graft-versus-host disease
HLA	Human leukocyte antigen
HCT	Hematopoietic cell transplantation
IL-2	Interleukin-2
iPSC	Induced pluripotent stem cell
MGH	Massachusetts General Hospital
MHC	Major histocompatibility complex
MMF	Mycophenolate mofetil
MSC	Mesenchymal stem cell
NAC	Nipple-areolar complex
NHP	Non-human primate
POD	Post-operative day
PSC	Pluripotent stem cell
scFv	Single-chain variable fragment
TAC	Tacrolimus
TBI	Total body irradiation
TCR	T-cell receptor
TESI	Tissue-engineered small intestine
Treg	Regulatory T cell
VBM	Vascularized bone marrow
VCA	Vascularized composite allograft

INTRODUCTION

Significant technical strides have been made in the last two decades in the area of reconstructive transplantation/vascularized composite allotransplantation (VCA) such that VCA is now a realistic option for patients with significant tissue loss.[1-4] Like solid organ transplantation, a major barrier to long-term VCA survival and function is control of the allogeneic immune response. Acute and chronic rejections pose significant clinical challenges particularly after VCA for several reasons.[5] First, unlike solid organs, VCAs are not subject to major histocompatibility complex (MHC) antigen matching due to the small donor pool.[6] Therefore, VCAs are often transplanted across MHC mismatched barriers, which increases the likelihood of an alloimmune response after transplantation. Second, the increased immunogenicity of skin relative to other tissues and organ types is well-documented, owing to an increased frequency of antigen presenting Langerhans cells which become activated upon antigenic stimulation to express MHC class II, proinflammatory cytokines, and adhesion molecules.[7] Illustrative of this relatively high immunogenicity, split tolerance, in which the skin component of the VCA (usually the epidermis) is rejected while the other components remain viable, is a commonly observed phenomenon in VCA immunologic tolerance research.[8]

In order to suppress the alloimmune response following VCA, potent immune suppressing agents are necessary, including steroids, calcineurin inhibitors, and T-cell depleting agents. The long-term sequelae of chronic immunosuppression are well-known and include increased risk of infection, malignancy, and medication side effects. Exposing VCA patients to these risks is particularly worrisome given the nature of VCA as a life-enhancing rather than a life-saving (such as a heart) allograft. Furthermore, despite the use of immunosuppressive agents, the risk of acute and chronic rejections following VCA is significantly higher than after solid organ transplantation. Strategies to modulate the immune system in favor of VCA tolerance or reduced requirement for high levels of immunosuppressive medications are of great clinical interest in order to prevent rejection episodes, minimize morbidity, and improve long-term graft outcomes. Herein, we will highlight several of these cell therapy immunomodulatory and tolerance-inducing strategies and their evolution from murine and large animal preclinical models to the clinic.

HEMATOPOIETIC CELL TRANSPLANTATION FOR MIXED CHIMERISM AND TOLERANCE INDUCTION

PRECLINICAL WORK

In preclinical murine and large animal models, hematopoietic cell transplantation (HCT) is a commonly employed strategy to induce mixed hematopoietic chimerism and confer immunological tolerance to a donor allograft, obviating the need for chronic immunosuppression. In some cases, these studies have successfully been translated to the clinic in the form of combined HCT and renal transplantation.[9–11] Ildstad and Sachs were among the first to demonstrate in a murine model that reconstitution of a recipient with allogeneic bone marrow (BM) facilitated donor-specific tolerance to a skin allograft.[12,13] These findings were then successfully translated to a variety of large animal swine and non-human primate (NHP) models by the Massachusetts General Hospital (MGH) group, in which either stable or transient mixed chimerism facilitated tolerance to a host of organs including kidney, composite "islet-kidneys", lung, and heart.[14–22] In a seminal 2008 report by Kawai et al., immune tolerance was achieved in humans following combined BM and kidney transplantation for end-stage renal disease (ESRD) secondary to multiple myeloma.[9] Four of five patients were successfully weaned off immunosuppression and maintained stable renal function. Subsequently, other groups validated the use of a non-myeloablative conditioning regimen and HCT as a practical and safe means of inducing mixed chimerism and immune tolerance in solid organ transplantation.[10,11]

As VCA has continued to emerge, the use of mixed chimerism has been studied in both murine and large animal models to prevent rejection and prolong graft survival. Tung et al. first evaluated a regimen consisting of T-cell depletion (CD4/CD8), costimulation blockade (anti-CD154), and donor bone marrow (DBM) infusion with or without low dose irradiation on VCA survival.[23,24] In both regimens (with and without irradiation), the addition of DBM induced transient mixed chimerism and prolonged graft survival but was not sufficient to induce true immunological tolerance. Histological analysis of rejected VCA grafts in recipients of DBM was consistent with a chronic rejection process.

Based on successful induction of tolerance to solid organ grafts in large animals, the mixed chimerism approach has been employed to induce VCA tolerance in several large animal models including canine, swine, and NHP. In a canine model, Mathes et al. demonstrated that recipients previously made mixed chimeric through dog leukocyte antigen (DLA) identical bone marrow transplant (BMT) were tolerant of VCA allografts transplanted between 52–90 weeks after BMT.[25] Given that clinical VCA grafts are derived from deceased donors, this time interval between BMT and VCA transplantation is not clinically feasible. As a result, Mathes et al. employed the same model to determine if simultaneous BMT + VCA could induce VCA tolerance.[26] All animals receiving simultaneous BMT + VCA were tolerant of their VCA grafts > 62 weeks, indicating that preexisting mixed chimerism and immune tolerance were not a prerequisite for induction of VCA tolerance. Finally, when this model was extended across a single MHC barrier (DLA haploidentical) to more accurately reflect a clinical scenario, only one of four recipients of combined BMT + VCA maintained VCA tolerance following cessation of immunosuppression.[27] Interestingly, all four recipients of cytokine "mobilized" HCT + VCA maintained long-term VCA tolerance, indicating that stem cell quality and differences in T-cell phenotyping within the grafts may be critical for VCA tolerance induction.[27]

Similar findings have been demonstrated in a haploidentical swine model. Leonard et al. reported the development of stable mixed chimerism across a haploidentical MHC barrier and tolerance to VCA grafts transplanted either simultaneously or after the establishment of chimerism.[28] In the same model, Shanmugarajah et al. studied the impact of MHC class I and II matching on VCA tolerance. In MHC class I mismatched recipients, VCA skin was rejected despite recipients remaining mixed chimeric and maintaining in vitro unresponsiveness to donor antigen. These findings suggest that local regulatory mechanisms are crucial to establishing and maintaining skin tolerance. Further, MHC class I antigen matching may be a clinical strategy to lower acute rejection rates and improve VCA survival.

Although canine and swine models have been integral in providing mechanistic insights into VCA tolerance, NHP may provide a more clinically relevant model for studies of mixed chimerism and VCA tolerance. Early studies in NHP worked to establish technically feasible and immunologically sound models that would allow for the study of immune modulating strategies.[29–31] Two subsequent studies evaluated the impact of vascularized bone marrow (VBM) and infused BM on VCA survival in NHP.[32,33] Murine studies have indicated that VBM is a crucial component of VCA for tolerance induction and that VBM as part of a VCA graft is capable of inducing significant levels of peripheral mixed chimerism (10–20%) in the setting of costimulation blockade (CoB) and total body irradiation (TBI).[34,35] In cynomolgus macaques, Barth et al. evaluated the immunological impact of VBM by incorporating the donor mandible in a facial segment VCA model. Tacrolimus (TAC) and mycophenolate mofetil (MMF) were used for post-grafting immunosuppression. VCA grafts without VBM experienced early acute rejection episodes and were uniformly rejected by post-operative day (POD) 42. Despite only receiving marrow in the form of vascularized donor mandible, recipients receiving VCA + VBM demonstrated evidence of transient macro chimerism in the peripheral blood (1–12%). VBM significantly prolonged VCA survival time to 267–462 days. However, transient macro chimerism was not sufficient to induce true immunological tolerance as VCA grafts were rejected upon discontinuation of immunosuppression. Future VCA + VBM studies may employ different immunosuppressive strategies, such as CoB and TBI, which have been shown in murine models to facilitate donor hematopoietic cell migration from the VBM niche and thymic engraftment with deletion of donor-reactive T-cell clones.[34]

Brazio et al. then compared the results achieved with VBM described by Barth to recipients receiving infused BM in the same model. Interestingly, despite a ~6x higher total BM cell dose, no animals receiving infused BM demonstrated evidence of mixed chimerism, and the median rejection-free survival time was no different than for NHP receiving VCA alone without BM. The absence of mixed chimerism in this model could be attributed to the lack of lymphocyte-depleting agents or the use of irradiation as part of the conditioning regimen, which may have impacted donor stem cell engraftment. Collectively, these observations suggest that VBM confers an immunological benefit in the setting of VCA transplant and may be superior to infused BM. Similar observations have been made in murine models.[35]

DELAYED TOLERANCE INDUCTION

As in humans, HCT in NHP induces transient chimerism rather than stable chimerism, which may be attributed to a more robust memory T-cell repertoire in NHP compared to other large animals. One strategy to overcome these memory T-cell responses in NHP and achieve tolerance induction has been the development of the "delayed BMT protocol", which involves organ transplantation using standard immunosuppression followed by delayed conditioning and BMT with cryopreserved donor BM after a period of two to four months. This protocol offers two advantages. First, in theory, this delay allows for a reduction in inflammation associated with the perioperative period, which may serve as an impediment to stem cell engraftment and tolerance induction. Second, a delayed BM protocol would significantly increase the donor pool by allowing the use of deceased donors. Due to the preconditioning prior to BMT, solid organ tolerance induction protocols have largely involved the use of living donors because of the difficulty in predicting when an organ may become available. By cryopreserving donor BM at the time of organ procurement, recipients can undergo preconditioning at a later time followed by BMT. This delayed BMT protocol has successfully induced tolerance to renal and lung allografts in NHP.[18,19] Lellouch et al. attempted to translate this model to induce VCA tolerance in cynomolgus macaques.[36] Recipients underwent either hand or face VCA allografts across both haploidentical and full MHC barriers and received standard triple immunosuppression and T-cell depletion with anti-thymocyte globulin (ATG). Despite this potent immunosuppression regimen, VCA allografts experienced acute rejection episodes in the interval between VCA transplant and BMT, a phenomenon not encountered in prior studies of renal or lung transplant. Subsequently, conditioning and BMT two months following VCA were unsuccessful in inducing mixed chimerism, and VCA grafts eventually succumbed to graft vasculopathy. An activated immune response in the setting of acute rejection episodes prior to BMT may have had a detrimental effect on chimerism and tolerance induction at the time of BMT. Collectively, these findings highlight the significant immunogenicity of VCA grafts relative to solid organ grafts and the need for further immune modulating strategies to induce chimerism and tolerance to VCA in NHP.

CLINICAL TOLERANCE STUDIES

Largely as a result of the success in swine models,[8] a trial of BM infusion was attempted in five human recipients of VCA (bilateral hand n = 2; unilateral hand n = 2; bilateral hand/forearm n = 1).[37] Patients received induction therapy with alemtuzumab and methylprednisolone and were maintained on TAC monotherapy posttransplant. At the time of procurement, BM was harvested from vertebral bodies and cryopreserved. On POD 14, unmodified BM cells were infused intravenously at a dose of $5–10 \times 10^8$ cells/kg body weight (CD34 dose was $\geq 2 \times 10^6$/kg). Overall, all five recipients were maintained on TAC monotherapy with 100% graft survival and acceptable function at one-year post-transplant. All five recipients experienced acute rejection episodes in the first-year post-transplant, but all episodes were successfully treated with either topical agents alone or a short course of steroids. TAC monotherapy represents a significant decrease in immunosuppression compared to historical controls of VCA allografts, which were often maintained using triple immunosuppression (TAC, MMF, steroids) post-transplantation. BM infusion with cryopreserved unmodified cells was safe and not associated with any side effects, including no evidence of graft-versus-host disease (GVHD). These promising results in a small cohort of patients justify further study of BM infusion in VCA transplantation.

CO-STIMULATORY BLOCKADE AND LOCAL IMMUNOSUPPRESSION TECHNOLOGIES

While hematopoietic cell transplant offers an opportunity to induce tolerance, other adjunctive strategies, including CoB-based immunosuppression, cellular therapies, and local immunosuppression, have been studied in an attempt to control rejection episodes and minimize immunosuppression. Freitas et al. compared standard calcineurin inhibition to CoB of the CD28-CD80/86 in an NHP VCA model and found that, overall, CoB prevented production of donor specific antibody (DSA) and conferred a survival benefit.[38] Given similar findings in clinical renal transplantation,[39] further study should be given to optimizing CoB-based therapies for VCA.

There is significant evidence demonstrating the rejection of skin VCA in the setting of mixed chimerism and in vitro donor unresponsiveness, suggesting that control of local allogeneic responses at the skin level may require a higher threshold. Local immunosuppression at the site of VCA may help control skin-directed allogeneic responses while minimizing the systemic effects of immunosuppression. Fries et al. studied the use of an enzyme responsive, TAC-eluting hydrogel in a swine limb VCA model.[40] Once implanted, the hydrogel releases the contained drug (TAC) in response to catalytic enzymes released during inflammation. This approach has been successfully used in rodent models to prolong VCA survival, while minimizing systemic levels of immunosuppression.[41,42] In swine, a single injection of the TAC hydrogel significantly prolonged survival time of VCAs transplanted across a single haplotype MHC barrier (56–93 days), compared to untreated controls (6 days). This proof-of-principle study demonstrated that local immunosuppression in the form of a drug eluting hydrogel may be a useful adjunct in clinical VCA.

MESENCHYMAL STEM CELLS AND REGULATORY DENDRITIC CELLS

Other cell therapies offer promising adjunctive additions to HCT and tolerance induction protocols. Compared to HCT alone, which can be associated with significant patient morbidity due to the harsh conditioning regimen, cellular therapies including regulatory dendritic cells (DCregs) and mesenchymal stem cells (MSCs) offer a targeted approach to modulating the immune system. Ezzelarab et al. studied the impact of DCregs, a regulatory cell type with immune modulating capabilities, on renal allograft survival in NHP.[43,44] The infusion of donor-derived DCregs prior to renal transplantation suppressed rejection and prolonged graft survival significantly.[43] Studies are currently underway to generate swine DCregs for use in a VCA model.[45] MSCs are multipotent adult stem cells found in multiple tissues and are capable of differentiating into several mesenchymal cell types.[46] MSCs do not express immunogenic costimulatory molecules such as CD40, B7-1, or B7-2, and MSCs have shown to have immunomodulatory effects, such as inhibiting T-cell activation and increasing regulatory T-cell populations.[47–49] In several studies by Kuo and colleagues, donor-derived MSCs were used as an adjunct to HCT to prolong VCA survival in swine models.[48,50,51] Interestingly, when MSCs were infused alone without concomitant immunosuppression, there was only a modest impact on allograft survival. However, when incorporated into an HCT regimen consisting of irradiation, calcineurin inhibition, and BMT, the impact of MSCs was augmented and VCA survival was significantly improved.

T CELLS IN RECONSTRUCTIVE TRANSPLANTATION

REGULATORY T CELLS

Regulatory T cells (Tregs) are a population of lymphocytes that play an essential role in suppressing autoimmunity, controlling inflammation, and maintaining peripheral T-cell tolerance. Of all regulatory cells, $CD4^+CD25^+Foxp3^+$ Tregs are particularly potent regulators.[52] Expression of the Foxp3 transcription factor is key for the development and function of Tregs,[52] and Tregs require costimulation by molecules such as CD28 to be fully functional.[53] Tregs mediate crucial immunoregulatory tasks by suppressing the function and expansion of conventional T cells and other immune cells, and utilize both contact-dependent and contact-independent mechanisms to do so.[54] One such contact-independent mechanism involves the release of suppressive cytokines including IL-10, transforming growth factor (TGF)-β, and IL-35.[55] In the context of transplantation, preclinical data has indicated that the immunosuppressive properties of Tregs are instrumental in the prevention of allograft rejection.[56] Moreover, Tregs represent a promising avenue for developing therapies for tolerance induction. Thus, extensive effort has been devoted to utilizing the immunosuppressive qualities of Tregs to induce tolerance in transplantation, including VCA,[57] HCT,[58] and solid organ transplantation.[59]

While Tregs are present in the peripheral blood and allograft of transplant recipients, the quantity of Tregs is not sufficient to effectively prevent allograft rejection following transplantation.[60] In fact, Tregs exist in particularly small quantities in the peripheral blood, with naturally occurring Tregs composing no more than 10% of peripheral CD4+ T cells.[61] Despite the insufficiency of naturally occurring Tregs, their immunosuppressive properties make them an attractive potential therapeutic option for inducing tolerance. Thus, in addition to exploring alternative sources of Tregs such as BM blood or umbilical blood, much of the effort to utilize Tregs for tolerance induction has been focused on expanding the recipient's Treg population.[62]

Treg therapy is currently in clinical development for the treatment of GVHD,[63] autoimmune disorders,[64,65] and allograft rejection.[56,66] Two established approaches to Treg therapy include (i) bringing about in vivo Treg expansion through the use of pharmacological strategies such as alloantigen infusion,[67] CoB,[68] and interleukin-2 (IL-2)[69] and (ii) utilizing ex vivo-expanded recipient or third-party Tregs for adoptive transfer or retransfer.[70] Studies utilizing in vivo expansion of or adoptive transfer of Tregs in animal models and clinical trials have shown to be safe and achieved encouraging results regarding tolerance induction.[71,72] Currently, the majority of ongoing clinical trials for Treg therapy utilize polyclonal Tregs with undetermined antigen specificity.[73] However, several major hurdles to the clinical implementation of polyclonal-Treg-based therapies for tolerance persist, including the need for Treg activation for enhanced suppressive functions, the requirement of Treg localization to the site of inflammation to minimize the risk of non-specific immunosuppression, and the large number of functional Tregs needed for effective therapy.[74]

ANTIGEN-SPECIFIC REGULATORY T CELLS

The use of antigen-specific (Ag-specific) Tregs presents a promising pathway for overcoming the challenges associated with polyclonal Treg therapy. Therapies utilizing Tregs specific for a desired antigen require fewer cells to prevent graft rejection and have reduced off-target effects due to more targeted suppression of the immune response.[66,75] Additionally, Ag-specific Tregs have shown to be functionally superior to polyclonal Tregs.[66] Clinical trials involving Ag-specific Tregs are currently in progress and significant research is underway focusing on developing techniques for the isolation, expansion, and engineering of Ag-specific Tregs.[76,77]

An established approach for generating Ag-specific Tregs involves the repetitive stimulation of polyclonal Tregs with donor antigen-presenting cells (APCs) to expand the population of Ag-specific Tregs among the original polyclonal Treg population.[67] While this approach effectively increases the quantity of Ag-specific Tregs, the method is inefficient as there are limited Ag-specific Tregs within the original population of polyclonal Tregs.[66] Another approach for generating Ag-specific Tregs utilizes the engineering of Tregs with T-cell receptors (TCR-Tregs). TCR-Tregs have shown to be more effective than polyclonal Tregs in preclinical models of hemophilia,[78] multiple sclerosis (MS),[79] and transplantation.[80] However, TCR-Tregs are MHC-restricted and thus limited in terms of their application.[81]

CHIMERIC ANTIGEN RECEPTOR T CELLS

One strategy for generating Ag-specific Tregs that overcome the MHC restrictions of TCR-Tregs involves the use of chimeric antigen receptor (CAR) technology. CAR-modified T cells (CAR-T cells) typically contain a single-chain variable fragment (scFv) derived from the monoclonal antibody, a transmembrane domain, an extracellular hinge, and an intracellular signaling region (Figure 1.1).[81]

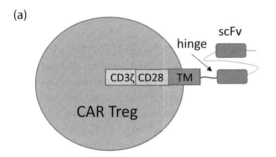

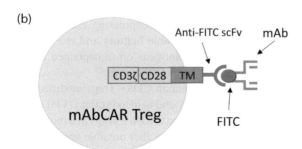

FIGURE 1.1 Schematic representation of a regulatory T cell (Treg) with a 2nd generation chimeric antigen receptor (CAR). The CAR-Treg consists of costimulatory domains (CD3ζ and CD28), a transmembrane domain (TM), an extracellular hinge, and a single-chain variable fragment (scFv) (a). Representation of a mAbCAR Treg expressing anti-FITC scFv with a FITC-conjugated mAb (b).

Currently, CAR-T cells are mainly used for cancer immunotherapy; CD19-targeted CAR-T cells have shown to be an effective therapy for treatment-resistant hematologic malignancies, and several CAR-T cell therapies have gained Food and Drug Administration (FDA) approval for use in clinical treatments.[82–84] As CARs have demonstrated their efficacy in animal models and the clinic, CAR technology has rapidly accumulated interest, and this interest has expanded to developing new CARs and broadening CAR-T cell therapies to treat solid tumors as well as for novel applications, such as autoimmunity and transplant tolerance. As tolerance-promoting cell therapies look to overcome the limitations of polyclonal Tregs and TCR-Tregs, Tregs expressing CARs tailored for disease-relevant antigens offer promise for transplantation.

MacDonald et al. engineered human Tregs with a CAR specific for human leukocyte antigen-A2 (HLA-A2), an antigen that is particularly prevalent among Caucasian donors and for which mismatching is associated with poor transplantation outcomes.[85,86] The group administered these A2-CAR-Tregs in vivo to treat xenogeneic GVHD induced by HLA-A2+ human cells in an immunodeficient mouse model.[35] Compared to mice receiving the control CAR-Tregs (stimulated only through the endogenous TCR), mice receiving A2-CAR-Tregs showed significant improvement in the prevention of xenogeneic GVHD and survival as the A2-CAR-Tregs resulted in stronger Ag-specific activation and proliferation.[86] Interestingly, unlike the control CAR-Tregs, the A2-CAR-Tregs could also stimulate IL-2 independent Treg proliferation in the short term.[86]

In addition to demonstrated efficacy for GVHD, A2-CAR-Tregs have also proven to be effective in the prevention of HLA-A2+ skin allograft rejection.[87] Injected A2-CAR-Tregs almost fully inhibited the allospecific immune reaction and prevented the killing of allogeneic targets in a mouse model, while control CAR-Tregs and unmodified Tregs inhibited the immune response to a smaller degree and had only a minor effect in preventing the killing of allogeneic targets.[87] Additionally, crucial to the success of Ag-specific or polyclonal Tregs is the homing of the regulatory cells to the graft.[88] Histologic testing indicated that the transferred A2-CAR-Tregs in this mouse model homed to the skin allografts and persisted within the graft long-term.[87] Another study found that, compared to polyclonal Tregs, A2-CAR-Tregs transmigrated through alloantigen-expressing endothelial cells significantly faster and demonstrated a more favorable homing and retention in allografts, suggesting that expression of targeted antigens on transplanted cells likely stimulates localization of Ag-specific CAR-Tregs to the graft.[89]

Interestingly, in a novel study, human CD8+ Tregs modified by CAR expression and directed toward HLA-A2 were found to also inhibit GVHD and solid organ graft rejection more effectively than polyclonal CD8+ Tregs in a mouse model.[90] Therefore, CAR-modified CD8+ Tregs may offer another possible approach to CAR-Treg based therapies as polyclonal CD8+ Tregs have shown to have a suppressive effect similar to that of CD4+ Tregs,[91] CD8+ Tregs have shown superior expansion in vitro compared to CD4+ Tregs,[91] and Ag-specific CD8+ Tregs have demonstrated efficacy in vitro and in animal models although they are yet to be tested in a clinical model.[90,92]

To better understand how CAR-modified CD4+ Tregs may alter the immune response and affect Ag-specific tolerance, Pierini et al. developed CAR-Tregs (referred to as mAbCAR) that express a FITC-targeted CAR and can be activated by various FITC-conjugated mAbs.[74] Mice receiving H-2D^d-mAbCAR Tregs targeted to an MHC-I antigen H-2D^d expressed by the allograft showed prolonged and enhanced islet allograft survival compared to mice receiving control mAbCAR Tregs or no Tregs after islet transplantation.[74] Importantly, although the expression of the CAR construct was transient, Treg localization and allograft tolerance persisted long-term, and the single introduction of transiently expressing CAR-Tregs led to persistent Ag-specific peripheral tolerance as mice receiving H-2Dd-mAbCAR Tregs later accepted MHC-matched secondary skin allografts while rejecting "third-party" grafts.[74] Furthermore, mAbCAR Tregs offer many advantages over the more rigid designs of earlier generation CAR-Tregs. Any monoclonal antibody can be recognized by mAbCAR Tregs through coupling the monoclonal antibody with FITC, thus permitting increasingly flexible and modular targeting of the CAR-Tregs.[74]

These numerous studies demonstrate the ability to redirect the specificity of human Tregs toward a transplant-relevant antigen using CAR, the efficacy of CAR-Tregs in inhibiting the immune response and preventing allograft rejection, the preferential homing of CAR-Tregs to the graft, and the potential lasting regulatory effects of transient CAR expression. Thus, these reports indicate that CAR-Tregs should indeed be further pursued as a potential Ag-specific cell therapy for clinical transplantation that overcomes the challenges associated with polyclonal Treg therapy and TCR-Treg therapy. However, the use of CAR-Tregs to promote allograft tolerance is a novel application with very limited clinical testing to date, and the approach could have a variety of pitfalls. A major concern with CAR-T cell therapies for cancer treatment is the risk of cytokine release syndrome,[93] and it is yet to be determined whether CAR-Treg therapies for transplant tolerance could induce a similar adverse reaction.[81] However, the reported risk of cytokine release syndrome in CAR-T cell clinical trials utilizing Tregs appears to be minor as Tregs do not release pro-inflammatory cytokines.[94] Even so, due to their potentially unstable phenotype, Tregs can actually lose their regulatory profile and take on an effector T-cell phenotype in inflammatory environments.[95] The formerly regulatory cells may begin to produce inflammatory cytokines rather than control the immune response, a devastating outcome that is a great concern with all Treg therapies.[95] Additionally, the long-term effect of repeated CAR stimulation on Tregs is yet to be determined,[77] as is the possibility of CAR-Treg exhaustion leading to limited suppression.

As investigators make progress with ongoing CAR-Treg therapies in animal models and early clinical trials, additional clinical trials evaluating CAR-Tregs for tolerance induction will emerge in the coming years. These necessary clinical trials will shed light on the potential of CAR-Tregs to be used independently or in conjunction with other therapies to promote allograft tolerance for multiple-tissue-type allografts and across MHC barriers, while also providing an enhanced understanding of what risks and challenges may arise with CAR-Treg therapies. Furthermore, the breadth of ongoing clinical trials using CAR technology for cancer immunotherapy will also support the development of CARs for transplantation tolerance as the advantages and limitations of CARs come to be better understood.

DECELLULARIZATION AND RECELLULARIZATION OF COMPOSITE TISSUE ALLOGRAFTS

THE AIM OF DECELLULARIZATION/RECELLULARIZATION TECHNOLOGY

Decellularization/recellularization (DE/RE) represents a promising pathway for overcoming many of the current challenges of transplantation, including tissue shortages and the long-term sequelae of chronic immunosuppression. Decellularization of organs and structures such as the liver, the heart, a whole limb, or the face can produce a non-immunogenic, biological scaffold that can undergo autologous recellularization and then be transplanted in such a way as to restore, maintain, or improve the function of the tissue or organ. Additionally, these scaffolds can potentially be repopulated with patient-derived cells, thus mitigating or eliminating the need for immunosuppression.[96] Furthermore, these cells can attach, proliferate, and execute specialized functions as they would in the original organ or structure, thus preserving the biological, mechanical, and geometric properties of the native tissue.[97]

The decellularization process allows the elimination of native cells while preserving the extracellular matrix (ECM). The resulting natural 3D scaffold offers many advantages over synthetic structures. These advantages include the preservation of the native tissue architecture, which is often difficult and costly to otherwise create on a large scale, and the preservation of the vascular network, which is currently impossible to reproduce using other techniques. The ECM also contains growth factors and cytokines that facilitate cell attachment and proliferation, and the ECM retains biochemical, physical, and biomechanical properties specific to the native specimen that mediate tissue remodeling following implantation.[96] Once the original cells have been removed, recellularization involves repopulating the decellularized tissue in order to render the construct viable and transplantable.

METHODS OF DECELLULARIZATION

Decellularization strategies aim to remove the cells in the tissue while preserving the three-dimensional ultrastructure of the ECM. Two different techniques used for decellularization include perfusion through the pedicle (artery and vein) and imbibition.[96] For solid organs, decellularization is performed using the perfusion approach by flushing the pedicle with detergent solutions.[98] Some commonly used chemical detergents include sodium dodecyl sulphate, Triton X-100, CHAPS, acids and bases, hypotonic and hypertonic solutions, alcohols, acetone, and tributyl phosphate. Perfusion through the vascular system is an effective method for homogenously delivering the detergent solution. However, the perfusion approach is not feasible for certain tissues such as the skin and tendons, and thus the imbibition technique is used in these circumstances.[99]

Other chemical strategies employed in the decellularization process include the use of enzymatic agents (nucleases, trypsin, collagenases), non-enzymatic agents, and chelating agents. The use of various physical agents (temperature, pressure, non-thermal irreversible electroporation) in the decellularization process has also been described.[99,100] Furthermore, induction of a pressure gradient across the tissue during

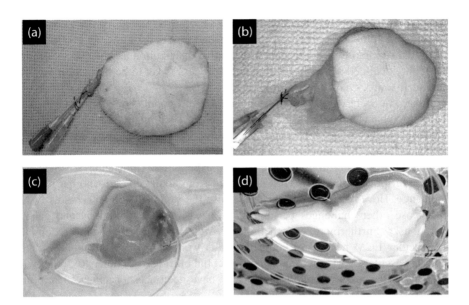

FIGURE 1.2 Swine fasciocutaneous flap before decellularization (a) and following decellularization (b). Rat hind limb before decellularization (c) and following decellularization (d).

decellularization has been used to supplement enzymatic treatment, resulting in improved preservation of the ultrastructure.[99] Another technique used for decellularization involves using supercritical fluid of carbon dioxide, which removes cellular residues when it passes through tissues at a controlled rate similar to that of critical point drying.[99]

While there are many different strategies for decellularization, the techniques employed for a specific graft depend on the clinical application, the tissue's properties, and the desired end product. Regardless of the technique used, effective removal of the native antigenic epitopes from the tissue is necessary in the decellularization process to avoid an adverse immune response from allogeneic or xenogeneic recipients of the ECM scaffold. However, complete decellularization of the tissue is not yet possible and most ECM scaffolds retain a small amount of residual DNA,[101] cytoplasmic material, and nuclear material of unknown immunogenicity.[102] The many chemical and physical techniques utilized in decellularization must balance efficiently, removing the cellular and nuclear material while not altering the composition of the ECM and causing ultrastructure disruption.

APPROACHES TO RECELLULARIZATION

The techniques used for recellularization of organ scaffolds include cell culture, tissue-engineering, cell-transplantation therapies, and isolated-organ perfusion. The process of recellularization involves two main steps: (i) cell seeding, in which selected cell populations are provided in order to repopulate the decellularized ECM, and then (ii) cell infusion, which is used to prepare the organ for an in vivo transplantation. A major challenge in cell seeding is providing the appropriate mixture and number of cells, and then placing these cells in the necessary niches within the scaffold in order to match the native distribution as much as possible.[96] While the ideal cell source for the seeding process is yet to be defined, many different cell sources have been studied.

Embryonic stem cells (ESCs) are an interesting population of clinically viable progenitors that can be used as a cell source for the seeding process because of their pluripotent characteristics. However, there are ethical and supply issues associated with using ESCs. Additionally, while once believed to be immune privileged, ESCs are now known to be immunogenic as they express HLA molecules on their surface.[103] Pluripotent stem cells (PSCs) derived from adult cells are another possible cell source. However, while PSCs do not raise the same ethical concerns as ESCs, PSCs pose other challenges pertaining to disease-related mutations and genetic alterations.[100] Furthermore, endothelial cells are also frequently used to repopulate the vascular ECM network. Endothelial cells work to prevent thrombosis of the exposed vascular ECM that can result in potential graft loss. Of note, no studies with vascular recellularization published to date have been able to achieve macro and micro vessel recellularization.

Depending on the cell type, cell infusion is performed using different techniques. One technique involves recellularization via the vascular network or another hollow structure (e.g. ureter, airway, intestinal lumen, or bile duct).[104] Cell infusion can also be performed via direct cellular injection into the parenchymal compartment.[104] Additionally, combinations of both techniques have been studied.[104] Cells are also delivered to the decellularized organ by perfusion using a bioreactor.[96] The bioreactor system is designed to provide a continuous flow of media (including growth factors and nutrients) and the selected cell populations. The bioreactor promotes tissue maturation and cell viability in order to prepare the organ for in vivo transplantation.

DECELLULARIZED SCAFFOLDS CURRENTLY IN CLINICAL USE AND UNDER INVESTIGATION

Biological scaffolds composed of decellularized ECM are used for the repair of various tissues, including skin,[105] bladder,[106,107] heart valves,[108,109] and vascular graft.[110] Several decellularized tissues have received FDA approval for clinical use in humans. Porcine heart valves (Synergraft®; Cryolife), dermal tissue (Alloderm®; LifeCell), and porcine bladder (bladder matrix; ACell) are commercially available.[111,112] However, while a number of skin substitutes and dermal matrices have been produced and commercialized, none thus far have truly functioned as full-thickness skin. Additionally, as of now, no DE/RE solid organs have been successfully re-implanted in humans.[113]

Beyond the applications of DE/RE currently being used in the clinic, there has been much success with pre-clinical models of DE/RE with various tissues and organs. In 2008, Ott et al. decellularized a heart, preserved the ECM, and then created functional heart valves, an intact vascular network, and a competent atrial and ventricular chamber geometry.[114] After maturing in a bioreactor system for eight days, the cardiac scaffolds of the decellularized rat were reseeded with neonatal rat cardiac and endothelial cells. The recellularized scaffold demonstrated contractile function and electrical responses to stimulation. In recent years, there has been considerable success with porcine hearts[115] and human myocardial tissue decellularization.[98,116] Moreover, two years after decellularizing rat hearts, Ott et al. and Petersen et al. decellularized rat lungs.[114,117] The bioengineered lungs were successfully transplanted into rats and effectively participated in gas exchange. The lungs were perfused with the recipient's circulation and ventilated using the recipient's airway and respiratory muscles, allowing for the in vivo gas exchange after transplantation. More recently, pig lungs[118] and human lungs[119] have been decellularized, and scaffolds of decellularized pig lungs have shown to have properties similar to those of human lungs.

Baptista et al. bioengineered a functional humanized rat liver using a bioreactor system to deliver human progenitor cells to acellular liver scaffolds.[120] The complete decellularization of pig livers was successful, as was the maintaining of the vascular network and important ECM proteins, but complete recellularization using all other liver cell types remains a challenge due to the availability of these cells.[121] To address the lack of a reliable cell source, researchers are generating hepatocytes using induced pluripotent stem cell (iPSC) technology.[122]

In 2013, Goh et al. seeded decellularized rat pancreas scaffolds with acinar and beta cell lines for up to five days.[123] The bioengineered pancreatic constructs showed successful cell engraftment and strong up-regulation of insulin expression, supporting the possibility of whole pancreas ECM being used as a scaffold for supporting and enhancing the function of pancreatic cells.[123] Mirmalek-Sani et al. created an intact porcine pancreas ECM scaffold, which was subsequently seeded with pancreatic islets and showed prolonged insulin secretion by the seeded islets compared to suspended islets.[124] Furthermore, in 2014, Costello et al. developed a synthetic 3D small intestine tissue scaffold which supported the attachment of intestinal cells and mimicked the native small intestine environment.[125]

In orthopedics, traumatic injuries and infections affecting bones, tendons, and ligaments typically require surgical reconstruction using autologous or allogenic grafting materials. Afflictions of this nature are a significant health and economic burden, and a major concern with surgical reconstruction is the need for subsequent suppression of the immune response. Thus, removal of allogeneic cellular and MHC components has emerged as a promising avenue for tissue engineering and regenerative medicine. Over thirty studies have investigated or are currently investigating different decellularization techniques that may be used for the bioengineering of bones, tendons, and ligaments.[126] While these studies propose many different decellularization protocols, decellularization of bones, tendons, and ligaments is generally achieved through a combination of chemical, enzymatic, and/or physical treatments. However, the immunogenicity of these grafts remains a major concern and obstacle to clinical translation.

VASCULARIZED COMPOSITE ALLOGRAFT DECELLULARIZATION

While decellularization and recellularization has shown much potential in solid organ transplantation, DE/RE for VCA has only recently been investigated. Given

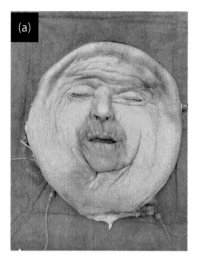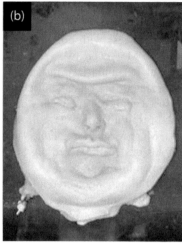

FIGURE 1.3 Human face composite allograft before decellularization (a) and following decellularization (b).

the life-enhancing rather than life-saving nature of VCAs, successful application of DE/RE techniques to VCA would be pivotal as this technology could potentially obviate the need for lifelong immunosuppression, a particularly limiting factor for elective procedures such as VCAs. Additionally, considering the increased immunogenicity of skin relative to other tissues and organ types, promising immuno-modulatory cell therapies are of great interest for VCA, as protocols that result in tolerance in solid organ transplantation may fail to prevent split tolerance or rejection of VCAs.

In 2017, Duisit et al.[127] showed the possibility of decellularizing a human face graft, producing decellularized partial and total faces from human cadaveric face grafts that maintained form and vascular perfusion while also allowing for cell engraftment.

In another proof-of-concept study, Gerli et al.[128] performed the decellularization of a full cadaveric human upper extremity, demonstrating that decellularization can be applied to produce large-scale, acellular human composite tissue scaffolds. In 2019, decellularization of a human penile specimen resulted in a complete penis scaffold in which the vascular networks and morphology of the native tissue was preserved.[129]

In another recent development, laryngeal grafts from human primary cells and decellularized laryngeal scaffolds were created, representing a significant step toward overcoming the challenges of engineering functional and viable grafts for laryngeal reconstruction.[130] Additionally, a decellularized human ovarian scaffold was produced using an optimized protocol involving a sodium lauryl ester sulfate-treated process.[131] Many other small specimens suitable for reconstruction and transplantation have been decellularized by immersion in detergent without infusion. For instance, Sano et al. proposes the use of decellularized human fat as injectable tissue fillers for use in reconstruction, suggesting that acellular adipose tissue may be useful for improving soft-tissue volume and shape in reconstructive surgeries without posing the risk of immune rejection.[132] Furthermore, to address the current challenge of nipple-areolar complex (NAC) reconstruction in breast cancer patients, for which there are limited options and variable outcomes, Pashos et al. developed a protocol for the decellularization of large animal nipples.[133] By keeping the micro and macro structures of the native tissue intact, the decellularized nipple would allow for the reconstruction of the NAC that aesthetically resembles the patient's pre-operative anatomy.

In conclusion, DE/RE technology is a promising approach for many tissue engineering/regenerative medicine applications, including solid organ transplantation and VCA. DE/RE is currently the only method for reproducing a natural 3D ECM. Additionally, decellularized vascular grafts may present a new option for patients with multiple co-morbidities such as diabetes mellitus for whom autografts may not be available.[134] However, due to the diversity of each tissue, there is no standardized method for DE/RE, and each application requires individual investigation. Nevertheless, considering the significant demonstrated potential of DE/RE and the novelty of this approach, it is not beyond the range of possibilities that solid organ and VCA constructs will eventually be routinely procured, cryopreserved, and then made available to match patients' specific reconstructive needs, thus granting surgeons access to a range of size-matched, tissue-specific grafting material readily available for rapidly repairing damaged tissue.

REFERENCES

1. Pomahac, B., Gobble, R. M. & Schneeberger, S. Facial and Hand Allotransplantation. *Cold Spring Harb. Perspect. Med.* **4**, 1–14 (2014).
2. Tasigiorgos, S. *et al.* Five-Year Follow-up after Face Transplantation. *N. Engl. J. Med.* **380**, 2579–2581 (2019).
3. Pomahac, B. *et al.* Three Patients with Full Facial Transplantation. *N. Engl. J. Med.* **366**, 715–722 (2012).
4. Cetrulo, C. L. *et al.* Penis Transplantation: First US Experience. *Ann. Surg.* **267**, 983–988 (2018).
5. Petruzzo, P. & Dubernard, J. M. The International Registry on Hand and Composite Tissue Allotransplantation. *Clin. Transpl.* 247–253 (2011).
6. Shanmugarajah, K. *et al.* The Effect of MHC Antigen Matching Between Donors and Recipients on Skin Tolerance of Vascularized Composite Allografts. *Am. J. Transplant. Off. J. Am. Soc. Transplant. Am. Soc. Transpl. Surg.* **17**, 1729–1741 (2017).
7. Chadha, R., Leonard, D. A., Kurtz, J. M. & Cetrulo, C. L. The Unique Immunobiology of the Skin: Implications for Tolerance of Vascularized Composite Allografts. *Curr. Opin. Organ Transplant.* **19**, 566–572 (2014).
8. Hettiaratchy, S. *et al.* Tolerance to Composite Tissue Allografts across a Major Histocompatibility Barrier in Miniature Swine. *Transplantation* **77**, 514–521 (2004).
9. Kawai, T. *et al.* HLA-Mismatched Renal Transplantation without Maintenance Immunosuppression. *N. Engl. J. Med.* **358**, 353–361 (2008).
10. Leventhal, J. *et al.* Chimerism and Tolerance without GVHD or Engraftment Syndrome in HLA-Mismatched Combined Kidney and Hematopoietic Stem Cell Transplantation. *Sci. Transl. Med.* **4**, 124ra28 (2012).
11. Busque, S. *et al.* Mixed Chimerism and Acceptance of Kidney Transplants after Immunosuppressive Drug Withdrawal. *Sci. Transl. Med.* **12**, 1–14 (2020).

12. Ildstad, S. T., Wren, S. M., Bluestone, J. A., Barbieri, S. A. & Sachs, D. H. Characterization of Mixed Allogeneic Chimeras. Immunocompetence, In Vitro Reactivity, and Genetic Specificity of Tolerance. *J. Exp. Med.* **162**, 231–244 (1985).

13. Ildstad, S. T. & Sachs, D. H. Reconstitution with Syngeneic Plus Allogeneic or Xenogeneic Bone Marrow Leads to Specific Acceptance of Allografts or Xenografts. *Nature* **307**, 168–170 (1984).

14. Kawai, T. *et al.* CD154 Blockade for Induction of Mixed Chimerism and Prolonged Renal Allograft Survival in Nonhuman Primates. *Am. J. Transplant. Off. J. Am. Soc. Transplant. Am. Soc. Transpl. Surg.* **4**, 1391–1398 (2004).

15. Kawai, T. *et al.* Effect of Mixed Hematopoietic Chimerism on Cardiac Allograft Survival in Cynomolgus Monkeys. *Transplantation* **73**, 1757–1764 (2002).

16. Kawai, T. *et al.* Mixed Allogeneic Chimerism and Renal Allograft Tolerance in Cynomolgus Monkeys. *Transplantation* **59**, 256–262 (1995).

17. Kimikawa, M. *et al.* Modifications of the Conditioning Regimen for Achieving Mixed Chimerism and Donor-Specific Tolerance in Cynomolgus Monkeys. *Transplantation* **64**, 709–716 (1997).

18. Yamada, Y. *et al.* Overcoming Memory T-cell Responses for Induction of Delayed Tolerance in Nonhuman Primates. *Am. J. Transplant. Off. J. Am. Soc. Transplant. Am. Soc. Transpl. Surg.* **12**, 330–340 (2012).

19. Tonsho, M. *et al.* Tolerance of Lung Allografts Achieved in Nonhuman Primates via Mixed Hematopoietic Chimerism. *Am. J. Transplant. Off. J. Am. Soc. Transplant. Am. Soc. Transpl. Surg.* **15**, 2231–2239 (2015).

20. Pathiraja, V. *et al.* Tolerance of Vascularized Islet-Kidney Transplants in Rhesus Monkeys. *Am. J. Transplant. Off. J. Am. Soc. Transplant. Am. Soc. Transpl. Surg.* **17**, 91–102 (2017).

21. Schwarze, M. L. *et al.* Mixed Hematopoietic Chimerism Induces Long-Term Tolerance to Cardiac Allografts in Miniature Swine. *Ann. Thorac. Surg.* **70**, 131–138; discussion 138–139 (2000).

22. Fuchimoto, Y. *et al.* Mixed Chimerism and Tolerance without Whole Body Irradiation in a Large Animal Model. *J. Clin. Invest.* **105**, 1779–1789 (2000).

23. Tung, T. H., Mackinnon, S. E. & Mohanakumar, T. Combined Treatment with CD40 Costimulation Blockade, T-cell Depletion, Low-Dose Irradiation, and Donor Bone Marrow Transfusion in Limb Allograft Survival. *Ann. Plast. Surg.* **55**, 512–518 (2005).

24. Tung, T. H., Mackinnon, S. E. & Mohanakumar, T. Prolonged Limb Allograft Survival with CD 40 Costimulation Blockade, T-cell Depletion, and Megadose Donor Bone-Marrow Transfusion. *Microsurgery* **25**, 624–631 (2005).

25. Mathes, D. W. *et al.* Tolerance to Vascularized Composite Allografts in Canine Mixed Hematopoietic Chimeras. *Transplantation* **92**, 1301–1308 (2011).

26. Mathes, D. W. *et al.* Simultaneous Transplantation of Hematopoietic Stem Cells and a Vascularized Composite Allograft Leads to Tolerance. *Transplantation* **98**, 131–138 (2014).

27. Chang, J. *et al.* Long-term Tolerance Toward Haploidentical Vascularized Composite Allograft Transplantation in a Canine Model Using Bone Marrow or Mobilized Stem Cells. *Transplantation* **100**, e120–e127 (2016).

28. Leonard, D. A. *et al.* Vascularized Composite Allograft Tolerance across MHC Barriers in a Large Animal Model. *Am. J. Transplant. Off. J. Am. Soc. Transplant. Am. Soc. Transpl. Surg.* **14**, 343–355 (2014).

29. Cendales, L. C. *et al.* Composite Tissue Allotransplantation: Development of a Preclinical Model in Nonhuman Primates. *Transplantation* **80**, 1447–1454 (2005).

30. Silverman, R. P. *et al.* A Heterotopic Primate Model for Facial Composite Tissue Transplantation. *Ann. Plast. Surg.* **60**, 209–216 (2008).

31. Barth, R. N. *et al.* Facial Subunit Composite Tissue Allografts in Nonhuman Primates: I. Technical and Immunosuppressive Requirements for Prolonged Graft Survival. *Plast. Reconstr. Surg.* **123**, 493–501 (2009).
32. Barth, R. N. *et al.* Vascularized Bone Marrow-Based Immunosuppression Inhibits Rejection of Vascularized Composite Allografts in Nonhuman Primates. *Am. J. Transplant. Off. J. Am. Soc. Transplant. Am. Soc. Transpl. Surg.* **11**, 1407–1416 (2011).
33. Brazio, P. S. *et al.* Infused Bone Marrow Fails to Prevent Vascularized Composite Allograft Rejection in Nonhuman Primates. *Am. J. Transplant. Off. J. Am. Soc. Transplant. Am. Soc. Transpl. Surg.* **15**, 2011–2012 (2015).
34. Oh, B. C. *et al.* Vascularized Composite Allotransplantation Combined with Costimulation Blockade Induces Mixed Chimerism and Reveals Intrinsic Tolerogenic Potential. *JCI Insight* **5** (2020).
35. Lin, C.-H. *et al.* The Intragraft Vascularized Bone Marrow Component Plays a Critical Role in Tolerance Induction after Reconstructive Transplantation. *Cell. Mol. Immunol.* (2019) doi:10.1038/s41423-019-0325-y.
36. Lellouch, A. G. *et al.* Toward Development of the Delayed Tolerance Induction Protocol for Vascularized Composite Allografts in Nonhuman Primates. *Plast. Reconstr. Surg.* **145**, 757e–768e (2020).
37. Schneeberger, S. *et al.* Upper-Extremity Transplantation Using a Cell-Based Protocol to Minimize Immunosuppression. *Ann. Surg.* **257**, 345–351 (2013).
38. Freitas, A. *et al.* Studies Introducing Costimulation Blockade for Vascularized Composite Allografts in Non-Human Primates. *Am. J. Transplant. Off. J. Am. Soc. Transplant. Am. Soc. Transpl. Surg.* **15**, 2240–2249 (2015).
39. Vincenti, F. *et al.* Belatacept and Long-Term Outcomes in Kidney Transplantation. *N. Engl. J. Med.* **374**, 333–343 (2016).
40. Fries, C. A. *et al.* Graft-Implanted, Enzyme Responsive, Tacrolimus-Eluting Hydrogel Enables Long-Term Survival of Orthotopic Porcine Limb Vascularized Composite Allografts: A Proof of Concept Study. *PLOS ONE* **14**, e0210914 (2019).
41. Gajanayake, T. *et al.* A Single Localized Dose of Enzyme-Responsive Hydrogel Improves Long-Term Survival of a Vascularized Composite Allograft. *Sci. Transl. Med.* **6**, 249ra110 (2014).
42. Dzhonova, D. V. *et al.* Local Injections of Tacrolimus-loaded Hydrogel Reduce Systemic Immunosuppression-related Toxicity in Vascularized Composite Allotransplantation. *Transplantation* **102**, 1684–1694 (2018).
43. Ezzelarab, M. B. *et al.* Regulatory Dendritic Cell Infusion Prolongs Kidney Allograft Survival in Nonhuman Primates. *Am. J. Transplant. Off. J. Am. Soc. Transplant. Am. Soc. Transpl. Surg.* **13**, 1989–2005 (2013).
44. Ezzelarab, M. B. *et al.* Renal Allograft Survival in Nonhuman Primates Infused with Donor Antigen-Pulsed Autologous Regulatory Dendritic Cells. *Am. J. Transplant. Off. J. Am. Soc. Transplant. Am. Soc. Transpl. Surg.* **17**, 1476–1489 (2017).
45. Comparative Analysis of Bone Marrow versus Blood Monocyte-Derived Regulatory Dendritic Cells for Evaluation in a Miniature Swine Vascular Composite Allotransplantation Model. *ATC Abstracts* https://atcmeetingabstracts.com/abstract/comparative-analysis-of-bone-marrow-versus-blood-monocyte-derived-regulatory-dendritic-cells-for-evaluation-in-a-miniature-swine-vascular-composite-allotransplantation-model/.
46. Pittenger, M. F. *et al.* Multilineage Potential of Adult Human Mesenchymal Stem Cells. *Science* **284**, 143–147 (1999).
47. Krampera, M. *et al.* Bone Marrow Mesenchymal Stem Cells Inhibit the Response of Naive and Memory Antigen-Specific T Cells to their Cognate Peptide. *Blood* **101**, 3722–3729 (2003).

48. Kuo, Y.-R. *et al.* Modulation of Immune Response and T-cell Regulation by Donor Adipose-Derived Stem Cells in a Rodent Hind-Limb Allotransplant Model. *Plast. Reconstr. Surg.* **128**, 661e–72e (2011).

49. Majumdar, M. K. *et al.* Characterization and Functionality of Cell Surface Molecules on Human Mesenchymal Stem Cells. *J. Biomed. Sci.* **10**, 228–241 (2003).

50. Kuo, Y.-R. *et al.* Immunomodulatory Effects of Bone Marrow-Derived Mesenchymal Stem Cells in a Swine Hemi-facial Allotransplantation Model. *PLOS ONE* **7**, e35459 (2012).

51. Kuo, Y.-R. *et al.* Mesenchymal Stem Cells Prolong Composite Tissue Allotransplant Survival in a Swine Model. *Transplantation* **87**, 1769–1777 (2009).

52. Khattri, R., Cox, T., Yasayko, S.-A. & Ramsdell, F. An Essential Role for Scurfin in CD4+CD25+ T Regulatory Cells. *Nat. Immunol.* **4**, 337–342 (2003).

53. Golovina, T. N. *et al.* CD28 Costimulation Is Essential for Human T Regulatory Expansion and Function. *J. Immunol.* **181**, 2855–2868 (2008).

54. Thornton, A. M. & Shevach, E. M. Suppressor Effector Function of CD4+CD25+ Immunoregulatory T Cells Is Antigen Nonspecific. *J. Immunol.* **164**, 183–190 (2000).

55. Bettini, M. & Vignali, D. A. A. Regulatory T Cells and Inhibitory Cytokines in Autoimmunity. *Curr. Opin. Immunol.* **21**, 612–618 (2009).

56. Xiao, F. *et al.* Ex Vivo Expanded Human Regulatory T Cells Delay Islet Allograft Rejection via Inhibiting Islet-Derived Monocyte Chemoattractant Protein-1 Production in CD34+ Stem Cells-Reconstituted NOD-scid IL2rγnull Mice. *PLOS ONE* **9**, e90387 (2014).

57. Fisher, J. D. *et al.* In Situ Recruitment of Regulatory T Cells Promotes Donor-Specific Tolerance in Vascularized Composite Allotransplantation. *Sci. Adv.* **6**, eaax8429 (2020).

58. Gaidot, A. *et al.* Immune Reconstitution is Preserved in Hematopoietic Stem Cell Transplantation Coadministered with Regulatory T Cells for GVHD Prevention. *Blood* **117**, 2975–2983 (2011).

59. Callaghan, C. J. *et al.* Abrogation of Antibody-Mediated Allograft Rejection by Regulatory CD4 T Cells with Indirect Allospecificity. *J. Immunol.* **178**, 2221–2228 (2007).

60. Wood, K. J. & Sakaguchi, S. Regulatory T Cells in Transplantation Tolerance. *Nat. Rev. Immunol.* **3**, 199–210 (2003).

61. Bahador, A. *et al.* Frequencies of CD4+ T Regulatory Cells and their CD25high and FoxP3high Subsets Augment in Peripheral Blood of Patients with Acute and Chronic Brucellosis. *Osong Public Health Res. Perspect.* **5**, 161–168 (2014).

62. Trenado, A. *et al.* Ex Vivo-Expanded CD4+CD25+ Immunoregulatory T Cells Prevent Graft-Versus-Host-Disease by Inhibiting Activation/Differentiation of Pathogenic T Cells. *J. Immunol. Baltim. Md 1950* **176**, 1266–1273 (2006).

63. Elias, S. & Rudensky, A. Y. Therapeutic Use of Regulatory T Cells for Graft-Versus-Host Disease. *Br. J. Haematol.* **187**, 25–38 (2019).

64. Kohm, A. P., Carpentier, P. A., Anger, H. A. & Miller, S. D. Cutting edge: CD4+CD25+ Regulatory T Cells Suppress Antigen-Specific Autoreactive Immune Responses and Central Nervous System Inflammation During Active Experimental Autoimmune Encephalomyelitis. *J. Immunol. Baltim. Md 1950* **169**, 4712–4716 (2002).

65. Tang, Q. *et al.* In Vitro-Expanded Antigen-Specific Regulatory T Cells Suppress Autoimmune Diabetes. *J. Exp. Med.* **199**, 1455–1465 (2004).

66. Sagoo, P. *et al.* Human Regulatory T Cells with Alloantigen Specificity Are More Potent Inhibitors of Alloimmune Skin Graft Damage than Polyclonal Regulatory T Cells. *Sci. Transl. Med.* **3**, 83ra42 (2011).

67. Peters, J. H., Hilbrands, L. B., Koenen, H. J. P. M. & Joosten, I. Ex Vivo Generation of Human Alloantigen-Specific Regulatory T Cells from CD4posCD25high T Cells for Immunotherapy. *PLOS ONE* **3**, e2233 (2008).

68. Wu, J. *et al.* In Vivo Costimulation Blockade-Induced Regulatory T Cells Demonstrate Dominant and Specific Tolerance to Porcine Islet Xenografts. *Transplantation* **101**, 1587–1599 (2017).
69. Levings, M. K., Sangregorio, R. & Roncarolo, M. G. Human CD25(+)CD4(+) T Regulatory Cells Suppress Naive and Memory T Cell Proliferation and Can Be Expanded In Vitro without Loss of Function. *J. Exp. Med.* **193**, 1295–1302 (2001).
70. Steiner, D., Brunicki, N., Blazar, B. R., Bachar-Lustig, E. & Reisner, Y. Tolerance Induction by Third-Party 'Off-the-Shelf' CD4+CD25+ Treg Cells. *Exp. Hematol.* **34**, 66–71 (2006).
71. Edinger, M. *et al.* CD4+CD25+ Regulatory T Cells Preserve Graft-Versus-Tumor Activity While Inhibiting Graft-Versus-Host Disease After Bone Marrow Transplantation. *Nat. Med.* **9**, 1144–1150 (2003).
72. Trzonkowski, P. *et al.* First-in-Man Clinical Results of the Treatment of Patients with Graft Versus Host Disease with Human Ex Vivo Expanded CD4+CD25+CD127- T Regulatory Cells. *Clin. Immunol. Orlando Fla.* **133**, 22–26 (2009).
73. Romano, M., Fanelli, G., Albany, C. J., Giganti, G. & Lombardi, G. Past, Present, and Future of Regulatory T Cell Therapy in Transplantation and Autoimmunity. *Front. Immunol.* **10**, article 43 (2019).
74. Pierini, A. *et al.* T Cells Expressing Chimeric Antigen Receptor Promote Immune Tolerance. *JCI Insight* **2**, e92865 (2017).
75. Putnam, A. L. *et al.* Clinical Grade Manufacturing of Human Alloantigen-Reactive Regulatory T Cells for Use in Transplantation. *Am. J. Transplant. Off. J. Am. Soc. Transplant. Am. Soc. Transpl. Surg.* **13**, 3010–3020 (2013).
76. Dawson, N. A. J., Vent-Schmidt, J. & Levings, M. K. Engineered Tolerance: Tailoring Development, Function, and Antigen-Specificity of Regulatory T Cells. *Front. Immunol.* **8**, 1460 (2017).
77. Dawson, N. A. *et al.* Systematic Testing and Specificity Mapping of Alloantigen-Specific Chimeric Antigen Receptors in Regulatory T Cells. *JCI Insight* **4**, e123672 (2019).
78. Kim, Y. C. *et al.* Engineered Antigen-Specific Human Regulatory T Cells: Immunosuppression of FVIII-Specific T- and B-Cell Responses. *Blood* **125**, 1107–1115 (2015).
79. Kim, Y. C. *et al.* Engineered MBP-Specific Human Tregs Ameliorate MOG-Induced EAE Through IL-2-Triggered Inhibition of Effector T Cells. *J. Autoimmun.* **92**, 77–86 (2018).
80. Tsang, J. Y.-S. *et al.* Conferring Indirect Allospecificity on CD4+CD25+ Tregs by TCR Gene Transfer Favors Transplantation Tolerance in Mice. *J. Clin. Invest.* **118**, 3619–3628 (2008).
81. Zhang, Q. *et al.* Chimeric Antigen Receptor (CAR) Treg: A Promising Approach to Inducing Immunological Tolerance. *Front. Immunol.* **9**, Article 2359 (2018).
82. Locke, F. L. *et al.* Phase 1 Results of ZUMA-1: A Multicenter Study of KTE-C19 Anti-CD19 CAR T Cell Therapy in Refractory Aggressive Lymphoma. *Mol. Ther. J. Am. Soc. Gene Ther.* **25**, 285–295 (2017).
83. Abramson, J. *et al.* High Cr Rates in Relapsed/Refractory (r/R) Aggressive B-Nhl Treated with the Cd19-Directed Car T Cell Product Jcar017 (transcend Nhl 001). *Hematol. Oncol.* **35**, 138–138 (2017).
84. Schuster, S. J. *et al.* Global Pivotal Phase 2 Trial of the Cd19-Targeted Therapy Ctl019 in Adult Patients with Relapsed or Refractory (r/R) Diffuse Large B-Cell Lymphoma (dlbcl)—an Interim Analysis. *Hematol. Oncol.* **35**, 27–27 (2017).
85. Verneris, M. R. *et al.* HLA-Mismatch Is Associated with Worse Outcomes after Unrelated Donor Reduced Intensity Conditioning Hematopoietic Cell Transplantation: An Analysis from the CIBMTR. *Biol. Blood Marrow Transplant. J. Am. Soc. Blood Marrow Transplant.* **21**, 1783–1789 (2015).

.

86. MacDonald, K. G. *et al.* Alloantigen-Specific Regulatory T Cells Generated with a Chimeric Antigen Receptor. *J. Clin. Invest.* **126**, 1413–1424 (2016).
87. Noyan, F. *et al.* Prevention of Allograft Rejection by Use of Regulatory T Cells with an MHC-Specific Chimeric Antigen Receptor. *Am. J. Transplant. Off. J. Am. Soc. Transplant. Am. Soc. Transpl. Surg.* **17**, 917–930 (2017).
88. Lamarche, C. & Levings, M. K. Guiding Regulatory T Cells to the Allograft. *Curr. Opin. Organ Transplant.* **23**, 106–113 (2018).
89. Boardman, D. A. *et al.* Expression of a Chimeric Antigen Receptor Specific for Donor HLA Class I Enhances the Potency of Human Regulatory T Cells in Preventing Human Skin Transplant Rejection. *Am. J. Transplant. Off. J. Am. Soc. Transplant. Am. Soc. Transpl. Surg.* **17**, 931–943 (2017).
90. Bézie, S. *et al.* Human CD8+ Tregs Expressing a MHC-Specific CAR Display Enhanced Suppression of Human Skin Rejection and GVHD in NSG Mice. *Blood Adv.* **3**, 3522–3538 (2019).
91. Bézie, S. *et al.* Ex Vivo Expanded Human Non-Cytotoxic CD8+CD45RClow/– Tregs Efficiently Delay Skin Graft Rejection and GVHD in Humanized Mice. *Front. Immunol.* **8**, Article 2014 (2018).
92. Bézie, S., Anegon, I. & Guillonneau, C. Advances on CD8+ Treg Cells and Their Potential in Transplantation. *Transplantation* **102**, 1467–1478 (2018).
93. Yáñez, L., Sánchez-Escamilla, M. & Perales, M.-A. CAR T Cell Toxicity: Current Management and Future Directions. *HemaSphere* **3**, e186 (2019).
94. Raffin, C., Vo, L. T. & Bluestone, J. A. Treg Cell-Based Therapies: Challenges and Perspectives. *Nat. Rev. Immunol.* **20**, 158–172 (2020).
95. Zhou, X. *et al.* Foxp3 Instability Leads to the Generation of Pathogenic Memory T Cells In Vivo. *Nat. Immunol.* **10**, 1000–1007 (2009).
96. Badylak, S. F., Taylor, D. & Uygun, K. Whole-Organ Tissue Engineering: Decellularization and Recellularization of Three-Dimensional Matrix Scaffolds. *Annu. Rev. Biomed. Eng.* **13**, 27–53 (2011).
97. Dhal, A., Brovold, M., Atala, A., & Soker, S. Principles of Organ Bioengineering. *Kidney Transplantation, Bioengineering and Regeneration*, Chapter 62, 873–876 (2017).
98. Guyette, J. P. *et al.* Perfusion Decellularization of Whole Organs. *Nat. Protoc.* **9**, 1451–1468 (2014).
99. Crapo, P. M., Gilbert, T. W. & Badylak, S. F. An Overview of Tissue and Whole Organ Decellularization Processes. *Biomaterials* **32**, 3233–3243 (2011).
100. Hillebrandt, K. H. *et al.* Strategies Based on Organ Decellularization and Recellularization. *Transpl. Int. Off. J. Eur. Soc. Organ Transplant.* **32**, 571–585 (2019).
101. Gilbert, T. W., Freund, J. M. & Badylak, S. F. Quantification of DNA in Biologic Scaffold Materials. *J. Surg. Res.* **152**, 135–139 (2009).
102. Cravedi, P. *et al.* Regenerative Immunology: The Immunological Reaction to Biomaterials. *Transpl. Int. Off. J. Eur. Soc. Organ Transplant.* **30**, 1199–1208 (2017).
103. Drukker, M. & Benvenisty, N. The Immunogenicity of Human Embryonic Stem-Derived Cells. *Trends Biotechnol.* **22**, 136–141 (2004).
104. Robertson, M. J., Dries-Devlin, J. L., Kren, S. M., Burchfield, J. S. & Taylor, D. A. Optimizing Recellularization of Whole Decellularized Heart Extracellular Matrix. *PLOS ONE* **9**, e90406 (2014).
105. Livesey, S. A., Herndon, D. N., Hollyoak, M. A., Atkinson, Y. H. & Nag, A. Transplanted Acellular Allograft Dermal Matrix. Potential as a Template for the Reconstruction of Viable Dermis. *Transplantation* **60**, 1–9 (1995).
106. Freytes, D. O., Badylak, S. F., Webster, T. J., Geddes, L. A. & Rundell, A. E. Biaxial Strength of Multilaminated Extracellular Matrix Scaffolds. *Biomaterials* **25**, 2353–2361 (2004).

107. Gilbert, T. W., Stolz, D. B., Biancaniello, F., Simmons-Byrd, A. & Badylak, S. F. Production and Characterization of ECM Powder: Implications for Tissue Engineering Applications. *Biomaterials* **26**, 1431–1435 (2005).

108. Schenke-Layland, K. *et al.* Impact of Decellularization of Xenogeneic Tissue on Extracellular Matrix Integrity for Tissue Engineering of Heart Valves. *J. Struct. Biol.* **143**, 201–208 (2003).

109. Naso, F. & Gandaglia, A. Different Approaches to Heart Valve Decellularization: A Comprehensive Overview of the Past 30 Years. *Xenotransplantation* **25**, E1234 (2018).

110. Urganci, E. *et al.* Implantation of a Decellularized Aortic Homograft in a Child. *Multimed. Man. Cardiothorac. Surg. MMCTS* **2020** (2020).

111. Gilbert, T. W., Sellaro, T. L. & Badylak, S. F. Decellularization of Tissues and Organs. *Biomaterials* **27**, 3675–3683 (2006).

112. Yang, Q. *et al.* A Cartilage ECM-Derived 3-D Porous Acellular Matrix Scaffold for In Vivo Cartilage Tissue Engineering with PKH26-Labeled Chondrogenic Bone Marrow-Derived Mesenchymal Stem Cells. *Biomaterials* **29**, 2378–2387 (2008).

113. Rajab, T. K., O'Malley, T. J. & Tchantchaleishvili, V. Decellularized Scaffolds for Tissue Engineering: Current Status and Future Perspective. *Artif. Organs*, **44**(10), 1031–1043 (2020) doi:10.1111/aor.13701.

114. Ott, H. C. *et al.* Perfusion-Decellularized Matrix: Using Nature's Platform to Engineer a Bioartificial Heart. *Nat. Med.* **14**, 213–221 (2008).

115. Wainwright, J. M. *et al.* Preparation of Cardiac Extracellular Matrix from an Intact Porcine Heart. *Tissue Eng. Part C Methods* **16**, 525–532 (2010).

116. Oberwallner, B. *et al.* Preparation of Cardiac Extracellular Matrix Scaffolds by Decellularization of Human Myocardium. *J. Biomed. Mater. Res. A.* **102**, 3263–3272 (2014).

117. Petersen, T. H. *et al.* Tissue-Engineered Lungs for In Vivo Implantation. *Science* **329**, 538–541 (2010).

118. O'Neill, J. D. *et al.* Decellularization of Human and Porcine Lung Tissues for Pulmonary Tissue Engineering. *Ann. Thorac. Surg.* **96**, 1046–1055; discussion 1055–1056 (2013).

119. Ren, X. *et al.* Engineering Pulmonary Vasculature in Decellularized Rat and Human Lungs. *Nat. Biotechnol.* **33**, 1097–1102 (2015).

120. Baptista, P. M. *et al.* The Use of Whole Organ Decellularization for the Generation of a Vascularized Liver Organoid. *Hepatol. Baltim. Md.* **53**, 604–617 (2011).

121. Ko, I. K. *et al.* Bioengineered Transplantable Porcine Livers with Re-endothelialized Vasculature. *Biomaterials* **40**, 72–79 (2015).

122. Jaramillo, M., Yeh, H., Yarmush, M. L. & Uygun, B. E. Decellularized Human Liver Extracellular Matrix (hDLM)-Mediated Hepatic Differentiation of Human Induced Pluripotent Stem Cells (hIPSCs). *J. Tissue Eng. Regen. Med.* **12**, e1962–e1973 (2018).

123. Goh, S.-K. *et al.* Perfusion-Decellularized Pancreas as a Natural 3D Scaffold for Pancreatic Tissue and Whole Organ Engineering. *Biomaterials* **34**, 6760–6772 (2013).

124. Mirmalek-Sani, S.-H. *et al.* Porcine Pancreas Extracellular Matrix as a Platform for Endocrine Pancreas Bioengineering. *Biomaterials* **34**, 5488–5495 (2013).

125. Costello, C. M. *et al.* Synthetic Small Intestinal Scaffolds for Improved Studies of Intestinal Differentiation. *Biotechnol. Bioeng.* **111**, 1222–1232 (2014).

126. Blaudez, F., Ivanovski, S., Hamlet, S. & Vaquette, C. An Overview of Decellularisation Techniques of Native Tissues and Tissue Engineered Products for Bone, Ligament and Tendon Regeneration. *Methods San Diego Calif.* **171**, 28–40 (2020).

127. Duisit, J. *et al.* Bioengineering a Human Face Graft: The Matrix of Identity. *Ann. Surg.* **266**, 754–764 (2017).

128. Gerli, M. F. M., Guyette, J. P., Evangelista-Leite, D., Ghoshhajra, B. B. & Ott, H. C. Perfusion Decellularization of a Human Limb: A Novel Platform for Composite Tissue Engineering and Reconstructive Surgery. *PLOS ONE* **13**, e0191497 (2018).

129. Tan, Y. *et al.* Complete Human Penile Scaffold for Composite Tissue Engineering: Organ Decellularization and Characterization. *Sci. Rep.* **9**, 16368 (2019).
130. Moser, P. T. *et al.* Creation of Laryngeal Grafts from Primary Human Cells and Decellularized Laryngeal Scaffolds. *Tissue Eng. Part A.* **26**, 543–555 (2020).
131. Hassanpour, A., Talaei-Khozani, T., Kargar-Abarghouei, E., Razban, V. & Vojdani, Z. Decellularized Human Ovarian Scaffold Based on a Sodium Lauryl Ester Sulfate (SLES)-Treated Protocol, as a Natural Three-Dimensional Scaffold for Construction of Bioengineered Ovaries. *Stem Cell Res. Ther.* **9**, 252 (2018).
132. Sano, H., Orbay, H., Terashi, H., Hyakusoku, H. & Ogawa, R. Acellular Adipose Matrix as a Natural Scaffold for Tissue Engineering. *J. Plast. Reconstr. Aesthetic Surg. JPRAS.* **67**, 99–106 (2014).
133. Pashos, N. C. *et al.* Characterization of an Acellular Scaffold for a Tissue Engineering Approach to Nipple—Areolar Complex Reconstruction. *Cells Tissues Organs* **203**, 183–193 (2017).
134. Natasha, G., Tan, A., Gundogan, B., Farhatnia, Y., Nayyer, L., Mahdibeiraghdar, S, Rajadas, J., De Coppi, P., Davies, A. H. & Seifalian, A. M. Tissue Engineering Vascular Grafts a Fortiori: Looking Back and Going Forward. *Expert Opin. Biol. Ther.* **15**, 231–244 (2015).

2 Novel T-Regulatory Cell-Based Therapies in Vascularized Composite Allotransplantation
Translational Implications

Yalcin Kulahci, Hulya Kapucu,
James D. Fisher, and Steven R. Little

CONTENTS

Introduction 27
The Possible Proposed Mechanisms for Tregs Inhibitory Effects
on Teff 28
Tregs: Classification and Subtypes 28
Tregs and Antigen Specificity: The Role of Donor Antigen-Specific
Tregs in Immunomodulation 29
Tregs and IL-2 Interaction 29
Tregs and Their Possible Role in Immunomodulation in VCA:
Overview 30
Immunosuppressive Drug Delivery System Using Degradable
Microparticles: Delivery of Rapamycin to Dendritic Cells 32
Treg Recruiting Microparticle Systems 32
Treg-Inducing Microparticle Systems 34
Tregs and Their Interaction with Immunosuppressive Drugs 35
The Clinical Applications of Tregs: Ex Vivo Expansion, Adoptive
Transfer, and Clinical Trials 35
Conclusions and Future Insight 36
References 37

INTRODUCTION

The ultimate goal of vascularized composite allotransplantation (VCA) is allograft survival and prevention of chronic rejection. T cells, expressing CD4, CD25,[1,2] and FoxP3,[3–5] are the dominant form of regulatory T cells (Tregs) and also the most commonly defined and widely studied regulator cells in the body. Their role in

DOI: 10.1201/9780429260179-3

autoimmune diseases and allotransplantations have been well-documented.[6,7] Moreover, the presence of Tregs in a long-term VCA recipient (up to 6 years) has also been shown in the literature.[8] Their cell-mediated tolerance induction and rejection control mainly depend on their T effector (Teff) cell inhibition.[9] Although during in vitro expansion there is a possibility of losing the immunosuppression function of Tregs, because it may be vulnerable, cumulative evidence in literature shows proofs of maintenance of their immunosuppressive functions.[10,11] Moreover, their effectiveness has also been shown in experimental VCA studies.[7,12]

Adjunctive rapamycin therapy increases the ability of human Tregs to inhibit vascular allograft rejection in a humanized mouse model of arterial transplantation.[13] Furthermore, when compared with conventional CD25^{hi}CD4+ Tregs, some subtypes of Tregs, CD4+CD25+CD127^{low}, are five times more potent in tolerance induction and immunosuppressive capability via inhibition of Teff cell function and graft invasion in an animal model of transplanted arteriosclerosis.[1,14]

When considering long-term allograft survival and immunotolerance, this finding would be promising because arteriosclerosis is one of the strong markers of chronic rejection. However, one study shows that Tregs may have limited prognostic value and does not predict outcomes with standard immunosuppressive protocols (tacrolimus and mycophenolate mofetil) used in a clinically relevant model of nonhuman primate (NHP) facial VCA.[1,15] Thus, in allograft transplant setting, although immunomodulation of host response with Tregs can be an open new area and its clinical application in VCA is possible, further studies are needed to reveal the specific role of Tregs in VCA and any role of Treg monitoring in clinical practice.[15] Thus, future advancement and refinement of this strategy would help to minimize or completely withdraw the current immunosuppressive regimens in VCA and also solid organ transplantation (SOT).

THE POSSIBLE PROPOSED MECHANISMS FOR Tregs INHIBITORY EFFECTS ON Teff

Tregs can exert their immunomodulatory effects on Teff via different mechanisms:

> Dendritic cell (DC) suppression; production inhibition of indoleamine 2,3-dioxygenase; lysis of Teff cells via granzyme A/B and perforin production; IL-2 deprivation; release of TGF-β, IL-10, and IL-35 (inhibitory cytokines); interfering Teff cell metabolism and production of cyclic adenosine monophosphate (cAMP).[1,16]

Tregs: CLASSIFICATION AND SUBTYPES

To date, three types of Tregs have been classified: Thymic Treg (tTreg) cells, peripherally induced Treg (pTreg) cells, and in vitro induced Treg (iTreg) cells.[17] It has been shown that in the presence of interleukin-2 (IL-2) and transforming growth factor-β (TGF-β), mice naive CD4+ CD25− T cells can be induced to express CD25+ Foxp3+ iTreg cells.[18,19] Other authors also show that the presence of retinoic acid (RA), IL-2, and TGF-β can induce human iTreg cells from peripheral blood mononuclear cells (PBMCs) in adults.[20]

Tregs AND ANTIGEN SPECIFICITY: THE ROLE OF DONOR ANTIGEN-SPECIFIC Tregs IN IMMUNOMODULATION

Another interesting concept is the importance of antigen specificity of Tregs because there is a possibility that naturally occurring polyclonal Tregs might cause systemic non-specific immunosuppression.[1] From this point, donor antigen-specific Tregs can demonstrate high efficacy by selectively inducing immune suppression against this antigen. This can be called "antigen-specific immune suppression".[10,21,22] It has been shown that after being previously exposed to certain antigens, Tregs can specifically accumulate within the graft and also in graft-draining lymph nodes and prevent the rejection of fully allogeneic skin grafts in mice.[23] However, it is not certain if this kind of immunosuppression is due to recognition of tissue-specific or omnipresent self-antigens. Hence, it can be concluded that the effect of antigen-specific Tregs on immunomodulation should be more than that of polyclonal Tregs.[24]

Donor antigen-specific Tregs can be produced by using DCs, B cells, and PBMCs.[25] It has been shown that when naive CD4+ T cells co-cultured with allogeneic antigen-presenting cells with TGF-β, RA, and IL-2, immunosuppressive function of alloantigen-specific Tregs can be induced in skin allografts.[26]

It has been shown that CD4+CD25+Foxp3+ Tregs, stimulated in vitro with alloantigens, induced long-term tolerance to bone marrow and subsequent skin and cardiac allografts. Although Tregs specific for directly presented donor antigens prevented only acute rejection, Tregs specific for directly and indirectly presented alloantigens prevented both acute and chronic rejection.[21] These findings emphasize the importance of donor antigen specificity in allograft survival and transplant tolerance.

Thus, antigen-specific Treg therapy would be the next promising step for immunomodulation in preclinical and clinical settings.[25,27]

In the context of this subtopic, it would be worth mentioning some new approaches related to donor antigen-specific Treg therapy: Chimeric antigen receptor (CAR) system and T cell receptor (TCR) gene modification. It has been shown that Tregs with human leukocyte antigen-2-specific CAR prevented xenogeneic graft-versus-host disease (GVHD) in mice model.[28] The immunosuppressive activity of this "CAR-Treg-cell-modulated donor antigen specifity" approach has been shown in some autoimmune diseases such as hemophilia A, encephalitis, and colitis.[29–31]

Teff cells can be converted into Tregs via FoxP3 overexpression. In fact, retroviral transduction of a TCR that recognizes an alloantigen, along with FoxP3 overexpression, should generate antigen-specific Tregs. Indirect donor antigen (major histocompatibility complex Class II) allospecific Tregs can be generated via TCR gene engineering, and this approach can be used for future tolerance induction studies in rat VCA.[32,33]

Tregs AND IL-2 INTERACTION

It has been shown that IL-2 blocks the differentiation of naive CD4+ T cells into pro-inflammatory TH17 cells,[34] and Tregs are naturally more sensitive to IL-2 than are Teff cells.[35] In 1993, it was discovered that IL-2[36] and IL-2R[37,38] signaling-deficient mice develop autoimmunity and inflammation, and this was attributed to defective Treg phenotype.[39] Furthermore, a massive expansion of Tregs has been observed in metastatic renal cancer patients receiving IL-2 treatment during phase I-II DC-based immunotherapy.[40]

In autoimmune and inflammatory diseases, early clinical benefits of low-dose IL-2 have been demonstrated via its capability of specifically activating Tregs.[41] Although Treg expansion and function can be promoted via low-dose IL-2,[41] this approach has some potential problems worth mentioning here. First of all, IL-2 has a short half-life and it may be even shorter in patients with autoimmune disorders, and there is a probability that IL-2 cannot evoke a signaling response in Tregs in these patients. Moreover, because of the difficulty of establishing a precise low-dose of IL-2 due to variable therapeutic window between the different inflammatory milieu, this can cause stimulation of the Teff cells in some cases.[42] Second, the threshold of high dose is very close to causing side effects in some patients.[42]

Tregs AND THEIR POSSIBLE ROLE IN IMMUNOMODULATION IN VCA: OVERVIEW

It has been known for years that Tregs have potential immunosuppressive effects related to autoimmunity, GVHD and even transplant rejection. Thus, the lack of adequate Tregs can be a main underlying factor for the development of inflammatory and autoimmune diseases.[43,44] From this point, it can be concluded that possible Treg enhancement strategies could be beneficial to suppress immunity towards autoantigens (as we see in autoimmune disorders) and even alloantigen (as we see allotransplantation settings).[43,45–47]

It is known that a wide variety of conditions such as autoimmunity,[43,48] dermatitis,[49] psoriasis,[50,51] periodontitis[52–54] and even transplant rejection[55,56] are closely associated with the absence of Tregs. FOXP3 gene mutations have been identified as an underlying cause of the immune dysregulation, polyendocrinopathy, enteropathy, X-linked (IPEX) syndrome.[57,58] The deficiency of CD25 also represents IPEX-like syndrome with impaired suppressive function of FoxP3 cells.[59,60]

Recently, the decreased number of FoxP3+ Tregs has been shown in class IV lupus nephritis and vasculitis patients.[61] The reduced number of Tregs has been found during the early phases of type 1 diabetes.[62] Furthermore, defects in IL-2R signaling have also been found as a contributing factor for diminished maintenance of FOXP3 expression in Tregs of type 1 diabetes patients.[63] Balandina et al. found a normal Treg number but a severe functional defect in their regulatory activity together with a decreased expression of FOXP3 in the thymus of patients with autoimmune myasthenia gravis.[64]

Although Thiruppathi et al. showed no alteration in the relative number of Tregs in myasthenia gravis patients, they demonstrated that Treg-mediated suppressive function was impaired in myasthenia gravis patients, and this was associated with a reduced expression of FOXP3 in isolated Tregs.[65] This impaired suppressive function could be reestablished using Tregs from healthy controls. These findings signify the potential therapeutic future of Tregs in autoimmune diseases like myasthenia gravis.[65]

Thus, increasing the local Treg count locally through Treg expansion or induction may be a potential therapeutic option for the treatment of these diseases. Besides, new drugs and biologics are also needed to develop to increase immunomodulatory function of Tregs.[66] However, Treg-based cellular therapies have their own challenges, and bio-based methods currently used for in vivo Treg expansion can cause many other undesirable side effects in addition to increasing the Treg numbers. First of all, these processes need Good Manufacturing Practice (GMP) facilities. In addition, isolating pure and homogenous populations of Tregs without Teff cells mixing is challenging. In addition, segregating large quantities of Tregs from the blood is also difficult. Truly, FOXP3, the best marker for Tregs, is not appropriate to refine viable cells by flow cytometry, and CD25, the other key and highly expressed membrane marker for Tregs, can also be temporarily expressed by Teff cells.[67]

Moreover, consistent maintenance of the Treg phenotype and suppressive function is also difficult.[68–70] Thus, the technology would increase numbers and/or the suppressive potency of Treg with providing avoidance from above-mentioned drawbacks and hurdles of in vitro expansion, and could promise clinical translation.[66]

The number of Tregs at local tissue sites can be enhanced by either ex vivo expansion followed by local or systemic administration or directly in vivo manipulation.[66] Local Treg induction may be preferred due to many disadvantages of the ex vivo expansion.[68–70] However, previous experiences with local induction agents have also shown some discouraging results related to their safety and mechanism of action (anti-IL-2 mAb,[71] superagonistic anti-CD28 mAb,[72] agonistic anti-CD4 mAb[73]), and failure in phase I clinical trials (anti-CD28 Ab) due to cytokine storm.[74]

In VCA, the supporting role of Tregs in long-term allograft survival or tolerance has also been a known fact. The presence of intragraft Foxp3+Tregs and suppressive cytokine profile have been shown in skin biopsies of hand transplant case at 6th year follow up.[9] Thus, in addition to indicating a critical role of Tregs in SOT and VCA tolerance, these studies also shed light upon future studies in this area.[75]

Currently, the applicability of Tregs has been extended to tolerance induction studies in connection with the VCA field.[76,77] Multiple studies show that peripheral allograft tolerance can be achieved by activation of Tregs,[43] and their absence can cause allograft rejection. Thus, Treg/Teff balance is crucial for allograft outcomes, rejection, and tolerance.[78–82] Yoshizawa et al. demonstrated that liver transplant recipients who have potent CD4+ CD25+ Tregs can be weaned from immunosuppression.[83] The degree of FOXP3+ expression showed significant positive correlation with the Banff grade of rejection in a primate kidney transplant model[9] and in clinical cardiac transplant patients, respectively.[84] Furthermore, the measurement of messenger RNA for FoxP3 in the urine of kidney transplant recipients also envisaged the outcome of acute rejection of renal allograft.[85] Hence, in the near future, fine-tuning of immunosuppressive drug dosage in allograft recipients would be possible with quantitative determination of the Treg/Teff balance.[75]

For these reasons, synthetic formulations that can locally increase and induce the Treg numbers (via locally immunosuppressive milieu) can be an alternative strategy to in vivo systemic induction strategies.[66] As described before, providing an environment which is rich in IL-2, TGF-β, and rapamycin is necessary to increase the ratio of Treg/Teff.[86-89] This kind of environment can be achieved via sustained release of this formulation using a poly(lactic-co-glycolic)acid (PLGA), a commonly used polymer.[66]

IMMUNOSUPPRESSIVE DRUG DELIVERY SYSTEM USING DEGRADABLE MICROPARTICLES: DELIVERY OF RAPAMYCIN TO DENDRITIC CELLS

Immunosuppressive drugs can be protected and released over time via degradable microparticles. In addition, if these microparticles are produced in an appropriate size, they can be phagocytosed by a DC, which has an important role in transplant rejection.[90,91]

Previously, we described a strategy to deliver an intracellular depot of rapamycin to DCs and demonstrated that DCs treated with rapamycin have the ability to suppress transplant rejection. A ~3.4 μm sized PLGA microparticle (rapaMP) was used to encapsulate the rapamycin. When compared with soluble rapamycin-treated DCs, T cell activation ability of DCs was significantly reduced following the phagocytosis of rapaMP. Thus, from the perspective of "DC function modulation", better efficacy of rapamycin has been achieved via DC-specific intracellular delivery of drug when compared with extracellular rapamycin.[91]

Treg RECRUITING MICROPARTICLE SYSTEMS

From this point, there is increasing demand to develop new techniques to increase this kind of specific immune cells. We were inspired from our extensive review of tumor biology because a wide range of tumors release the CCL22, and tumor-specific immune evasion is a well-known reality. First of all, we developed a microscale controlled-release system of CCL22 for the recruitment of Tregs.[92,93] Then we fabricated and reported other innovative Treg-inducing synthetic formulations of IL-2, TGF-β, and rapamycin, which are capable of providing a 3- to 4-week controlled release.[91,94] In this section, we present and discuss ideas and innovations behind the development of this technology and our current groundbreaking in vivo experiences with Treg-inducing systems.

As mentioned, our aim was to focus on in vivo controlled release of CCL22 to achieve local recruitment of Treg.[95] As a first attempt, we designed a release vehicle suitable for the steady release of CCL22 and achieved this goal with release of CCL22 without any periods of lag.[95] To achieve sustained release within a 3- to 8-week period, the polymer PLGA was used. In addition, the particles were produced to be large enough to escape from phagocytosis and impede their passage through the vascular endothelium. Thus, finally we observed that in vivo used CCL22MP particles remained immobilized at the site of injection and site-specific recruitment of Tregs leading to local modulation of immune responses can be achieved.[95]

We tested the ability of CCL22MP to attract Treg via fluorescently labeled CCL22MP, which were injected into the triceps muscle of normal FVB mice followed by intravenous infusion of ex vivo-alloactivated Treg (AATreg).[96] The hind limb muscles were chosen as the site for MP injections because distal sites are not expected to produce large quantities of CCL22. Finally, we observed that a significantly greater number of AATreg was recruited to the site of CCL22MP injection compared to blank microparticles lacking CCL22.[95]

In the literature, authors report that even small local increase in the ratio of Treg to Teff cells is enough to change the immune responses.[55] As a parallel to this report, we also demonstrate that CCL22MP are able to delay the rejection of transplanted allogeneic cells.[95]

It has been suggested that freshly isolated or ex vivo-expanded Treg infusion can suppress autoimmune diseases and even prevent transplant rejection.[3,43,97] However, it should be kept in mind that CCR4, a receptor for CCL22, is expressed in both Treg and Teff cells[98] and CCL22 can be attracted to these two cell populations. However, Tregs in tumors[92,99] or long-surviving allografts[68] suggest that CCL22 production change the balance on behalf of Tregs and immunotolerance.[95] This could be due to markedly more CCR4 expression of Tregs than Teff cells.[99]

In our previous study using models of periodontitis, CCL22 microspheres have been shown to reduce the inflammation and disease symptoms via recruitment of endogenous Tregs.[54]

Furthermore, we currently tested Treg-recruiting microspheres, CCL22 particles, in a murine model of dry eye disease, which is a well-known model of destructive inflammation and autoimmunity.[100] In this study, CCL22 microparticles were capable of overwhelming the immunological disproportion of Tregs and CD4+ IFN− γ+ cells in the lacrimal gland and alleviate the symptoms of dry eye disease as measured by different evaluating methods such as corneal epithelial integrity, tear clearance, and goblet cell density.[100]

Effective local immunosuppression can be achieved by optimal balance between Treg/Teff and not a complete absence of Teff cells.[3,101] Besides the Treg recruiting properties, CCL22MP can also be modified to simultaneous release of ultra-low-dose immunosuppressive drugs (rapamycin etc.)[102] to impede Teff and support Treg functions.[95] Thus, to assist the Treg and provide more control to undesirable immune responses,[92,93] we fabricated and reported other innovative Treg-inducing synthetic formulation of IL-2, TGF-β, and rapamycin.

We extended our experience with "CCL22 Treg recruiting microparticle systems" in rodent hind-limb model of VCA in order to achieve donor-specific immune tolerance and reduce the need for systemic immunosuppression. VCA offers a new potential era to restore appearance and function of extensively damaged tissues such as hand and face with the donor allograft tissue which has the same texture and function. However, current lifelong systemic immunosuppression regimens needed for exact rejection control consist of multiple drug combinations and unfortunately have considerable adverse effects in the long-term follow up. We showed that prolonged hindlimb allograft survival over 200 days and donor-specific tolerance induction has been achieved with this Treg-recruiting microparticle systems. We observed the enriched Treg populations in allograft skin and draining lymph nodes and enhanced Treg function without affecting the proliferative capacity of conventional T cells. We also showed that synthetic human CCL22 induced preferential migration of human Treg in vitro. These results suggest that local enrichment of immunomodulatory Treg cells via CCL22 microparticles promotes donor-specific tolerance induction.[103]

Treg-INDUCING MICROPARTICLE SYSTEMS

We fabricated and reported a Treg-inducing synthetic formulation capable of providing a 3- to 4-week controlled release of IL-2, TGF-β, and rapamycin, which is named as TRI microparticles (TRI-MP) in vitro using mouse cells.[91,94]

Moreover, we also demonstrated that these release formulations can induce high expression of FoxP3+ in human Tregs.[66] Additionally, via this Treg-inducing formulation, in vitro Tregs keep their proliferative capacity and functional ability and express their phenotypic surface characteristic markers (soluble factor induced Treg).[66] It has also been shown that this formulation works even under inflammatory milieu.[86–88] The main obstacle is the sustainable maintenance of this formulation in tissue site, and this can be overcome with controlled-release vehicles.[66] Furthermore, we observed that the microparticles do not have any adverse effects on Tregs even if there were contact with each other.[66] According to these data, we suggested that in vivo local Treg induction can be used to mitigate autoimmunity and also transplant rejection. Thus, these microparticulate formulations could be an 'off-the-shelf' therapy for local immunosuppressive strategies.[66]

We also tested TRI-MP in a murine inflammatory model of dry eye disease for preventing the key signs of dry eye disease such as aqueous tear secretion, conjunctival goblet cells, and epithelial corneal integrity and showed the alleviation of the disease for symptoms via shifting the balance of Treg/Teff cells and reducing the pro-inflammatory cytokine environment in the tissue.[104]

Furthermore, we showed that teaching the immune system to tolerate contact allergens is possible by expanding allergen-specific Tregs. These microparticles have been shown to effectively prevent or reverse allergic contact dermatitis in an allergen-specific manner (by expanding allergen-specific Tregs and reducing pro-inflammatory Teff cells) in previously sensitized mice.[105]

These promising results with TRI-MP led us to test their feasibility in one of the most challenging VCA model: the rodent hind-limb allotransplantation model. Thus, more recently, these Treg-inducing microparticle systems, engineered to sustainably release TGF-β1, IL-2, and rapamycin to enrich Tregs, were used in the well-known VCA model of rat hind limb allotransplantation model. We showed that TRI-MP prolonged allograft survival over 300 days without long-term systemic immunosuppression. Besides, in allograft tissue, we observed that inflammatory mediators' expression was reduced, and Treg-associated cytokine expression was increased. Moreover, in allograft-draining lymph nodes, we found that Treg was enriched and inflammatory Th1 populations were reduced with local TRI-MP application. Furthermore, beyond the local immunomodulation, as an evidence of achievement of systemic donor-specific tolerance, recipient rats accepted secondary skin grafts from the same donor but rejected skin grafts from a third-party donor. We can conclude that Treg-inducing microparticle systems could be considered as a new emerging tool for management of autoimmune diseases and also for mitigating allotransplant rejection without facing the detrimental effects of systemic immunosuppressive agents.[106]

Tregs AND THEIR INTERACTION WITH IMMUNOSUPPRESSIVE DRUGS

The activation, proliferation, and immune regulatory functions of Tregs in VCA can interact with conventional immunosuppressive drugs. Thus, meticulous evaluation of these effects is crucial to develop immunomodulatory approaches in transplantation tolerance.

The mammalian target of rapamycin (Sirolimus) (mTOR) signaling pathway activation is essential for development of Th17 effector lineages. However, the absence of this signaling pathway led to naive T cells specially differentiating into Tregs. Rapamycin is a specific inhibitor of mTOR and inhibition of mTOR with rapamycin can suppress Teff cell function and also improve the inflammatory response control ability of Tregs.[107] It has been reported that Treg and CD8+ memory T cell populations were expanded and IL-4 and IL-17 production inhibited by rapamycin.[108] Furthermore, it has been shown that rapamycin can help the maintenance of the sustainability, function, and proliferative ability of Tregs in allotransplantation settings. The long-term rejection-free survival of cardiac allograft transplant with antigen-specific Tregs along with rapamycin has been reported in rodents.[55] Besides, rapamycin also induces Tregs in healthy volunteers and type I diabetes mellitus (DM) cases.[109]

Calcineurin inhibitors, specifically cyclosporin A, have negative effect on Tregs by interfering with their development suppressive activity.[75,110] Tacrolimus even promotes human Tregs.[111] Although the low doses of cyclosporine inhibit Treg activity, tacrolimus could be more advantageous than cyclosporine in controlling rejection by relatively enhanced proliferation of Tregs in association with altered gene expression levels of TCR signaling molecules (Foxp3-regulated TCR signal related-genes, PTPN22 and Itk) in human Tregs.[111,112]

Methylprednisolone, a corticosteroid, inhibits T and B cell proliferation and may help Treg cell function via its anti-inflammatory effects. The combination of mycophenolate mofetil with 1,25-dihydroxyvitamin D3 (1,25(OH)2D3), the biologically active metabolite of vitamin D3, stimulates the Tregs and tolerance induction.[75]

Histone deacetylases inhibitors such as HDAC6 are expressed at higher levels in Tregs than in Tconv cells. It has been shown that these inhibitors selectively increase Treg cell function in lupus-prone mice and protect them from lupus nephritis.[113,114]

In addition, Tregs in HDAC6-deficient mice had improved suppressive activity, poor antibody responses to antigen,[115] and reduced autoimmune and inflammatory responses.[116]

THE CLINICAL APPLICATIONS OF Tregs: EX VIVO EXPANSION, ADOPTIVE TRANSFER, AND CLINICAL TRIALS

The isolation, ex vivo expansion, and adoptive transfer of Tregs have been attractive aims for their future routine clinical applicability.[117] However, for clinical application, they have to be produced under GMP conditions with the highest Foxp3 marker purity and lacking pro-inflammatory cytokine secretion.[68] In vivo expansion protocols for polyclonal and antigen-specific Treg cells have been published.[10,11,118,119]

So far, in vitro Treg cell proliferation has been successfully stimulated by IL-2 induction in combination with TCR and CD28 facilitated stimulation.[11] Currently, CD4+CD25++ or CD4+ CD25+CD127– Tregs have been used in adoptive transfer studies. Besides, it has been shown that CD4+ CD25highCD45RA+ Tregs are ideal population for generation of homogeneous and stable Tregs.[120] Immunomodulator functions of expanded human iTreg cells have been shown in GVHD.[47] Indeed, it has been shown that following allogeneic hematopoietic stem cell transplantation, GVHD has worsened if there is Treg cell depletion and this condition can be controlled via Treg cell infusion.[121,122]

Although more than 300 clinical trials have been conducted with polyclonal or donor antigen-specific Tregs including GVHD, type I DM, kidney and liver transplantation, and autoimmune diseases, there is no ongoing clinical trials related to VCA.[27]

In regard to their direct allospecificity, donor antigen-specific Tregs have a promising situation in clinical allotransplantation setting.[123] In this context, allograft acceptance would be also depending on some other factors such as infusion time, the ratio of Treg/Teff cells, and accompanied immunosuppressive agents or strategies.[1]

CONCLUSIONS AND FUTURE INSIGHT

Prevention of allograft rejection and providing long-term survival are entire goals in VCA. Considering the high antigenicity of VCA, which is more than 85% of patients experience acute rejection episode within a year, new immunomodulation strategies need to be focused on rejection control without undesirable side effects of current lifelong immunosuppressive protocols. Recently, one of the most popular concepts in allotransplantation is local immunomodulation via some topical vehicles like microparticles, which can provide ultra-low-dose, slow-releasing immunosuppressive drugs and/or immunomodulatory cytokines to elicit local recruitment of Tregs.[103,106]

Tregs have been broadly hyped as central mediators for peripheral self-tolerance induction and maintenance. Although Tregs-based therapies seem to promise great perspective in the near future, there are some limitations such as logistical, financial, and even scientific hurdles which need to be addressed before their routine clinical application. The adoptive transfer of Tregs needs GMP facilities to produce desired quality of Foxp3+ Tregs.[42]

First of all, cytokines, other mediators, surgical trauma and ischemia-reperfusion injury would have significant effects on Tregs and also on immunity regulation and tolerance induction. For instance, even Tregs are expanded ex-vivo with high IL-2 concentration; they would become immediately unstable, not exert their suppressive function and even die in case of possible low dosage of in-vivo IL-2. Moreover, following the infusion, the inhibitory activity of Tregs can change and Teff response can increase, and this can cause new inflammatory milieu.[42] Thus, it has been suggested that maximum mitigation of ischemia-reperfusion injury would be crucial in tolerance induction.[75]

Secondly, due to difference between human and murine Tregs, information produced in mice may not be completely clinically translational. As such, some subsets of human Tregs have no suppressive function in contrast to more homogeneous murine Tregs. Thirdly, elevated numbers of Teff cells may have already been found in patients previously diagnosed with autoimmune disease, and it can be difficult for Tregs to exert their immunomodulatory effects in these inflammatory environments such as rheumatoid arthritis[124] and systemic lupus erythematosus.[125,126] In other words, enormous number of Tregs would be needed to suppress these Teff cells in such a condition. Moreover, under these kinds of inflammatory milieu, Tregs can be easily transformed into Tconv cells and even Teff cells and can further increase the present inflammation. Thus, exploring new methods to decrease the number and effectiveness of already activated alloreactive Teff cells would be another helpful approach before Treg application.[42]

Thus, understanding the main functional properties of different Tregs and their characteristic markers is crucial to success. The next step will be to determine the manipulation methods of specific Treg populations to roll the critical balance between immune boosting and tolerance induction.[75] To utilize these cells for further clinical application such as via adoptive therapy, ex vivo investigation of function and downstream effects of specific Treg populations is needed.

Although Treg cell-based therapies have been applied in some clinical trials of SOT and autoimmune diseases, there is no known ongoing trials related to VCA.[1] One step ahead in Treg cell-based therapies would be "donor antigen-specific Treg cell-based therapies", and this seems to be a new emerging field in solid and vascularized composite allotransplantation.[1] Besides, development of new tools for determining the amount of engrafted Tregs and predicting the possible upcoming rejection based on this engraftment would also be a great accomplishment in the field of VCA.

REFERENCES

1. Sakaguchi, S., et al., Immunologic tolerance maintained by CD25+ CD4+ regulatory T cells: their common role in controlling autoimmunity, tumor immunity, and transplantation tolerance. *Immunol Rev*, 2001. **182**(1): p. 18–32.
2. Sakaguchi, S., et al., Immunologic self-tolerance maintained by activated T cells expressing IL-2 receptor alpha-chains (CD25). Breakdown of a single mechanism of self-tolerance causes various autoimmune diseases. *J Immunol*, 1995. **155**(3): p. 1151–1164.
3. Hori, S., Control of regulatory T cell development by the transcription factor Foxp3. *Science*, 2003. **299**(5609): p. 1057–1061.
4. Fontenot, J.D., M.A. Gavin, and A.Y. Rudensky, Foxp3 programs the development and function of CD4+CD25+ regulatory T cells. *Nat Immunol*, 2003. **4**(4): p. 330–336.
5. Khattri, R., et al., An essential role for Scurfin in CD4+CD25+ T regulatory cells. *Nat Immunol*, 2003. **4**(4): p. 337–342.
6. Sakaguchi, S., Naturally arising CD4+ regulatory T cells for immunologic self-tolerance and negative control of immune responses. *Annu Rev Immunol*, 2004. **22**: p. 531–562.
7. Issa, F. and K.J. Wood, The potential role for regulatory T-cell therapy in vascularized composite allograft transplantation. *Curr Opin Organ Transplant*, 2014. **19**(6): p. 558–565.
8. Eljaafari, A., et al., Isolation of regulatory T cells in the skin of a human hand-allograft, up to six years posttransplantation. *Transplantation*, 2006. **82**(12): p. 1764–1768.
9. Yang, J.H. and S.C. Eun, Therapeutic application of T regulatory cells in composite tissue allotransplantation. *J Transl Med*, 2017. **15**(1): p. 218.

10. Tang, Q., et al., In vitro-expanded antigen-specific regulatory T cells suppress autoimmune diabetes. *J Exp Med*, 2004. **199**(11): p. 1455–1465.
11. Hoffmann, P., et al., Large-scale in vitro expansion of polyclonal human CD4+CD25high regulatory T cells. *Blood*, 2004. **104**(3): p. 895–903.
12. Safinia, N., et al., Promoting transplantation tolerance; adoptive regulatory T cell therapy. *Clin Exp Immunol*, 2013. **172**(2): p. 158–168.
13. Hester, J., et al., Low-dose rapamycin treatment increases the ability of human regulatory T cells to inhibit transplant arteriosclerosis in vivo. *Am J Transplant*, 2012. **12**(8): p. 2008–2016.
14. Issa, F., A. Schiopu, and K.J. Wood, Role of T cells in graft rejection and transplantation tolerance. *Expert Rev Clin Immunol*, 2010. **6**(1): p. 155–169.
15. Brazio, P.S., et al., Regulatory T cells are not predictive of outcomes in a nonhuman primate model of vascularized composite allotransplantation. *Transplantation*, 2013. **96**(3): p. 267–273.
16. Josefowicz, S.Z., L.-F. Lu, and A.Y. Rudensky, Regulatory T cells: mechanisms of differentiation and function. *Annu Rev Immunol*, 2012. **30**: p. 531–564.
17. Abbas, A.K., et al., Regulatory T cells: recommendations to simplify the nomenclature. *Nat Immunol*, 2013. **14**(4): p. 307–308.
18. Chen, W., et al., Conversion of peripheral CD4+CD25- naive T cells to CD4+CD25+ regulatory T cells by TGF-beta induction of transcription factor Foxp3. *J Exp Med*, 2003. **198**(12): p. 1875–1886.
19. Zheng, S.G., et al., IL-2 is essential for TGF-β to convert naive CD4+CD25− cells to CD25+Foxp3+ regulatory T cells and for expansion of these cells. *J Immunol*, 2007. **178**(4): p. 2018–2027.
20. Lu, L., et al., Characterization of protective human CD4CD25 FOXP3 regulatory T cells generated with IL-2, TGF-β and retinoic acid. *PLOS ONE*, 2010. **5**(12): p. e15150.
21. Joffre, O., et al., Prevention of acute and chronic allograft rejection with CD4+CD25+Foxp3+ regulatory T lymphocytes. *Nat Med*, 2008. **14**(1): p. 88–92.
22. Hoffmann, P., et al., Donor-type CD4(+)CD25(+) regulatory T cells suppress lethal acute graft-versus-host disease after allogeneic bone marrow transplantation. *J Exp Med*, 2002. **196**(3): p. 389–399.
23. Karim, M., et al., CD25+CD4+ regulatory T cells generated by exposure to a model protein antigen prevent allograft rejection: antigen-specific reactivation in vivo is critical for bystander regulation. *Blood*, 2005. **105**(12): p. 4871–4877.
24. Dawson, N.A.J. and M.K. Levings, Antigen-specific regulatory T cells: are police CARs the answer? *Transl Res*, 2017. **187**: p. 53–58.
25. Safinia, N., et al., Regulatory T cells: serious contenders in the promise for immunological tolerance in transplantation. *Front Immunol*, 2015. **6**: p. 438.
26. Moore, C., et al., Alloreactive regulatory T cells generated with retinoic acid prevent skin allograft rejection. *Eur J Immunol*, 2014. **45**(2): p. 452–463.
27. Jeffery, H.C., et al., Clinical potential of regulatory T cell therapy in liver diseases: an overview and current perspectives. *Front Immunol*, 2016. **7**: p. 334.
28. MacDonald, K.G., et al., Alloantigen-specific regulatory T cells generated with a chimeric antigen receptor. *J Clin Invest*, 2016. **126**(4): p. 1413–1424.
29. Fransson, M., et al., CAR/FoxP3-engineered T regulatory cells target the CNS and suppress EAE upon intranasal delivery. *J Neuroinflammation*, 2012. **9**: p. 112.
30. Blat, D., et al., Suppression of murine colitis and its associated cancer by carcinoembryonic antigen-specific regulatory T cells. *Mol Ther*, 2014. **22**(5): p. 1018–1028.
31. Yoon, J., et al., FVIII-specific human chimeric antigen receptor T-regulatory cells suppress T- and B-cell responses to FVIII. *Blood*, 2017. **129**(2): p. 238–245.
32. Tsang, J.Y.-S., et al., Conferring indirect allospecificity on CD4+CD25+ Tregs by TCR gene transfer favors transplantation tolerance in mice. *J Clin Invest*, 2008. **118**(11): p. 3619–3628.

33. Berdien, B., et al., TALEN-mediated editing of endogenous T-cell receptors facilitates efficient reprogramming of T lymphocytes by lentiviral gene transfer. *Gene Ther*, 2014. **21**(6): p. 539–548.

34. Laurence, A., et al., Interleukin-2 signaling via STAT5 constrains T helper 17 cell generation. *Immunity*, 2007. **26**(3): p. 371–381.

35. Yu, A., et al., A low interleukin-2 receptor signaling threshold supports the development and homeostasis of T regulatory cells. *Immunity*, 2009. **30**(2): p. 204–217.

36. Sadlack, B., et al., Ulcerative colitis-like disease in mice with a disrupted interleukin-2 gene. *Cell*, 1993. **75**(2): p. 253–261.

37. Suzuki, H., et al., Deregulated T cell activation and autoimmunity in mice lacking interleukin-2 receptor beta. *Science*, 1995. **268**(5216): p. 1472–1476.

38. Willerford, D.M., et al., Interleukin-2 receptor α chain regulates the size and content of the peripheral lymphoid compartment. *Immunity*, 1995. **3**(4): p. 521–530.

39. Malek, T.R., et al., CD4 regulatory T cells prevent lethal autoimmunity in IL-2Rβ-deficient mice. *Immunity*, 2002. **17**(2): p. 167–178.

40. Lemoine F.M., et al., Massive expansion of regulatory T-cells following interleukin 2 treatment during a phase I-II dendritic cell-based immunotherapy of metastatic renal cancer. *Int J Oncol*, 2009. **35**(3): p. 569–581.

41. Klatzmann, D. and A.K. Abbas, The promise of low-dose interleukin-2 therapy for autoimmune and inflammatory diseases. *Nat Rev Immunol*, 2015. **15**(5): p. 283–294.

42. Sharabi, A., et al., Regulatory T cells in the treatment of disease. *Nat Rev Drug Discov*, 2018. **17**(11): p. 823–844.

43. Sakaguchi, S., et al., Regulatory T cells and immune tolerance. *Cell*, 2008. **133**(5): p. 775–787.

44. Wing, K. and S. Sakaguchi, Regulatory T cells exert checks and balances on self tolerance and autoimmunity. *Nat Immunol*, 2009. **11**(1): p. 7–13.

45. Campbell, D.J. and M.A. Koch, Phenotypical and functional specialization of FOXP3+ regulatory T cells. *Nat Rev Immunol*, 2011. **11**(2): p. 119–130.

46. Brunstein, C.G., et al., Infusion of ex vivo expanded T regulatory cells in adults transplanted with umbilical cord blood: safety profile and detection kinetics. *Blood*, 2011. **117**(3): p. 1061–1070.

47. Hippen, K.L., et al., Generation and large-scale expansion of human inducible regulatory T cells that suppress graft-versus-host disease. *Am J Transplant*, 2011. **11**(6): p. 1148–1157.

48. de Kleer, I.M., et al., CD4+CD25bright regulatory T cells actively regulate inflammation in the joints of patients with the remitting form of juvenile idiopathic arthritis. *J Immunol*, 2004. **172**(10): p. 6435–6443.

49. Robinson, D.S., M. Larché, and S.R. Durham, Tregs and allergic disease. *J Clin Invest*, 2004. **114**(10): p. 1389–1397.

50. Wang, H., et al., TGF-β–dependent suppressive function of Tregs requires wild-type levels of CD18 in a mouse model of psoriasis. *J Clin Invest*, 2008. **118**(7): p. 2629–2639.

51. Jorn Bovenschen, H., et al., Foxp3+ regulatory T cells of psoriasis patients easily differentiate into IL-17A-producing cells and are found in lesional skin. *J Invest Dermatol*, 2011. **131**(9): p. 1853–1860.

52. Garlet, G.P., et al., Actinobacillus actinomycetemcomitans-induced periodontal disease in mice: patterns of cytokine, chemokine, and chemokine receptor expression and leukocyte migration. *Microbes Infect*, 2005. **7**(4): p. 738–747.

53. Garlet, G.P., et al., Regulatory T cells attenuate experimental periodontitis progression in mice. *J Clin Periodontol*, 2009. **37**(7): p. 591–600.

54. Araujo-Pires, A.C., et al., IL-4/CCL22/CCR4 axis controls regulatory T-cell migration that suppresses inflammatory bone loss in murine experimental periodontitis. *J Bone Miner Res*, 2015. **30**(3): p. 412–422.

55. Raimondi, G., et al., Mammalian target of rapamycin inhibition and alloantigen-specific regulatory T cells synergize to promote long-term graft survival in immuno-competent recipients. *J Immunol*, 2010. **184**(2): p. 624–636.

56. Lee, I., et al., Recruitment of Foxp3+ T regulatory cells mediating allograft tolerance depends on the CCR4 chemokine receptor. *J Exp Med*, 2005. **201**(7): p. 1037–1044.

57. Torgerson, T.R. and H.D. Ochs, Immune dysregulation, polyendocrinopathy, enteropathy, X-linked: Forkhead box protein 3 mutations and lack of regulatory T cells. *J Allergy Clin Immunol*, 2007. **120**(4): p. 744–750.

58. Bennett, C.L., et al., The immune dysregulation, polyendocrinopathy, enteropathy, X-linked syndrome (IPEX) is caused by mutations of FOXP3. *Nat Genet*, 2001. **27**(1): p. 20–21.

59. Malek, T.R., The biology of interleukin-2. *Annu Rev Immunol*, 2008. **26**(1): p. 453–479.

60. Malek, T.R. and A.L. Bayer, Tolerance, not immunity, crucially depends on IL-2. *Nat Rev Immunol*, 2004. **4**(9): p. 665–674.

61. Afeltra, A., et al., The involvement of T regulatory lymphocytes in a cohort of lupus nephritis patients: a pilot study. *Intern Emerg Med*, 2015. **10**(6): p. 677–683.

62. Marwaha, A.K., et al., Cutting edge: increased IL-17-secreting T cells in children with new-onset type 1 diabetes. *J Immunol*, 2010. **185**(7): p. 3814–3818.

63. Long, S.A., et al., Defects in IL-2R signaling contribute to diminished maintenance of FOXP3 expression in CD4(+)CD25(+) regulatory T-cells of type 1 diabetic subjects. *Diabetes*, 2010. **59**(2): p. 407–415.

64. Balandina, A., et al., Functional defect of regulatory CD4(+)CD25+ T cells in the thymus of patients with autoimmune myasthenia gravis. *Blood*, 2005. **105**(2): p. 735–741.

65. Thiruppathi, M., et al., Impaired regulatory function in circulating CD4(+)CD25(high) CD127(low/-) T cells in patients with myasthenia gravis. *Clin Immunol*, 2012. **145**(3): p. 209–223.

66. Jhunjhunwala, S., et al., Controlled release formulations of IL-2, TGF-β1 and rapamycin for the induction of regulatory T cells. *J Control Release*, 2012. **159**(1): p. 78–84.

67. Trzonkowski, P., et al., Hurdles in therapy with regulatory T cells. *Sci Transl Med*, 2015. **7**(304): p. 304ps18.

68. Riley, J.L., C.H. June, and B.R. Blazar, Human T regulatory cell therapy: take a billion or so and call me in the morning. *Immunity*, 2009. **30**(5): p. 656–665.

69. Safinia, N., et al., Adoptive regulatory T cell therapy: challenges in clinical transplantation. *Curr Opin Organ Transplant*, 2010. **15**(4): p. 427–434.

70. Wieckiewicz, J., R. Goto, and K.J. Wood, T regulatory cells and the control of alloimmunity: from characterisation to clinical application. *Curr Opin Immunol*, 2010. **22**(5): p. 662–668.

71. Webster, K.E., et al., In vivo expansion of Treg cells with IL-2–mAb complexes: induction of resistance to EAE and long-term acceptance of islet allografts without immunosuppression. *J Exp Med*, 2009. **206**(4): p. 751–760.

72. Beyersdorf, N., et al., Selective targeting of regulatory T cells with CD28 superagonists allows effective therapy of experimental autoimmune encephalomyelitis. *J Exp Med*, 2005. **202**(3): p. 445–455.

73. Deal watch: Boosting TRegs to target autoimmune disease. *Nat Rev Drug Discov*, 2011. **10**(8): p. 566.

74. Suntharalingam, G., et al., Cytokine storm in a phase 1 trial of the anti-CD28 monoclonal antibody TGN1412. *N Engl J Med*, 2006. **355**(10): p. 1018–1028.

75. Gorantla, V.S., et al., T regulatory cells and transplantation tolerance. *Transplant Rev (Orlando)*, 2010. **24**(3): p. 147–159.

76. LeGuern, C., et al., Intracellular MHC class II controls regulatory tolerance to allogeneic transplants. *J Immunol*, 2010. **184**(5): p. 2394–2400.

77. Scalea, J.R., et al., Abrogation of renal allograft tolerance in MGH miniature swine: the role of intra-graft and peripheral factors in long-term tolerance. *Am J Transplant*, 2014. **14**(9): p. 2001–2010.

78. Kingsley, C.I., et al., CD25+CD4+ regulatory T cells prevent graft rejection: CTLA-4- and IL-10-dependent immunoregulation of alloresponses. *J Immunol*, 2002. **168**(3): p. 1080–1086.

79. Cobbold, S. and H. Waldmann, Infectious tolerance. *Curr Opin Immunol*, 1998. **10**(5): p. 518–524.

80. Graca, L., S.P. Cobbold, and H. Waldmann, Identification of regulatory T cells in tolerated allografts. *J Exp Med*, 2002. **195**(12): p. 1641–1646.

81. Zheng, X.X., et al., The balance of deletion and regulation in allograft tolerance. *Immunol Rev*, 2003. **196**(1): p. 75–84.

82. Sánchez-Fueyo, A., et al., Tracking the immunoregulatory mechanisms active during allograft tolerance. *J Immunol*, 2002. **168**(5): p. 2274–2281.

83. Yoshizawa, A., et al., The roles of CD25+CD4+ regulatory T cells in operational tolerance after living donor liver transplantation. *Transplant Proc*, 2005. **37**(1): p. 37–39.

84. Dijke, I.E., et al., FOXP3 mRNA expression analysis in the peripheral blood and allograft of heart transplant patients. *Transpl Immunol*, 2008. **18**(3): p. 250–254.

85. Muthukumar, T., et al., Messenger RNA for FOXP3 in the urine of renal-allograft recipients. *N Engl J Med*, 2005. **353**(22): p. 2342–2351.

86. Haxhinasto, S., D. Mathis, and C. Benoist, The AKT–mTOR axis regulates de novo differentiation of CD4+Foxp3+ cells. *J Exp Med*, 2008. **205**(3): p. 565–574.

87. Kopf, H., et al., Rapamycin inhibits differentiation of Th17 cells and promotes generation of FoxP3+ T regulatory cells. *Int Immunopharmacol*, 2007. **7**(13): p. 1819–1824.

88. Cobbold, S.P., et al., Infectious tolerance via the consumption of essential amino acids and mTOR signaling. *Proc Natl Acad Sci U S A*, 2009. **106**(29): p. 12055–12060.

89. Thomson, A.W., H.R. Turnquist, and G. Raimondi, Immunoregulatory functions of mTOR inhibition. *Nat Rev Immunol*, 2009. **9**(5): p. 324–337.

90. Jhunjhunwala, S. and S.R. Little, Microparticulate systems for targeted drug delivery to phagocytes. *Cell Cycle*, 2011. **10**(13): p. 2047–2048.

91. Jhunjhunwala, S., et al., Delivery of rapamycin to dendritic cells using degradable microparticles. *J Control Release*, 2009. **133**(3): p. 191–197.

92. Curiel, T.J., et al., Specific recruitment of regulatory T cells in ovarian carcinoma fosters immune privilege and predicts reduced survival. *Nat Med*, 2004. **10**(9): p. 942–949.

93. Wei, S., I. Kryczek, and W. Zou, Regulatory T-cell compartmentalization and trafficking. *Blood*, 2006. **108**(2): p. 426–431.

94. Eghtesad, S., et al., Rapamycin ameliorates dystrophic phenotype in mdx mouse skeletal muscle. *Mol Med*, 2011. **17**(9–10): p. 917–924.

95. Jhunjhunwala, S., et al., Bioinspired controlled release of CCL22 recruits regulatory T cells in vivo. *Adv Mater*, 2012. **24**(35): p. 4735–4738.

96. Rothstein, S.N., W.J. Federspiel, and S.R. Little, A unified mathematical model for the prediction of controlled release from surface and bulk eroding polymer matrices. *Biomaterials*, 2009. **30**(8): p. 1657–1664.

97. Haribhai, D., et al., Regulatory T cells dynamically control the primary immune response to foreign antigen. *J Immunol*, 2007. **178**(5): p. 2961–2972.

98. Takamura, K., et al., Regulatory role of lymphoid chemokine CCL19 and CCL21 in the control of allergic rhinitis. *J Immunol*, 2007. **179**(9): p. 5897–5906.

99. Brusko, T.M., A.L. Putnam, and J.A. Bluestone, Human regulatory T cells: role in autoimmune disease and therapeutic opportunities. *Immunol Rev*, 2008. **223**(1): p. 371–390.

100. Ratay, M.L., et al., Treg-recruiting microspheres prevent inflammation in a murine model of dry eye disease. *J Control Release*, 2017. **258**: p. 208–217.

101. Bromley, S.K., T.R. Mempel, and A.D. Luster, Orchestrating the orchestrators: chemokines in control of T cell traffic. *Nat Immunol*, 2008. **9**(9): p. 970–980.

102. Mailloux, A.W. and M.R.I. Young, NK-dependent increases in CCL22 secretion selectively recruits regulatory T cells to the tumor microenvironment. *J Immunol*, 2009. **182**(5): p. 2753–2765.

103. Fisher, J.D., et al., In situ recruitment of regulatory T cells promotes donor-specific tolerance in vascularized composite allotransplantation. *Sci Adv*, 2020. **6**(11): p. eaax8429.

104. Ratay, M.L., et al., TRI microspheres prevent key signs of dry eye disease in a murine, inflammatory model. *Sci Rep*, 2017. **7**(1): p. 17527.

105. Balmert, S.C., et al., In vivo induction of regulatory T cells promotes allergen tolerance and suppresses allergic contact dermatitis. *J Control Release*, 2017. **261**: p. 223–233.

106. Fisher, J.D., et al., Treg-inducing microparticles promote donor-specific tolerance in experimental vascularized composite allotransplantation. *Proc Natl Acad Sci U S A*, 2019. **116**(51): p. 25784–25789.

107. Delgoffe, G.M., et al., The mTOR kinase differentially regulates effector and regulatory T cell lineage commitment. *Immunity*, 2009. **30**(6): p. 832–844.

108. Lai, Z.W., et al., Sirolimus in patients with clinically active systemic lupus erythematosus resistant to, or intolerant of, conventional medications: a single-arm, open-label, phase 1/2 trial. *Lancet*, 2018. **391**(10126): p. 1186–1196.

109. Battaglia, M., et al., Rapamycin and interleukin-10 treatment induces T regulatory type 1 cells that mediate antigen-specific transplantation tolerance. *Diabetes*, 2005. **55**(1): p. 40–49.

110. Kang, H.G., et al., Effects of cyclosporine on transplant tolerance: the role of IL-2. *Am J Transplant*, 2007. **7**(8): p. 1907–1916.

111. Kogina, K., et al., Tacrolimus differentially regulates the proliferation of conventional and regulatory CD4(+) T cells. *Mol Cells*, 2009. **28**(2): p. 125–130.

112. Miroux, C., et al., In vitro effects of cyclosporine A and tacrolimus on regulatory T-cell proliferation and function. *Transplantation*, 2012. **94**(2): p. 123–131.

113. Hancock, W.W., et al., HDAC inhibitor therapy in autoimmunity and transplantation. *Ann Rheum Dis*, 2012. **71**(Suppl 2): p. i46–i54.

114. Regna, N.L., et al., Specific HDAC6 inhibition by ACY-738 reduces SLE pathogenesis in NZB/W mice. *Clin Immunol*, 2016. **162**: p. 58–73.

115. Zhang, Y., et al., Mice lacking histone deacetylase 6 have hyperacetylated tubulin but are viable and develop normally. *Mol Cell Biol*, 2008. **28**(5): p. 1688–1701.

116. de Zoeten, E.F., et al., Histone deacetylase 6 and heat shock protein 90 control the functions of Foxp3(+) T-regulatory cells. *Mol Cell Biol*, 2011. **31**(10): p. 2066–2078.

117. Tang, Q. and J.A. Bluestone, Regulatory T-cell therapy in transplantation: moving to the clinic. *Cold Spring Harb Perspect Med*, 2013. **3**(11): p. a015552.

118. Brunstein, C.G., et al., Umbilical cord blood-derived T regulatory cells to prevent GVHD: kinetics, toxicity profile, and clinical effect. *Blood*, 2016. **127**(8): p. 1044–1051.

119. Godfrey, W.R., et al., Cord blood CD4+CD25+-derived T regulatory cell lines express FoxP3 protein and manifest potent suppressor function. *Blood*, 2005. **105**(2): p. 750–758.

120. Hoffmann, P., R. Eder, and M. Edinger, Polyclonal expansion of human CD4(+)CD25(+) regulatory T cells. *Methods Mol Biol*, 2011. **677**: p. 15–30.

121. Taylor, P.A., C.J. Lees, and B.R. Blazar, The infusion of ex vivo activated and expanded CD4+CD25+ immune regulatory cells inhibits graft-versus-host disease lethality. *Blood*, 2002. **99**(10): p. 3493–3499.

122. Cohen, J.L., et al., CD4(+)CD25(+) immunoregulatory T Cells: new therapeutics for graft-versus-host disease. *J Exp Med*, 2002. **196**(3): p. 401–406.

123. Sagoo, P., et al., Human regulatory T cells with alloantigen specificity are more potent inhibitors of alloimmune skin graft damage than polyclonal regulatory T cells. *Sci Transl Med*, 2011. **3**(83): p. 83ra42.
124. Herrath, J., et al., The inflammatory milieu in the rheumatic joint reduces regulatory T-cell function. *Eur J Immunol*, 2011. **41**(8): p. 2279–2290.
125. Vargas-Rojas, M.I., et al., Quantitative and qualitative normal regulatory T cells are not capable of inducing suppression in SLE patients due to T-cell resistance. *Lupus*, 2008. **17**(4): p. 289–294.
126. Chowdary Venigalla, R.K., et al., Reduced CD4+,CD25− T cell sensitivity to the suppressive function of CD4+,CD25high,CD127−/lowregulatory T cells in patients with active systemic lupus erythematosus. *Arthritis Rheum*, 2008. **58**(7): p. 2120–2130.

.

Section II

Unique Considerations and Emerging Indications in Reconstructive Transplantation

3 Invasive and Non-Invasive Surrogates for Chronic Rejection in Vascularized Composite Allotransplantation
Claims and Controversies

Nicholas L. Robbins and Warren C. Breidenbach

CONTENTS

Introduction 47
Defining Chronic Rejection in 2019 48
Invasive Surrogate Techniques 49
Non-Invasive Surrogate Techniques 50
Discussion: Claims and Controversies 52
    Invasive Surrogate Claims and Controversies 52
    Non-Invasive Surrogate Claims and Controversies 56
Conclusion 56
References 57

INTRODUCTION

The first successful vascularized composite allotransplantation (VCA) was a hand transplant performed by Dubernard et al. in 1998 and the second by Breidenbach et al. in 1999.[1,2] We are now beyond the 20-year mark of hand transplantation survival with a subsequent 100 plus upper extremity transplants and 30 plus face transplants in varying states of survival. With these first successful VCAs, we demonstrated that skin, muscle, bone, and arteries could be transplanted with varying degrees of motor function return.[1,3] These first successful cases indicated that long-term survival of a VCA is obtainable. That being said, given sufficient time, we expected the VCA to fail due to chronic rejection (CR), as we know lasting tolerance has not been achieved in any human transplantation to date.[4]

Recent seminal publications indicate apparent CR presence in two of the French team's face transplantation patients.[5–7] In both of these cases, it appears that CR manifested initially as intimal hyperplasia (IH) in the deep arteries. This led to poor

DOI: 10.1201/9780429260179-5

circulation in the muscle and skin of the transplants, causing necrosis of the skin and deeper tissues. Both patients' deaths were attributed to primary tumor development, not from the transplants. Likewise, Kaufman et al. reported the first case of CR in hand transplantation in 2012, and many more cases were discussed in the 2017 International Society of VCA (ISVCA) meeting from various international teams.[8,9]

What are we to conclude from these outcomes? We believe the best strategy for us at this point is to proceed with the assumption that CR is present in VCA despite variations in management, and we further believe more cases will develop as time elapses. Therefore, the purpose of this paper is to review the current definition and etiology of CR while reviewing the most current diagnostic tools employed over the last three years of clinical experience.

DEFINING CHRONIC REJECTION IN 2019

The field of VCA has been limited by its understanding of CR. The current accepted comprehensive definition of CR was first published by Kanitakis et al. in 2016 and has since been referenced by many teams during the 2017 ISVCA congress, as well as the Morelon et al. manuscript published in August 2018. The clinical and histopathological definition can be seen in Table 3.1.[6,10,11]

From 1998 to 2011, there were no reported cases of CR in VCA. In 2012, Kaufman et al. claimed to have seen the first case of CR out of Louisville in a hand transplant patient.[12] Since then, many teams have further defined clinical cases of CR based on the clinical and histopathological grading seen in Table 3.1 with and without the

---

TABLE 3.1

Most Common Non-Specific Clinicopathological Findings Used to Define Chronic Rejection in VCA as of September 2018

Clinical	Pathological
Scaly psoriasiform cutaneous lesions	Graft vasculopathy
Purpuric cutaneous lesions	Epidermal and adnexal atrophy
Necrotic skin ulceration	Dermal sclerosis
Skin sclerosis	Capillary thrombosis
Dyschromia	Tertiary lymphoid organ-like follicles
Finger thinning	
Nail loss	
Pain	

Sources: Kanitakis J, Petruzzo P, Badet L, et al. Chronic rejection in human vascularized composite allotransplantation (hand and face recipients): an update. *Transplantation.* 2016;100(10):2053–2061. Morelon E, Petruzzo P, Kanitakis J. Chronic rejection in vascularized composite allotransplantation. *Curr Opin Organ Transplant.* 2018;23(5):582–591. Cendales L, Kaufman C. Chronic rejection in VCA; definition, follow up, diagnosis and therapy. Paper presented at: 13th Congress of the International Society of Vascularized Composite Allotransplantation; October 27, 2017; Salzburg, Austria.

presence of donor-specific antibodies (DSA).[5,10,13–15] The first re-transplantation of a face due to CR was performed by Lantieri et al. in January 2018.[16,17]

Because of the growing presence of CR-induced graft failure in a multitude of VCA patients, the need for precise definition, mechanism, and site of injury is required to diagnose and treat CR as it arises. As the clinical cases have been few to date, the extent of invasive and non-invasive clinically applied diagnostic instrumentation and tissue markers have been limited. Below is a summary of the surrogate techniques utilized in the literature over the last three years to diagnose and direct treatment.

INVASIVE SURROGATE TECHNIQUES

Since the emergence of the field in 1998, to date, superficial cutaneous biopsy has remained the key diagnostic tool for VCA patients. These "protocol biopsies" have been recommended to be performed weekly for the first month followed by 2, 3, 6, 9, 12, 18, 24, 30, and 36 months. After the graft has reached 3-year post-operative survival, the biopsies can be performed biannually per protocol biopsy assessment.[18] The 2007 Banff scale continues to be used as the gold standard in the field to evaluate these biopsies for both acute and chronic rejection.[14,19] As shown in Table 3.2, the definition of histopathologic and immunohistochemical findings continue to be expanded upon as the tissue database in VCA grows.[20] Additionally, many have included superficial biopsies in their description of the assessment of CR, noting capillary thrombosis in dermal networks, with and without the finding of C4d deposition in the endothelium, along with epidermal and adnexal atrophy, and dermal sclerosis.[6,10,21]

TABLE 3.2

Banff 2007 Grading Classification for Protocol and for-Cause Skin Biopsies in Human VCA

Grade	Inflammatory Infiltrate	Involvement of Epithelium (Epidermis or Adnexa)
0 (no rejection)	None/rare	None
I (mild rejection)	Mild perivascular	None
II (moderate rejection)	Moderate to severe perivascular	Mild (limited to spongiosis or lymphocytic exocytosis
III (severe rejection)	Dense	Apoptosis, dyskeratosis, and/
IV (acute necrotizing rejection)	Frank necrosis of the epidermis or dermis	or keratinolysis

Note: This diagnostic scale has been used for 12 years, evaluating immune response findings at the epidermis and superficial dermis. Note that it is a technique that alleviates deep dermal and cutis findings, as well as muscular, large vasculature, and boney tissue results. Significant adaptation of this scale will be required to translate to the CR VCA patient.

Sources: Cendales L. Histopathology workshop and Banff. Paper presented at: 13th Congress of the International Society of Vascularized Composite Allotransplantation; October 26, 2017; Salzburg, Austria. Cendales LC, Kanitakis J, Schneeberger S, et al. The Banff 2007 working classification of skin-containing composite tissue allograft pathology. *Am J Transplant.* 2008;8(7):1396–1400.

The key diagnostic tool many treating teams have incorporated since the emergence of the field has been the "for-cause" skin biopsy. This is generally a superficial cutaneous biopsy, which allows for histological examination confirming skin, dermal, and superficial subcutaneous rejection based on the Banff scale.[18] The use of the Banff grading scale remains the gold standard diagnostic tool for acute cellular rejection (Banff grade I or greater). It is a technique that allows for early intervention of rejection but continues to recommend against the treatment of subclinical rejection. This has historically been due to its lack of sensitivity toward CR.[18] This recommendation continues to persist, despite the findings published by Diefenbeck et al. noting synovial arterioles with IH as early as 18 months post-transplantation.[22] This team described a knee VCA that went on to complete loss at 36 months and perhaps is the first case of CR failure reported in the VCA literature.[23]

As CR is seen in a growing number of patients, the use of deep wide biopsy (DWB) has expanded, as exemplified in the Louisville, Polish, and French teams' cases of reported CR.[5,8,24] Despite its ability to evaluate deep dermal and subcutaneous structures, the use of DWB has largely been limited by the treating VCA teams to avoid extensive aesthetic and cosmetic dysmorphic outcomes to the transplant. Thus, this technique has been reserved by many as a last resort tool for diagnosing CR.

Finally, biomarkers have become a standard assessment in the broad field of transplantation, which has carried over into the VCA community for diagnosing the possible presence of CR. Traditional assessment in CR has been in the presence of DSA as well as a phenotypic cellular immune response (CD4+, CD3+, and CD8+).[6] Beyond this, serum biomarker assessment in the field has yet to apply further specific markers of CR. In VCA, the assessment of DSA-positive patients has been at best inconsistent when a diagnosis of CR is reported, despite being seen as a leading indicator of CR in solid organ transplantation (SOT).[10,15,25] This technique continues to expand in the basic science research literature and is a desirable precise technique as it requires a simple skin or mucosal swab, avoiding the invasive procedure.

NON-INVASIVE SURROGATE TECHNIQUES

As discussed in a 2012 publication by Kaufman et al., **ultrasound biomicroscopy** could be used as a potential non-invasive tool for diagnosing CR by monitoring the development of IH in the donor vessel (facial artery, radial artery, etc.).[8] In 2015, Kueckelhaus et al. designed and developed an expanded donor to recipient vessel assessment in five face transplant patients.[26] A ratio of facial artery to radial artery was used to evaluate the relationship of native recipient IH to donor vessel IH development. In this study, a 48 MHz ultrasound transducer was used to measure the donor facial arteries divided by the recipient radial arteries. At the conclusion of the study, controls indicated a ratio value of 1.00 compared to 0.87 in VCA recipients, with a P-value of 0.58. The lack of statistical significance was attributed to mean age difference between the two cohorts (face transplant patients 46 years old vs. control age 26 years).

Flow magnetic resonance imaging (*flow*MRI) is another non-invasive surrogate that was used during the work up of the French team's first face transplant patient.

Although this imaging technique was not specifically intended to assess and diagnose CR, the team found severe IH development on microscopic examination, which corroborated the decrease in flow seen on the *flow*MRI. In contrast, the team performed a Computed Tomography–Angiography (CT-A), which indicated a patent vascular pedicle. If the team had only assessed with the CT-A, they would have missed the severely decreased blood flow seen in the *flow*MRI due to IH in the donor facial artery.[5,7]

Recently, our team presented a hypothesis based on the review of seven VCA cases describing a vascular-functional diagnosis of CR.[8,27,28] This hypothesis is predicated on the well-documented rejection process in the arteries and capillaries initially outlined by the French team.[6,10,21] Capillary destruction is referenced as the first step to the formation of IH in numerous papers describing SOT rejection, but it has not been explored in the VCA literature.[29] Learning from the work of our colleagues in SOT, and the extensive clinical experience of our team in VCA, we believe that the capillaries are a primary inciting structure infiltrated by the immune system to initiate the development of IH in the arteries that leads to failure.[30]

The foundation of this hypothesis is the application of well-known fluid dynamic formulas and principles in a VCA, namely the detrimental impact of IH development on the Windkessel effect. The relationship can be appreciated when reviewing the formulas in Table 3.3. The formulas listed define the relationship of flow

---

TABLE 3.3

Representative Formulas of Vascular Flow through a Non-Ideal State as Outlined by Robbins et al.

Mathematical Explanation for Vascular Rejection in a VCA	
Formula	**Rationale**
$Q = \dfrac{\Delta P}{R}$	Resistance (R) indirectly related to flow (Q).
$R = \dfrac{8L\eta}{\pi r4}$	Length (L) of the vascular pedicle and radius (r^4) are the only two variables altered by transplantation.
$C = \dfrac{\Delta V}{\Delta P}$	Compliance (C) is indirectly related to resistance (R), thereby a decrease in radius directly affects compliance by a factor of 4.
$P(t) = P(td)e\left(-\dfrac{t}{RC}\right)$	Resistance (R) and compliance (C) and the time of diastolic flow only relevant variable in Windkessel effect.
$PWV = \sqrt{\dfrac{V \times \Delta P}{\rho \times \Delta V}}$	Pulse wave velocity (PWV) measured is inversely proportional to compliance (C).

Abbreviations: Q = flow; ΔP = change in pressure; R = resistance; L = length; r = radius; C = vessel compliance; ΔV = change in volume; t = time; td = diastolic time; PWV = pulse wave velocity; ρ = whole blood viscosity; η, π, = mathematical constants

Note: for a theoretical cause, clinical finding, and diagnostic measure of chronic rejection. More importantly, it possesses the observation of functional decline and therefore ischemia, cellular apoptosis, necrosis and failure of the VCA.

Source: Robbins NL, Wordsworth MJ, Parida BK, et al. A flow dynamic rationale for accelerated vascularized composite allotransplant rejection. *Plast Reconstr Surg.* 2019;143(3):637e–643e.

(Q) and resistance (R) found in the cardiac and peripheral vascular systems.[31] Postoperatively, the radius (r) is primarily affected by development of IH due to the vessels response from insult of the immune system and any damage to the external vasa vasorum during procurement. As the VCA undergoes rejection, i.e. IH development, an inherent loss of vessel elasticity and compliance (C) will occur.[32] With this decrease in C, the vessels lose the ability to maintain appropriate diastolic pressure and the ability to propagate the diastolic vascular flow in the graft, leading to a near no-flow phenomenon. This will result in ischemia and failure of the VCA.

In addition, the mathematical relationship between wall compliance and vascular flow allows for the use of a non-invasive monitor. Namely, pulse wave velocity (PWV) measurements are inversely proportional to C. Thus, by measuring PWV, these mathematical equations can be utilized to indirectly evaluate VCA rejection.[27]

Lastly, there are multiple emerging techniques for rejection monitoring, including, but not limited to, fluorine MRI, nanotechnology, biosensors, and extended evaluation of biomarkers such as genetic markers of expression (RNA, mRNA, etc.). These techniques have not been expanded into the clinical realm and hence are beyond the scope of this manuscript but could emerge as a viable option as CR is defined further.

DISCUSSION: CLAIMS AND CONTROVERSIES

As described by Etra et al. and Morelon et al., as of 2018, the field has, and will continue to experience, various states of rejection in VCA patients.[10,33] The complexity of the rejection phases are vast in a multi-tissue transplant such as a VCA, whether acute cellularly mediated, DSA and antibody-mediated rejection, and the less defined phases of CR.[33] In a field with less than 200 total transplants performed over the last 20 years, the number of CR cases remains small and hence becomes difficult to standardize. A series of one to five patients is a good start for the field, but not enough to entirely validate a particular technique due to multiple confounding factors, including patient compliance, care, and the variability in the diagnostic technique being utilized. It should be cautioned that claims for novel techniques to definitively diagnose CR, particularly in the absence of an agreed upon definition, should be heavily peer reviewed to allow the field to progress on scientifically founded outcomes.

INVASIVE SURROGATE CLAIMS AND CONTROVERSIES

The **Banff grading scale** has been the work horse for routine monitoring of acute and chronic rejection development since the first VCA case was performed in 1998. It has been an invaluable tool to indicate acute T-cell-mediated rejection requiring immunological intervention. However, the scale is limited in its ability to assess the VCA as a complete unit, and many published cases have shown differences between biopsies of the graft, biopsies of a sentinel graft, and as seen in Figure 3.1, the immunologic findings in the deeper tissue.[28,34] Further, the local invasiveness of the biopsy itself is inherently stimulatory to an immune response. This has been a known result when using this technique, but little research has been conducted on what the level of immune response this causes locally in the graft. At the very least, there is concern

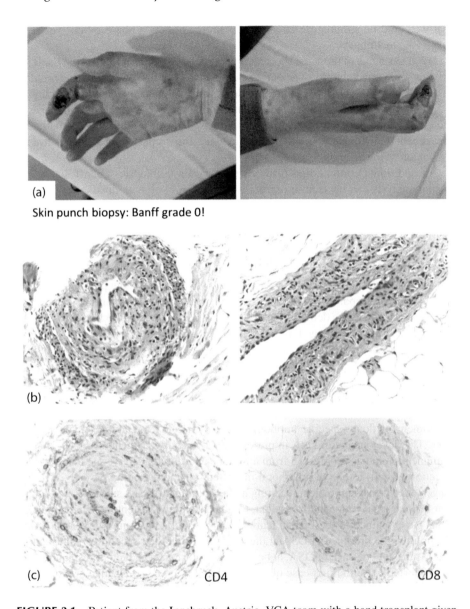

FIGURE 3.1 Patient from the Innsbruck, Austria, VCA team with a hand transplant given a clinical diagnosis of CR at 7 years despite finding of Banff Grade 0. (a) A clinical photo taken representing many of the findings listed in Table 3.1 that lead to the diagnosis of CR. (b) H&E histopathology representing intimal and medial hyperplasia and fibrosis development in the deep vessels at 7 years. (c) Immunohistochemistry staining indicating findings of CD4 and CD8 within the wall of the vessel, representing a result of rejection primarily of the vasculature during CR, whereas the punch biopsy of the epidermis and dermis were inert on the classic Banff grading scale established 12 years ago. (From Grahammer J, Weissenbacher, A, Wolfram-Raunicher, D, et al. A case report: graft loss 7 years after hand transplantation. Paper presented at: International Society of Vascularized Composite Allotransplantation Meeting; October 26–27, 2017; Salzburg, Austria.)

that we could be stimulating an acute on chronic rejection phase by our very own diagnostic techniques.

DWB has many of the same shortcomings as described above when using the Banff grading scale punch biopsy. The purpose of its invasive use is to rule out the presence of deep tissue involvement. The greatest downsides to this method are in its additional painful surgical procedures to the patient, poor cosmetic dysmorphic outcomes to the graft, and inciting local inflammatory effects. This, unfortunately, is a method of assessment that will be required until the field has fully replaced the need for invasive evaluation of the deep tissues.

An additional confounding result of invasive tissue biopsies (Banff and DWB) during analysis can be seen in reports by Kaufman et al. and Unadkat et al.[35,36] In these reports, the histopathologic hematoxylin and eosin (H&E) stains of failed VCA arteries indicate that IH development led to occlusion in the arteries and therefore caused loss of circulation to the VCA.[8,36] This hypothesis would lead one to assume that IH development progressed to the point of complete loss of blood flow, i.e. occlusion. In this setting, the skin would likely be lost at an alarming rate due to severe ischemia necrosis; however, this was not the observed result. One potential explanation for this discrepancy could be in the processing of the histopathological slides. H&E is known to cause dehydration of the tissue during prep of the vessel, which can create a false-positive image for complete occlusion as opposed to the likely stenotic state the vessel was in (i.e. decreased blood blow rather than no flow, thrombosis versus collapse).

The discussion of **biomarkers** is loosely referred to as an invasive surrogate assessment simply due to the need for serum collection from the patient. The only biomarker discussed to date in the clinical literature of VCA patients has been the assessment of donor-specific antibodies (DSA) directed to human leukocyte antigens. The development of DSA in pre-operatively negative patients indicates that the immune system has progressed from an innate and initial adaptive mediated state of rejection (T-cell) to one of a humoral mediated rejection (memory B-cell). With the longest face transplant patient reaching a maximum of 10 years survival and the current 20-year surviving hand transplant, CR has been inconsistent in its assessment of DSA. As explained in the French team's face transplant outcomes, their first patient exemplified the presence of DSA at the time of CR but their second patient exemplified a transient presence of DSA, at best.[6,7] The Kaufman et al. hand transplant patient was reported to be the first case of CR, but noted to be DSA negative at the time of diagnosis.[8] Berglund and Weissenbacher et al. expressed, during the ISVCA meeting in 2017, that their teams' hand transplant patient had begun to express positive DSA in what appears to be a clinical picture of progressive CR (Figure 3.2).[25]

Given the variability seen in VCA to date, we do not believe that the field can rule out the use of the standard transplant biomarker assessment of serum DSA as the field data points are too few to make this assertion. The SOT literature's experience supports the claim that monitoring patients for DSA presence is essential in the VCA patient where there is concern for CR. Assessing and recording DSA over the next 10 years of clinical practice could prove to be a key indicator of what defines the timeline of CR, bringing us to a closer understanding of how and when it occurs.

(a)

Association of HLA-mismatch at antigen class I loci HLA-A and HLA-B, and class II locus HLA-DR and acute rejection and antibody development. Statistical significance evaluated with Chi-square test.				
	AR incidence in the first year^x of transplant (%)	**P-value**	**Antibody development (%)**	**P-value**
HLA-A				
0 mismatch (n=5)	80% (n=4)		60% (n=3, one presens.)	
1 mismatch (n=15)	93% (n=14)	0.714	60% (n=9)	0.998
2 mismatch (n=23)	91% (n=21)		61% (n=14, two presens.)	
HLA-B				
0 mismatch (n=1)	100% (n=1)		0%	
1 mismatch (n=8)	100% (n=8)	0.371	88% (n=7, one presens.)	0.081
2 mismatch (n=34)	88% (n=30)		56% (n=19, two presens.)	
HLA-DR				
0 mismatch (n=0)				
1 mismatch (n=14)	93% (n=13)	1.000	36% (n=5, one presens.)	0.044*
2 mismatch (n=29)	90% (n=26)		72% (n=21, two presens.)	

^{x}Three out of the 43 patients had a total duration of follow-up of less than one year (160, 278, and 330 days). Abbreviations: Acute rejection (AR), Human leukocyte antigen (HLA). *Statistical significance, p-value < 0.05.

(b)

Patient	Time Post Tx	ACR	Evidence of CR in Skin?	Significant Vasculopathy?	Donor Specific Antibody	Capillary Thrombosis in Upper Dermis
1	18 years	Quiet course	No	No	No	Not found
2	16 years	Multiple >15		No	No	Yes, Grade 2.3
3	10 years	Multiple >15	Yes	Yes	No	Yes Day 58 forward
4	9 months	One (Grade 2)	No	Yes	No	Only days prior to amputation in Grade 0 biopsy
5	8 years	Quiet year 1-7 multiple recent episodes	Yes	Yes	Yes	Yes, Grade 1-3
7	6 years	Quiet course	No	No	Yes	Found in Grade 1 biopsy
8	5 years	Quiet course	No	No	No	Not found (yet)
10	1 year	None to date	No	No	No	No, but year 1 biopsy pending

FIGURE 3.2 Tables above were presented by two separate international VCA teams (Louisville, KY, and Innsbruck, Austria) at the 2017 ISVCA congress. (a) represents a table presented by Weissenbacher et al. indicating the development of DSA in patients primarily associated with HLA-DR which were found to have a higher rate of acute rejection I and II episodes early on and projected to establish CR diagnosis earlier due to these findings. Compared to (b) Kaufman et al. demonstrating two separate patients from a cohort of 10 that have undergone a hand transplantation. Patient no. 3 and Patient no. 5 in the table indicate patients that have been diagnosed by the treating team with CR. Patient no. 3 was found to have no DSA present and Patient no. 5 was found to have DSA present. While both appear to have had very different acute rejection episode occurrences, both were diagnosed with CR at 10 and 8 years, respectively. (From Kaufman C, Zaring R, Chilton PM, et al. Evidence of capillary thrombosis prior to development of chronic rejection in a hand transplant recipient. Paper presented at: 13th Congress of the International Society of Vascularized Composite Allotransplantation; October 26, 2017; Salzburg, Austria; Berglund E, Ljungdahl MA, Bogdanovic D, et al. Clinical significance of alloantibodies in hand transplantation: impact on rejection and functional outcome. Paper presented at: 13th Congress of the International Society of Vascularized Composite Allotransplantation; October 27, 2017; Salzburg, Austria.)

Non-Invasive Surrogate Claims and Controversies

As initially shown by Kaufman et al. followed by Kueckelhaus et al. and Petruzzo et al., ultrasound biomicroscopy could be a promising clinical tool for the future. That being said, the current technology has too great a risk of user variability during measurement to provide a non-invasive surrogate that can be validated for CR diagnosis. From the first published use in 2012 for diagnosis of IH and CR in VCA, Kueckelhaus et al. appeared to reduce the user variability with a slightly more powerful transducer (25 MHz vs. 48 MHz). This study in 2015 showed a statistical difference in IH formation in the facial artery in the VCA patient compared to the healthy control patient; however, the facial-to-radial artery ratio evaluation showed no statistically significant difference between the VCA patient and the control (P = 0.57).[37] The authors concluded this technique could be used for IH assessment and therefore for CR development and diagnosis in VCA patients despite being statistically unsupported by their results.

Beyond the variability seen by these team's results, we believe an even greater set of questions exists around this technique. When does the presence of IH appear? Is IH an acute rejection complication and/or a CR complication? At what level of IH development can we truly say CR is present based off of a static ultrasound image? And lastly, at what level of IH development is the basic function of the vasculature compromised, and thus leads to VCA failure? The ultrasound biomicroscope is an instrument that could assess structural change in the arterial intima without any indication of its functional change, and it is much more likely that IH is caused by a continuum of rejection in the VCA. What should matter most is the detriment to the basic function of the vascular system in a VCA as opposed to the mere existence of *vasculopathy*. Until we know at what specific depth IH formation leads to functional loss, the knowledge of only IH presence places the treating team one step behind in properly managing rejection.

Finally, our team's published hypothesis, as described above, could be utilized to assess the functional loss, and thereby the structural change of the arterial tree in a VCA.[27] The transcutaneous measurement of the PWV across the primary recipient and donor arteries, in addition to interstitial fluid pressure measurements, allows the treating physician to evaluate the graft's vascular function in its entirety. This provides a local assessment of the vessel's pathologic development of IH indirectly and, more importantly, allows for the direct assessment of the function of the VCA that leads to a classic clinical picture of CR. And though the *flow*MRI as shown by Morelon et al. was able to indicate functional change in the failed face transplant due to CR, i.e. a decrease in blood flow, the cost of this imaging modality remains less efficient compared to these transcutaneous techniques.[5] Again, for a claim such as this, a thorough validation by the field as a whole is mandatory to progress.

CONCLUSION

In the VCA field's infancy, CR was a predicted outcome, but the understanding of immediate success of a composite tissue transplant followed by acute rejection recognition and management was a more immediate and tangible diagnosis of concern. Twenty years later, after the longest surviving hand transplant was performed, the diagnosis of CR continues to remain incompletely understood. The exact cellular mechanisms, underlying clinical findings, have been at best inconsistent across all centers. Many diagnostic technologies have been implemented, both invasive and non-invasive, with less than ideal outcomes. Initially, individual centers attempted to diagnose CR based on individual patient results. But, as of 2017, international teams have begun to collaboratively address this question in order to advance the field for the benefit of the patient.

Financial Disclosure Statement: None of the authors has a financial interest in any of the products, devices, or drugs mentioned in this manuscript.

Grant: No funding was received for this article.

REFERENCES

1. Dubernard JM, Owen E, Herzberg G, et al. Human hand allograft: report on first 6 months. *Lancet.* 1999;353(9161):1315–1320.
2. Jones JW, Gruber SA, Barker JH, Breidenbach WC. Successful hand transplantation. One-year follow-up. Louisville Hand Transplant Team. *N Engl J Med.* 2000;343(7):468–473.
3. Breidenbach WC, Gonzales NR, Kaufman CL, Klapheke M, Tobin GR, Gorantla VS. Outcomes of the first 2 American hand transplants at 8 and 6 years posttransplant. *J Hand Surg Am.* 2008;33(7):1039–1047.
4. Cetrulo CL, Jr., Drijkoningen T, Sachs DH. Tolerance induction via mixed chimerism in vascularized composite allotransplantation: is it time for clinical application? *Curr Opin Organ Transplant.* 2015;20(6):602–607.
5. Morelon E, Petruzzo P, Kanitakis J, et al. Face transplantation: partial graft loss of the first case 10 years later. *Am J Transplant.* 2017;17(7):1935–1940.
6. Kanitakis J, Petruzzo P, Badet L, et al. Chronic rejection in human vascularized composite allotransplantation (hand and face recipients): an update. *Transplantation.* 2016;100(10):2053–2061.
7. Petruzzo P, Kanitakis J, Testelin S, et al. Clinicopathological findings of chronic rejection in a face grafted patient. *Transplantation.* 2015;99(12):2644–2650.
8. Kaufman CL, Ouseph R, Blair B, et al. Graft vasculopathy in clinical hand transplantation. *Am J Transplant.* 2012;12(4):1004–1016.
9. Weissenbacher A, Cendales L, Morelon E, et al. Meeting report of the 13th congress of the International Society of Vascularized Composite Allotransplantation. *Transplantation.* 2018;102(8):1250–1252.
10. Morelon E, Petruzzo P, Kanitakis J. Chronic rejection in vascularized composite allotransplantation. *Curr Opin Organ Transplant.* 2018;23(5):582–591.
11. Cendales L, Kaufman C. Chronic rejection in VCA; definition, follow up, diagnosis and therapy. Paper presented at: 13th Congress of the International Society of Vascularized Composite Allotransplantation; October 27, 2017; Salzburg, Austria.
12. Kanitakis J, Karayannopoulou G, Lanzetta M, Petruzzo P. Graft vasculopathy in the skin of a human hand allograft: implications for diagnosis of rejection of vascularized composite allografts. *Transpl Int.* 2014;27(11):e118–123.
13. Grahammer J, Weissenbacher, A, Wolfram-Raunicher, D, Zelger, BG, Zelger, B, Mühlbacher, A, Pierer, G, Öfner-Velano, D, Schneeberger, S. A case report: graft loss 7 years after hand transplantation. Paper presented at: International Society of Vascularized Composite Allotransplantation Meeting; October 26–October 27, 2017; Salzburg, Austria.

14. Cendales L. Histopathology workshop and Banff. Paper presented at: 13th Congress of the International Society of Vascularized Composite Allotransplantation; October 26, 2017; Salzburg, Austria.

15. Kaufman C, Zaring R, Chilton PM, et al. Evidence of capillary thrombosis prior to development of chronic rejection in a hand transplant recipient. Paper presented at: 13th Congress of the International Society of Vascularized Composite Allotransplantation; October 26, 2017; Salzburg, Austria.

16. Rosenburg E. The world's first recipient of a second face transplant? A 43-year-old who says he feels 22 again. Accessed April 17, 2018. Washington Post. https://www.washingtonpost.com/news/to-your-health/wp/2018/04/17/the-worlds-first-recipient-of-a-second-face-transplant-a-43-year-old-who-says-he-feels-22-again/

17. Garrel-Jaffrelot T. Frenchman is first in world to get 2 full face transplants. Accessed October 2, 2018. NY Times. https://www.nytimes.com/2018/04/19/world/europe/jerome-hamon-face-transplant-france.html

18. Sicard A, Kanitakis J, Dubois V, et al. An integrated view of immune monitoring in vascularized composite allotransplantation. *Curr Opin Organ Transplant.* 2016;21(5):516–522.

19. Cendales LC, Kanitakis J, Schneeberger S, et al. The Banff 2007 working classification of skin-containing composite tissue allograft pathology. *Am J Transplant.* 2008;8(7):1396–1400.

20. Schneider M, Cardones AR, Selim MA, Cendales LC. Vascularized composite allotransplantation: a closer look at the Banff working classification. *Transpl Int.* 2016;29(6):663–671.

21. Kanitakis J, Petruzzo P, Gazarian A, et al. Capillary thrombosis in the skin: a pathologic hallmark of severe/chronic rejection of human vascularized composite tissue allografts? *Transplantation.* 2016;100(4):954–957.

22. Diefenbeck M, Wagner F, Kirschner MH, Nerlich A, Muckley T, Hofmann GO. Management of acute rejection 2 years after allogeneic vascularized knee joint transplantation. *Transpl Int.* 2006;19(7):604–606.

23. Diefenbeck M, Wagner F, Kirschner MH, Nerlich A, Muckley T, Hofmann GO. Outcome of allogeneic vascularized knee transplants. *Transpl Int.* 2007;20(5): 410–418.

24. Petruzzo P, Kanitakis J, Badet L, et al. Long-term follow-up in composite tissue allotransplantation: in-depth study of five (hand and face) recipients. *Am J Transplant.* 2011;11(4):808–816.

25. Berglund E, Ljungdahl MA, Bogdanovic D, et al. Clinical significance of alloantibodies in hand transplantation: impact on rejection and functional outcome. Paper presented at: 13th Congress of the International Society of Vascularized Composite Allotransplantation; October 27, 2017; Salzburg, Austria.

26. Kueckelhaus M, Fischer S, Seyda M, et al. Vascularized composite allotransplantation: current standards and novel approaches to prevent acute rejection and chronic allograft deterioration. *Transpl Int.* 2016;29(6):655–662.

27. Robbins NL, Wordsworth MJ, Parida BK, et al. A flow dynamic rationale for accelerated vascularized composite allotransplant rejection. *Plast Reconstr Surg.* 2019;143(3):637e–643e.

28. Diefenbeck M, Nerlich A, Schneeberger S, Wagner F, Hofmann GO. Allograft vasculopathy after allogeneic vascularized knee transplantation. *Transpl Int.* 2011;24(1): e1–5.

29. Meehan SM, Limsrichamrern S, Manaligod JR, et al. Platelets and capillary injury in acute humoral rejection of renal allografts. *Hum Pathol.* 2003;34(6):533–540.

30. Xenos ES, Pacanowski JP, Ragsdale J, et al. Histopathological study of renal transplant artery stenosis: role of rejection and cold ischaemia time in the pathogenesis of intimal hyperplasia in an arterial allograft. *Clin Transplant.* 2003;17(9):27–30.

31. Valanis KC, Sun CT. Poiseuille flow of a fluid with couple stress with applications to blood flow. *Biorheology.* 1969;6(2):85–97.

32. Missaridis TX, Shung KK. The effect of hemodynamics, vessel wall compliance and hematocrit on ultrasonic Doppler power: an in vitro study. *Ultrasound Med Biol.* 1999;25(4):549–559.

33. Etra JW, Raimondi G, Brandacher G. Mechanisms of rejection in vascular composite allotransplantation. *Curr Opin Organ Transplant.* 2018;23(1):28–33.

34. Kanitakis J, Badet L, Petruzzo P, et al. Clinicopathologic monitoring of the skin and oral mucosa of the first human face allograft: Report on the first eight months. *Transplantation.* 2006;82(12):1610–1615.

35. Unadkat JV, Schneeberger S, Horibe EH, et al. Composite tissue vasculopathy and degeneration following multiple episodes of acute rejection in reconstructive transplantation. *Am J Transplant.* 2010;10(2):251–261.

36. Unadkat JV, Schneeberger S, Goldbach C, et al. Investigation of antibody-mediated rejection in composite tissue allotransplantation in a rat limb transplant model. *Transplant Proc.* 2009;41(2):542–545.

37. Sass C, Herbeth B, Chapet O, Siest G, Visvikis S, Zannad F. Intima-media thickness and diameter of carotid and femoral arteries in children, adolescents and adults from the Stanislas cohort: effect of age, sex, anthropometry and blood pressure. *J Hypertens.* 1998;16(11):1593–1602.

4 Reperfusion Injury in Vascularized Composite Tissue Allografts
Impact on Graft Outcomes and Preventive Strategies

Kagan Ozer

CONTENTS

Introduction and Mechanism of Reperfusion Injury 61
Reperfusion Injury Mediated Tissue Damage in Vascularized
Composite Tissue Allografts 62
Prevention and Treatment of Ischemia/Reperfusion Injury
in Vascularized Allotransplantation 64
Future Directions 69
References 70

INTRODUCTION AND MECHANISM OF REPERFUSION INJURY

Under aerobic conditions, cells on average produce 10–100 million molecules of adenosine triphosphate (ATP) per second[1]. The energy currency of the cell, ATP is primarily produced after glucose molecules are transported into the cell. Each glucose molecule gives rise to approximately 38 molecules of ATP in the presence of oxygen. Under anaerobic conditions, this number goes down to two ATP molecules and a lactate. Overall, lactate accumulation in any given cell is tolerated until ATP stores are depleted. Depletion of ATP at the cellular level first results in dysregulation of ATP-dependent membrane ion exchangers, leading to potassium ion leak into extracellular space and causing sodium ion concentration to increase in the cell (Na^+/K^+ ATPase). Cellular swelling results in disruption of calcium-dependent exchangers (Ca^{+2}/Na^+ ATPase), increase in intracellular Ca^{+2}, and eventually membrane disruption[2–4]. If the blood flow is not restored at that stage, cells will either undergo apoptosis or necrosis. How quickly these events occur depends on the mitochondrial content, or the energy expenditure and dependence of the cell. In vascularized composite allografts (VCAs), muscle and endothelial cells are the most susceptible tissues to ischemia.

DOI: 10.1201/9780429260179-6

61

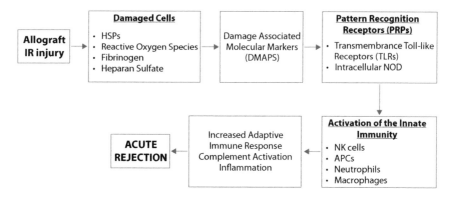

FIGURE 4.1 Factors activating the immune system leading to acute rejection.

During the reperfusion phase, further oxygen influx aggravates cellular injury via mitochondrial disintegration and intracellular iron overload, which amplifies the rate of reactive oxygen species (ROS) (Figure 4.1). This type of tissue damage results in the release of a wide variety of proteins collectively known as danger/damage-associated molecular patterns (DAMPs)[5]. Some of these include heat shock protein, oxidized proteins, ROS, fibrinogen, cathelicidin, heparan sulfate, and defensin. DAMPs are recognized by pattern recognition receptors (PRRs) expressed on cells of the innate immune response, which results in strong inflammation caused by reperfusion injury. In particular, toll-like receptors (TLRs), a subgroup of PRRs, are expressed on macrophages, neutrophils, and natural killer cells, and trigger a non-specific immune response[3,6]. The direct result of this activation is the upregulation of proinflammatory cytokines, chemokines, and adhesion molecules further attracting other components of the immune system and thrombocytes[7]. The cascade of events up until this point are necessary steps for tissue repair/replacement and commonly seen after revascularization of autografts (as in replantation) or allografts (as in transplantation). TLRs, however, play another important role and activate antigen-presenting cells, resulting in an increase in effector T-cells[8]. The activation of the innate and adaptive immune systems results in high incidence of acute and chronic rejection episodes in solid organ transplantation[9]. It is now well established that prolonged ischemia results in higher incidences of acute and chronic rejection and vasculopathy in kidney, liver, heart, and lung allografts[10–12].

REPERFUSION INJURY MEDIATED TISSUE DAMAGE IN VASCULARIZED COMPOSITE TISSUE ALLOGRAFTS

Ischemia is inevitable following organ or limb procurement. As stated earlier, muscle and endothelial cells are the tissues most susceptible to ischemic damage. Reperfusion injury in particular begins at the microcirculatory level with endothelial dysfunction[13]. Normal endothelial cells are covered by glycocalyx, a layer preventing the exposure of proinflammatory mediators. Ischemia results in partial loss of the glycocalyx. Shedding of proinflammatory mediators into microcirculation results in leukocyte activation, leading to increased numbers of rolling, adhering, and transmigrating leukocytes[14,15]. The magnitude of this immune response depends on the duration of ischemia and reperfusion. Increased vascular permeability in muscle cells leads to edema, increased extracellular tissue pressure, and acute compartment syndrome. Subsequent rhabdomyolysis and myoglobin release results in disseminated intravascular coagulopathy, generalized inflammation, and systemic multiorgan dysfunction.

In muscle ischemia, irreversible changes begin to occur as early as in 3 hours and become complete within 6 hours of warm ischemia[4]. Cold ischemia time (CIT) appears to prolong viability with a set of consequences of its own. In an experimental study of tourniquet ischemia model, hind limbs were exposed to 2, 10, and 30 hours of cold ischemia followed by 10 days of reperfusion[16]. Muscle histology in 2 hours of CIT group showed perivascular infiltration without necrosis and fibrosis. Those exposed to 10 and 30 hours of CIT demonstrated diffuse inflammatory infiltration, vasculopathy of small vessels, and high degree of mitochondrial degeneration. Nerve tissue was affected even more adversely than the muscle, showing a high degree of separation and vacuolization of myelin lamellae because of Wallerian degeneration regardless of the duration of the CIT. Compared to muscle and nerve tissues, skin was affected only to a minor degree at 2 and 10 hours, but extensively at 30 hours group[16]. In another experimental study on syngeneic rat hind limb transplantation model, we demonstrated that rat hind limbs exposed to 6 hours CIT did not recover in terms of muscle and nerve function, although limbs were still viable at 12 weeks following surgery[17]. Similarly, sciatic nerve myelination was also impaired as seen in histology and nerve conduction studies[18]. On allogeneic rat skin flap and graft models, investigators demonstrated increased acute rejection episodes with increasing ischemia times prior to transplantation[19,20]. Strong correlation between the duration of cold ischemia and extent of chronic rejection was also demonstrated on rodent hind limb allografts[21,22].

Finding conclusive evidence between prolonged ischemia time and the frequency of acute rejection episodes is more challenging in the clinical setting as multiple factors affect the acute rejection in the host. However, in a unique case of a bilateral hand transplantation, declining allograft function was attributed to differing CITs resulting in a gradual development of ischemic flexion contracture and coagulative myonecrosis[23].

It is clear that limb allografts begin to suffer from irreversible muscle damage without circulation as early as in 3 hours and develop severe functional deficits on cold ischemia beyond 6 hours. The standard of care in the current practice (static cold storage) has detrimental effects on survival and long-term function of the allograft. Immunologic issues associated with static cold storage results in higher rejection rates and impairs functional recovery. Strategies to improve tissue (muscle, nerve, and endothelium) ischemic tolerance have the greatest potential to advance the field.

PREVENTION AND TREATMENT OF ISCHEMIA/REPERFUSION INJURY IN VASCULARIZED ALLOTRANSPLANTATION

Strategies to block or mitigate the adverse effects of reperfusion injury are focused at two levels: prevention (preinjury) and treatment (postinjury) (Figure 4.2). Preservative solutions, antioxidants, immunotherapy, and donor pretreatment to induce chimerism have all been used with limited success. From mechanistic standpoint, these methods are considered static measures, designed to neutralize by products of reperfusion injury, or to preserve existing structures through one-time administration. In general, treatment of reperfusion injury (during post-injury phase) has limited success in prolonged ischemia. The use of antioxidants, such as heme oxygenase 1, Tempol, and coenzyme Q10, was shown to improve mitochondrial dysfunction, reduce infarct size, and reduce tissue damage[24–26]. Currently, these molecules are not standard parts of the clinical practice.

During the pre-injury phase, static methods using preservative solutions and dynamic methods using machine perfusion (MP) have been extensively studied in solid organ transplantation and adapted to VCAs. Preservative solutions were primarily developed for solid organ transplantations and were designed to reduce the detrimental effects of warm and cold ischemic injury. Organ preservation solutions such as University of Wisconsin[27–29], Euro Collins[30–33] as well as lactated ringers[31], mannitol[34], and saline[35] were all used with limited success in keeping limb allografts viable. Promising use of preservative solutions in liver and other solid organ transplants did not lead to successful results in VCAs due to viscosity issues and the differences in the circulatory structure and microcirculation[36,37]. The delivery of oxygen directly into the microcirculation using artificial oxygen carriers and

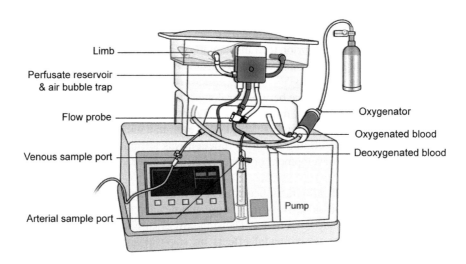

FIGURE 4.2 Swine forelimb perfusion system consists of a temperature-controlled limb chamber, an oxygenator (Baby Capiox® RX, Terumo, Tokyo, Japan), a pulsatile perfusion pump (Waters Medical Systems, Minneapolis, MN), perfusate reservoir for open drainage, and heat exchanger to maintain temperature at 27–32°C.

hyperbaric oxygen have also been tried with some positive end results, but never translated into clinical practice due to concerns over their toxicity and setup[29,38–41].

Based on experience gathered from solid organ transplantation, dynamic preservation modalities, namely MP, were adapted to VCAs, both in the experimental and clinical settings. Unlike static methods, pulsatile perfusion or MP delivers oxygen and other nutrients into the microcirculation while clearing toxic substances. MP was first introduced by Carrell in the early 20th century while experimenting on lower extremity specimens[42], and later used to transplant a kidney in 1968[43,44]. Over the course of the last 5 decades, MP has been perfected and successfully used in solid organ transplantations[45–47]. As VCA transplantation became a reality, MP was adapted to VCA preservation in order to extend preservation times and mitigate the effects of reperfusion injury.

MP, also known as ex-situ, ex-vivo, or extracorporeal perfusion, offers dynamic clearance of the microcirculation from toxic metabolites while maintaining the vasoactive tone and delivering oxygen along with other nutrients. Constantinescu et al. compared static cold storage to 12 hours of ex-situ perfusion using autologous blood at near-normothermic temperatures (27–32°C) and demonstrated minimal reperfusion injury 7 days after heterotopic replantation of porcine extremities[48,49]. These promising results were furthered by our group. We developed three experimental models on swine, rodents, and human forearm to study both the upper limits of viability and the long-term effects of ex-situ perfusion on extremity preservation. We conducted our first experiments on orthotopic swine forelimb transplantation model[50,51] (Figure 4.2). Amputated swine forelimbs were perfused using pulsatile ex-situ MP and diluted red blood cells at 27–32°C at increasing perfusion times of 6, 12, 18, 24, 36, and 48 hours[50]. Compared to contralateral limbs preserved at 4°C, perfused limbs showed excellent preservation of neuromuscular excitability up to 36 hours. Single muscle fiber contractility testing, muscle and nerve histology showed minimal signs of reperfusion injury up to 24 hours of ex-situ perfusion[51]. We also found that ex-situ perfusion beyond 36 hours resulted in significant edema and increase in limb weight, both of which are signs of extensive reperfusion injury. Neuromuscular excitability was lost after 50 hours on ex-situ perfusion with significant drops in perfusate pH and lactic acidosis. While the extension of survival up to 24 hours on MP is an unprecedented finding, ex-situ perfusion also had limits in keeping limbs viable under this protocol.

In the next step, we engineered the first portable ex-situ perfusion device for human use (Figure 4.3)[52]. Swine forelimb transplantation had many similarities to human forearm in terms of the structure of macro and microcirculations, skeletal muscle composition, ischemic tolerance, and cardiac output. Types of pumps, oxygenators, and tubing used for swine can easily be adapted to a portable machine designed for hand transplantation. In this experiment, we tested five human forearms procured from deceased donors on mechanical ventilation. Forearms were disarticulated at the elbow, immediately cannulated and flushed with heparin solution, and connected to MP. Diluted red blood cells obtained from the blood bank were used at 27–32°C in a pulsatile fashion to perfuse limbs for 24 hours. In this feasibility study with no transplantations performed, we found minimal limb weight increase, excellent neuromuscular contractility on large and small

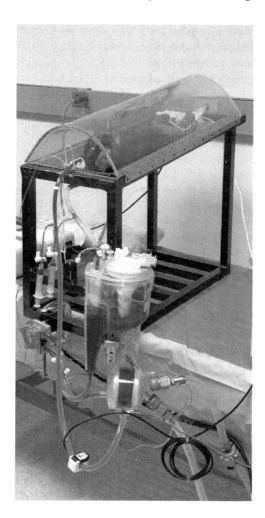

FIGURE 4.3   Limb chamber consists of a custom-made frame, fiberglass lid with 15° inclination to collect blood draining openly. Pulse oximetry was used continuously to monitor oxygen saturation. Circuit flows were controlled through the pump (Shiley Roller Pump; Stockert Instruments, Munich, Germany or M pump; MC3, Ann Arbor, MI), with target flow set to 6–8% of the donor's estimated cardiac output. Systolic pressure was maintained at 110 mmHg; circuit flow was adjusted, when necessary, to stay below this limit. Temperature within the chamber is maintained at 30–33°C. The sweep gas was a combination of oxygen (40–60% by concentration), carbon dioxide (5–10%), with the balance nitrogen. The perfusate was plasma-based with packed red blood cells added to achieve a hemoglobin concentration of 4–6 g/dL. Additives to the perfusate included concentrated albumin, sodium bicarbonate, tromethamine, calcium chloride, and sodium heparin. Dextrose was added as needed to maintain perfusate glucose greater than 100 mg/dL, while regular insulin was administered if the glucose concentration was greater than 300 mg/dL. Antibiotics were added to cover skin flora. Total perfusate volume in the circuit was 250–300 mL. Partial perfusate exchange was performed every 3–5 hours.

diameter motor nerves (including median, ulnar, and radial nerves, and motor branch of the median nerve), and no barotrauma on muscle structure with a gradual increase in lactate levels in the perfusate suggesting ongoing viability of the skeletal muscle (Figure 4.4)[52]. Other groups also achieved extension of survival up to 24 hours on ex-situ perfused swine forelimb allografts using autologous blood at normothermic temperatures[53] and human forelimbs using acellular solution at hypothermic temperatures[54].

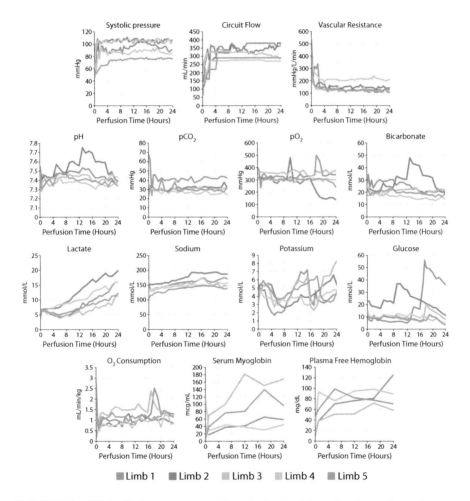

FIGURE 4.4 All five limbs were procured from brain-dead, heart-beating patients. Average cold ischemia time was 75 minutes between procurement and beginning of the perfusion. Donors of limb no. 1 (blue) and no. 2 (orange) had diabetes with partial insulin resistance resulting in unexpected increases in blood glucose. Hemodynamic variables remained stable throughout 24 hours of ex-situ perfusion. Lactate increase over time was controlled with perfusate exchange as there was no filter within the circuit. Despite a gradual increase in lactate, pH remained steady. (Adapted from Werner NL, Alghanem F, Rakestraw SL, et al. Ex situ perfusion of human limb allografts for 24 hours. *Transplantation*. 2017;101(3):e68-e74.)

Based on these results on human and swine forelimbs, it became clear that when pulsatile perfusion is used to deliver glucose and other nutrients at near-normothermic temperatures, and red blood cells are used as the oxygen carrier, microcirculation remains open with a steady oxygen consumption seen on blood gas analysis. This effect lasts up to 36 hours until cells shift from aerobic to anaerobic respiration as seen in higher levels of lactate accumulating within the perfusate. This is detrimental for survival of muscle cells, and potentially triggers an immune response leading to acute rejection. Even in the presence of oxygen and other nutrients at physiologic temperatures optimum for tricarboxylic acid cycle enzymes, overall shift from aerobic to anaerobic respiration suggest a microcirculatory dysfunction and deserves further investigation.

Studies of ex-situ perfusion on limb preservation only reported the short-term effects of reperfusion injury on muscle and nerve viability due to limitations in experimental designs and animal models. Long-term effects of ex-situ perfusion on muscle and nerve regeneration and functional recovery were not investigated until recently. To address these limitations and to answer other questions, we adapted our system to a small animal model. Rat hind limb transplantation is an established animal model to monitor long-term neuromuscular recovery in a cost-effective manner (Figure 4.5). Once we tested the feasibility to use an ex-situ perfusion system on rat hind limbs[55], we conducted a series of experiments to determine the best perfusate and temperature for optimum long-term neuromuscular recovery. In these experiments, amputated rat hind limbs were immediately perfused using ex-situ perfusion system and transplanted to another recipient within the same species[55]. This type of limb transfer is syngeneic and does not require immunosuppression within the same rat species. This allowed us to see the effects of reperfusion injury directly on limb survival and function excluding effects of the immune system. All experimental groups were compared to static cold storage group preserved at 4°C using muscle and nerve histology, nerve conduction studies, and muscle metabolomics after 12 weeks of sciatic nerve regeneration. Interestingly, our previously developed near-normothermic perfusion modality using diluted red blood cells as the perfusate failed, with no surviving recipients on the second postoperative day due to severe reperfusion injury. This was likely due to rodents' limited ability to clear waste products and higher metabolic rate per muscle cell. In order to reduce the metabolic rate, and lessen the reperfusion injury, we experimented with lower temperatures to find the optimum temperature along with other types of perfusates. In the end, we had long-term survival in two groups including hypothermic (10–15°C) perfusion using histidine-tryptophan-ketoglutarate (HTK) solution and sub-normothermic (20–22°C) perfusion using red blood cells and plasma, which was filtered from another animal in real-time to enrich the perfusate. Hypothermic ex-situ perfusion using HTK, although performed better than the static cold storage, failed to restore normal muscle strength[56]. Limbs ex-situ perfused with red blood cells and plasma at sub-normothermic temperature (20–22°C) demonstrated the best functional recovery with no statistically significant difference seen between immediately transplanted limbs with 1 hour of ischemia (unpublished data). This is the first time we achieved near normal muscle and nerve function following ex-situ perfusion. This result is likely to be attributed to the protective effects of the fresh plasma and successful preservation of energy stores at lower temperatures. The protective effects of plasma in endothelial stabilization has recently

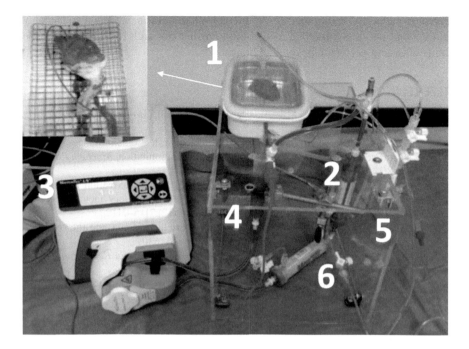

FIGURE 4.5 Figure shows mini ex-situ perfusion system including; (1) VCA chamber (Leak-proof Container, SE-560, Steeltainer, Quebec, CA), (2) a coiled glass heat exchanger connected to a cardiopulmonary bypass heat regulator (TCM 400 MR, Terumo Sarns TCM II Heater Cooler, Sarns, Tokyo, Japan), (3) peristaltic roller pump (Masterflex L/S peristaltic pump w/easy-load 3 pump head, Pump: HV-07528, Pump head: HV-77800, Cole-Parmer, IL, USA), (4) venous reservoir (Luer-Lok 30 mL syringe, 302832, Becton Dickinson and Company, NJ, USA), (5) silicone membrane oxygenator (PDMSXA-1000, PermSelect, MI, USA), (6) hemofilter (Minntech Hemocor, HPH-Junior, Medtronic) with plasma outflow and inflow pumps (Alaris Infusion Pump, 7230, version 4.54, Alaris/Carefusion, CA, USA), and 22G IV cannula for arterial cannulation (Inset). All components were connected using 1/8-inch internal diameter (ID) PVC tubing (Nalgene™ 180 Clear Plastic PVC Tubing, ThermoFisher, 8000-9020, MA, USA) and barbed tubing connectors (Harvard Apparatus, 72–1406, MA, USA). All other parts were commercially available and can be sterilized using ethyline oxide. (Adapted from Gok E, Alghanem F, Moon R, et al. Development of an ex-situ limb perfusion system for a rodent model. *ASAIO J.* 2019;65(2):167–172.)

gained interest after successful mitigation of reperfusion injury and improved survival in hemorrhagic shock[57–61]. We are currently working on the analysis of the component of the plasma critical for endothelial stabilization to improve the perfusate.

FUTURE DIRECTIONS

Multiple methods available to prevent or mitigate the reperfusion injury are yet to be tested on an acute rejection model across a major histocompatibility complex (MHC) barrier. It is unclear at this point if these methods will reduce the incidence of acute rejection episodes in VCAs. Currently tested ex-situ perfusion modalities appear to support viability up to 24 hours on limb allografts. Widespread use of MP will depend on its commercial availability. Further research is required to explore limits of ex-situ perfusion beyond 24 hours.

REFERENCES

1. Flamholz A, Phillips R, Milo R. The quantified cell. *Mol Biol Cell.* 2014;25(22): 3497–3500.
2. Duehrkop C, Rieben R. Ischemia/reperfusion injury: effect of simultaneous inhibition of plasma cascade systems versus specific complement inhibition. *Biochem Pharmacol.* 2014;88(1):12–22.
3. Zhai Y, Shen XD, O'Connell R, et al. Cutting edge: TLR4 activation mediates liver ischemia/reperfusion inflammatory response via IFN regulatory factor 3-dependent MyD88-independent pathway. *J Immunol.* 2004;173(12):7115–7119.
4. Blaisdell FW. The pathophysiology of skeletal muscle ischemia and the reperfusion syndrome: a review. *Cardiovasc Surg.* 2002;10(6):620–630.
5. Matzinger P. Tolerance, danger, and the extended family. *Annu Rev Immunol.* 1994; 12:991–1045.
6. Mannon RB. Macrophages: contributors to allograft dysfunction, repair, or innocent bystanders? *Curr Opin Organ Transplant.* 2012;17(1):20–25.
7. Land WG. The role of postischemic reperfusion injury and other nonantigen-dependent inflammatory pathways in transplantation. *Transplantation.* 2005;79(5):505–514.
8. Akira S, Takeda K, Kaisho T. Toll-like receptors: critical proteins linking innate and acquired immunity. *Nat Immunol.* 2001;2(8):675–680.
9. Land WG. Injury to allografts: innate immune pathways to acute and chronic rejection. *Saudi J Kidney Dis Transpl.* 2005;16(4):520–539.
10. Tullius SG, Reutzel-Selke A, Egermann F, et al. Contribution of prolonged ischemia and donor age to chronic renal allograft dysfunction. *J Am Soc Nephrol.* 2000; 11(7):1317–1324.
11. Halloran PF, Homik J, Goes N, et al. The "injury response": a concept linking nonspecific injury, acute rejection, and long-term transplant outcomes. *Transplant Proc.* 1997;29(1–2):79–81.
12. Boucek MM, Aurora P, Edwards LB, et al. Registry of the International Society for Heart and Lung Transplantation: tenth official pediatric heart transplantation report–2007. *J Heart Lung Transplant.* 2007;26(8):796–807.
13. Ozer K, Adanali G, Zins J, Siemionow M. In vivo microscopic assessment of cremasteric microcirculation during hindlimb allograft rejection in rats. *Plast Reconstr Surg.* 1999;103(7):1949–1956.
14. Ozer K, Zielinski M, Unsal M, Siemionow M. Development of mouse cremaster transplantation model for intravital microscopic evaluation. *Microcirculation.* 2002;9(6):487–495.
15. Ozer K, Adanali G, Siemionow M. Late effects of TNF-alpha-induced inflammation on the microcirculation of cremaster muscle flaps under intravital microscopy. *J Reconstr Microsurg.* 2002;18(1):37–45.
16. Hautz T, Hickethier T, Blumer MJ, et al. Histomorphometric evaluation of ischemia-reperfusion injury and the effect of preservation solutions histidine-tryptophan-ketoglutarate and University of Wisconsin in limb transplantation. *Transplantation.* 2014;98(7):713–720.
17. Gok E, Rojas-Pena A, Bartlett RH, Ozer K. Rodent skeletal muscle metabolomic changes associated with static cold storage. *Transplant Proc.* 2019;51(3):979–986.

18. Gok E, Kubiak CA, Guy E, Kemp SWP, Ozer K. Effect of static cold storage on skeletal muscle after vascularized composite tissue allotransplantation. *J Reconstr Microsurg.* 2020;36(1):9–15.

19. Pradka SP, Ong YS, Zhang Y, et al. Increased signs of acute rejection with ischemic time in a rat musculocutaneous allotransplant model. *Transplant Proc.* 2009;41(2): 531–536.

20. Shimizu F, Okamoto O, Katagiri K, Fujiwara S, Wei FC. Prolonged ischemia increases severity of rejection in skin flap allotransplantation in rats. *Microsurgery.* 2010;30(2):132–137.

21. Bonastre J, Landin L, Bolado P, Casado-Sanchez C, Lopez-Collazo E, Diez J. Effect of cold preservation on chronic rejection in a rat hindlimb transplantation model. *Plast Reconstr Surg.* 2016;138(3):628–637.

22. Datta N, Devaney SG, Busuttil RW, Azari K, Kupiec-Weglinski JW. Prolonged cold ischemia time results in local and remote organ dysfunction in a murine model of vascularized composite transplantation. *Am J Transplant.* 2017;17(10):2572–2579.

23. Landin L, Cavadas PC, Garcia-Cosmes P, Thione A, Vera-Sempere F. Perioperative ischemic injury and fibrotic degeneration of muscle in a forearm allograft: functional follow-up at 32 months post transplantation. *Ann Plast Surg.* 2011;66(2):202–209.

24. Katori M, Busuttil RW, Kupiec-Weglinski JW. Heme oxygenase-1 system in organ transplantation. *Transplantation.* 2002;74(7):905–912.

25. Tran TP, Tu H, Pipinos, II, Muelleman RL, Albadawi H, Li YL. Tourniquet-induced acute ischemia-reperfusion injury in mouse skeletal muscles: Involvement of superoxide. *Eur J Pharmacol.* 2011;650(1):328–334.

26. Bolcal C, Yildirim V, Doganci S, et al. Protective effects of antioxidant medications on limb ischemia reperfusion injury. *J Surg Res.* 2007;139(2):274–279.

27. Gordon L, Levinsohn DG, Borowsky CD, et al. Improved preservation of skeletal muscle in amputated limbs using pulsatile hypothermic perfusion with University of Wisconsin solution. A preliminary study. *J Bone Joint Surg Am.* 1992;74(9):1358–1366.

28. Norden MA, Rao VK, Southard JH. Improved preservation of rat hindlimbs with the University of Wisconsin solution and butanedione monoxime. *Plast Reconstr Surg.* 1997;100(4):957–965.

29. Tsuchida T, Kato T, Yamaga M, et al. The effect of perfusion with UW solution on the skeletal muscle and vascular endothelial exocrine function in rat hindlimbs. *J Surg Res.* 2003;110(1):266–271.

30. Arai K, Hotokebuchi T, Miyahara H, et al. Successful long-term storage of rat limbs. The use of simple immersion in Euro-Collins solution. *Int Orthop.* 1993;17(6):389–396.

31. Hicks TE, Boswick JA, Jr., Solomons CC. The effects of perfusion on an amputated extremity. *J Trauma.* 1980;20(8):632–648.

32. Tsuchida T, Kato T, Yamaga M, et al. Effect of perfusion during ischemia on skeletal muscle. *J Surg Res.* 2001;101(2):238–241.

33. Kuroda Y, Fujino Y, Morita A, et al. Successful 96-hour preservation of the canine pancreas. *Transpl Int.* 1992;5(Suppl 1):S388–S390.

34. Domingo-Pech J, Garriga JM, Toran N, et al. Preservation of the amputated canine hind limb by extracorporeal perfusion. *Int Orthop.* 1991;15(4):289–291.

35. Mehl RL, Paul HA, Shorey WD, Schneewind JH, Beattie EJ, Jr. Patency of the microcirculation in the traumatically amputated limb–a comparison of common perfusates. *J Trauma.* 1964;4:495–505.

36. Garcia-Gil FA, Serrano MT, Fuentes-Broto L, et al. Celsior versus University of Wisconsin preserving solutions for liver transplantation: postreperfusion syndrome and outcome of a 5-year prospective randomized controlled study. *World J Surg.* 2011;35(7):1598–1607.

37. Russo L, Gracia-Sancho J, Garcia-Caldero H, et al. Addition of simvastatin to cold storage solution prevents endothelial dysfunction in explanted rat livers. *Hepatology.* 2012;55(3):921–930.
38. Rosen HM, Slivjak MJ, McBrearty FX. The role of perfusion washout in limb revascularization procedures. *Plast Reconstr Surg.* 1987;80(4):595–605.
39. Usui M, Sakata H, Ishii S. Effect of fluorocarbon perfusion upon the preservation of amputated limbs. An experimental study. *J Bone Joint Surg Br.* 1985;67(3):473–477.
40. Yabe Y, Ishiguro N, Shimizu T, Tamura Y, Wakabayashi T, Miura T. Morphologic and metabolic study of the effect of oxygenated perfluorochemical perfusion on amputated rabbit limbs. *J Reconstr Microsurg.* 1994;10(3):185–191.
41. Edwards RJ, Im MJ, Hoopes JE. Effects of hyperbaric oxygen preservation on rat limb replantation: a preliminary report. *Ann Plast Surg.* 1991;27(1):31–35.
42. Carrel A. Landmark article, Nov 14, 1908: Results of the transplantation of blood vessels, organs and limbs. By Alexis Carrel. *JAMA.* 1983;250(7):944–953.
43. Carrel A, Lindbergh CA. The culture of whole organs. *Science.* 1935;81(2112): 621–623.
44. Belzer FO, Ashby BS, Gulyassy PF, Powell M. Successful seventeen-hour preservation and transplantation of human-cadaver kidney. *N Engl J Med.* 1968;278(11):608–610.
45. Moers C, Smits JM, Maathuis MH, et al. Machine perfusion or cold storage in deceased-donor kidney transplantation. *N Engl J Med.* 2009;360(1):7–19.
46. Schlegel A, Kron P, Dutkowski P. Hypothermic machine perfusion in liver transplantation. *Curr Opin Organ Transplant.* 2016;21(3):308–314.
47. St Peter SD, Imber CJ, Friend PJ. Liver and kidney preservation by perfusion. *Lancet.* 2002;359(9306):604–613.
48. Constantinescu MA, Knall E, Xu X, et al. Preservation of amputated extremities by extracorporeal blood perfusion; a feasibility study in a porcine model. *J Surg Res.* 2011;171(1):291–299.
49. Muller S, Constantinescu MA, Kiermeir DM, et al. Ischemia/reperfusion injury of porcine limbs after extracorporeal perfusion. *J Surg Res.* 2013;181(1):170–182.
50. Ozer K, Rojas-Pena A, Mendias CL, Bryner B, Toomasian C, Bartlett RH. Ex situ limb perfusion system to extend vascularized composite tissue allograft survival in swine. *Transplantation.* 2015;99(10):2095–2101.
51. Ozer K, Rojas-Pena A, Mendias CL, Bryner BS, Toomasian C, Bartlett RH. The effect of ex situ perfusion in a swine limb vascularized composite tissue allograft on survival up to 24 hours. *J Hand Surg.* 2016;41(1):3–12.
52. Werner NL, Alghanem F, Rakestraw SL, et al. Ex situ perfusion of human limb allografts for 24 hours. *Transplantation.* 2017;101(3):e68–e74.
53. Fahradyan V, Said SA, Ordenana C, et al. Extended ex vivo normothermic perfusion for preservation of vascularized composite allografts. *Artif Organs.* 2020;44(8):846–855.
54. Haug V, Kollar B, Tasigiorgos S, et al. Hypothermic ex situ perfusion of human limbs with acellular solution for 24 hours. *Transplantation.* 2020;104(9):e260–e270.
55. Gok E, Alghanem F, Moon R, et al. Development of an ex-situ limb perfusion system for a rodent model. *ASAIO J.* 2019;65(2):167–172.
56. Gok E, Kubiak CA, Guy E, et al. Long-term effects of hypothermic ex situ perfusion on skeletal muscle metabolism, structure, and force generation after transplantation. *Transplantation.* 2019;103(10):2105–2112.
57. Imam AM, Jin G, Duggan M, et al. Synergistic effects of fresh frozen plasma and valproic acid treatment in a combined model of traumatic brain injury and hemorrhagic shock. *Surgery.* 2013;154(2):388–396.
58. Imam AM, Jin G, Sillesen M, et al. Early treatment with lyophilized plasma protects the brain in a large animal model of combined traumatic brain injury and hemorrhagic shock. *J Trauma Acute Care Surg.* 2013;75(6):976–983.

59. Pati S, Potter DR, Baimukanova G, Farrel DH, Holcomb JB, Schreiber MA. Modulating the endotheliopathy of trauma: Factor concentrate versus fresh frozen plasma. *J Trauma Acute Care Surg.* 2016;80(4):576–584; discussion 584–575.
60. Peng Z, Pati S, Potter D, et al. Fresh frozen plasma lessens pulmonary endothelial inflammation and hyperpermeability after hemorrhagic shock and is associated with loss of syndecan 1. *Shock.* 2013;40(3):195–202.
61. Wataha K, Menge T, Deng X, et al. Spray-dried plasma and fresh frozen plasma modulate permeability and inflammation in vitro in vascular endothelial cells. *Transfusion.* 2013;53(Suppl 1):80S–90S.

5 Pediatric Upper Extremity Vascularized Composite Allotransplantation
Progress and Insights

Kevin J. Zuo, Anna Gold, Randi Zlotnik Shaul,
Emily S. Ho, Gregory H. Borschel,
and Ronald M. Zuker

CONTENTS

Introduction 76
Worldwide Experience to Date 76
Considerations for and Management of Pediatric VCA Recipients 80
  Etiology of Amputation 80
  Failed Trial of Prostheses 81
  Allograft Size, Selection, and Transport 81
  Allograft Growth 82
  Patient Rehabilitation 82
  Functional Reinnervation 83
  Cortical Plasticity 84
  Immunosuppression 85
  Outcomes Assessment Tools 86
Psychosocial Issues 86
  Individual Child Factors 89
    Expectations and Functionality 89
    Self-Image: Integration and Acceptance of Limb 89
    Treatment Adherence 89
  Family and Caregiver Factors 89
    Family-Centered Care 89
  Community and Societal Factors 90
Ethical Considerations 90
  Weighing Risks and Benefits to the Patient 90
  Consent 91
Indications for Pediatric Upper Extremity Allotransplantation 91
Conclusions 92
Compliance with Ethical Standards 92

DOI: 10.1201/9780429260179-7

Conflict of Interest...92
Human and Animal Rights and Informed Consent 92
References...92

INTRODUCTION

It has been over 20 years since the first successful adult upper limb transplant, a milestone that heralded the modern era of vascularized composite allotransplantation (VCA) (1). Since then, over 120 upper extremities, 50 uteruses, and 40 faces have been transplanted around the world, including a pediatric recipient of bilateral upper limb allografts (2). Reminiscent of the first kidney and heart solid organ transplantations, VCA has generated both fascination and condemnation within the medical community and in the public. The controversies surrounding VCA have become exponentially magnified as the list of potential candidates has expanded to include children. Despite these challenges, advancements in clinical care and translational research portend hope for pediatric VCA to become a standard treatment to restore form and function for well-selected candidates. The objective of this chapter is to summarize the worldwide experience with transplantation of vascularized composite upper extremities in children and to examine the unique considerations facing potential pediatric VCA recipients.

WORLDWIDE EXPERIENCE TO DATE

To date, three successful pediatric composite extremity transplantations have been performed (Table 5.1). Two cases involved transplantation of vascularized composite isografts from a monozygotic twin, which negated the need for systemic immunosuppression therapy, and one case involved transplantation of vascularized composite upper extremity allografts, which required immunosuppression post-operatively.

In 2000 in Malaysia, a 28-day-old girl with congenital transverse absence of the distal forearm received an above elbow vascularized composite isograft from her twin who had an unsurvivable congenital meningomyolocele. Given her aplastic forearm anatomy, a transhumeral transplantation was performed to optimize neuromuscular reconstruction of a functioning elbow, wrist, and fingers. Thumb extension was noted at 2 months post-surgery, and at 8 months, the child had prehensile grasp and pinch. At 18 months, full active elbow and wrist motion was documented with comparable growth to the intact contralateral upper limb; however, intrinsic hand function did not recover (3).

In 2005 in Canada, a 3-month-old ischiopagus twin infant received a lower limb vascularized composite isograft from her twin sister who had an unsurvivable congenital cardiac anomaly (4). Like the first case, no systemic immunosuppression was required for isograft maintenance. At 6-year follow-up, she had good motor and sensory recovery with minimal functional impairment. Functional magnetic resonance imaging (MRI) demonstrated cortical integration of the transplanted limb, suggesting that children born without a normal limb may successfully develop somatotopic control of a transplanted limb due to cortical plasticity (5).

To date, only one child has successfully received upper extremity allografts requiring maintenance systemic immunosuppression. In 2015, Zion, an 8-year-old boy in the USA with quadrimembral amputations due to septic shock underwent bilateral forearm VCA (Figure 5.1). Of note, he had previously received a living-related donor kidney allograft at age 5 maintained without steroid therapy on FK506 and

TABLE 5.1

Worldwide Pediatric (<18 years) Composite Transplantation Experience

Year	Location	Surgical Lead	Patient Age	Organ	Type	Follow-up	Motor Outcome	Sensory Outcome	Functional Outcome
2000	Kuala Lumpur, Malaysia	V. Pathmanathan	28 days	Unilateral above elbow upper limb	Isograft from monozygotic twin (VCI)	18 months			Good functional and aesthetic outcome
2005	Toronto, Canada	Ronald Zuker	3 months	Unilateral lower limb	Isograft from monozygotic twin (VCI)		Hip flexion MRC3 Knee extension MRC3 Knee flexion MRC4 Ankle dorsiflexion MRC0 Ankle plantarflexion MRC0	Reduced light touch sensation more evident proximally than distally No chronic or neuropathic pain	SF-36 66.9% -General health 85% -Physical functioning 70% -Emotional wellbeing 68% -Social functioning 100% LEFS 86.25% Attends regular stream school Does not feel left behind by peers
2010	Mexico City, Mexico	Martin Iglesias	17 years	Bilateral above elbow upper limb	Allograft (VCA)	Immediate post-operative period	Severe complications and death		

(Continued)

TABLE 5.1 (Continued)
Worldwide Pediatric (<18 years) Composite Transplantation Experience

Year	Location	Surgical Lead	Patient Age	Organ	Type	Follow-up	Motor Outcome	Sensory Outcome	Functional Outcome
2015	Philadelphia, USA	L. Scott Levin	8 years	Bilateral below elbow upper limb (forearm)	Allograft (VCA)	18 months	Intrinsic recovery at 8 months (right) and 10 months (left) Motor evoked potentials of APB and FDI by 7 months (right) and 10 months (left)	Semmes Weinstein monofilament 4.08 on both dorsal and palmar surfaces bilaterally (above protective sensation threshold) Tactile stimulation elicited large amplitude somatosensory evoked fields in primary sensory cortex on MEG	Box and Block test -Surpassed preoperative scores by 8 months Nine-hole peg test -Unable to complete preoperatively; able to complete with transplanted hands
2019	Poland	Adam Maciejewski	6 years	Composite neck (tongue, larynx, throat, esophagus)	Allograft (VCA)	9 months	Able to swallow and learning to speak		

Abbreviation: VCI = vascularized composite isotransplantation; VCA = vascularized composite allotransplantation; SF-36 = Short form-36 Questionnaire; LEFS = lower extremity functional scale; APB = abductor pollicis brevis; FDI = first dorsal interosseous; MEG = magnetoencephalography.

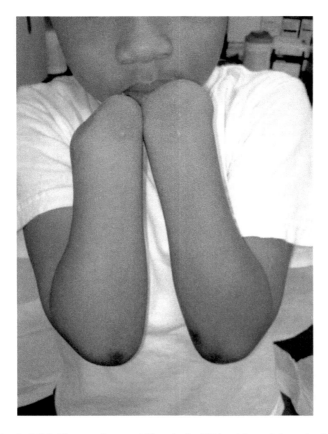

FIGURE 5.1   In 2015, Zion, an 8-year-old boy in the USA with quadrimembral amputations due to septic shock underwent bilateral forearm vascularized composite allotransplantation. (Reprinted with permission of Elsevier from Amaral S, Kessler SK, Levy TJ, Gaetz W, McAndrew C, Chang B, et al. 18-month outcomes of heterologous bilateral hand transplantation in a child: a case report. *Lancet Child Adolesc Health*. 2017;1(1):35–44.)

mycophenolate mofetil immunosuppression. His bilateral forearm allografts were revascularized after 208 minutes of cold ischemia time and a surgical operating time of 10 hours and 40 minutes (6). Post-operatively, he experienced multiple episodes of acute mild to severe allograft rejection, and his pre-transplant immunosuppression regimen was necessarily intensified with addition of corticosteroids and sirolimus to mitigate FK506's nephrotoxicity. Bimanual coordination was possible after 8 months, he gained protective sensation of his hands and could toilet himself independently after 12 months (Figure 5.2). After 18 months, his performance on the Box and Block and Nine-Hole Peg Tests surpassed his pre-transplant scores, with evidence of cortical somatosensory reintegration on magnetoencephalography (Table 5.1) (7).

In addition to these cases, a 17-year-old recipient of bilateral above elbow allografts in Mexico in 2010 died in the immediate post-operative period due to severe medical complications (8). The cause for death was not unclear but may have been due to transfusion-related acute lung injury, ischemic reperfusion syndrome, or

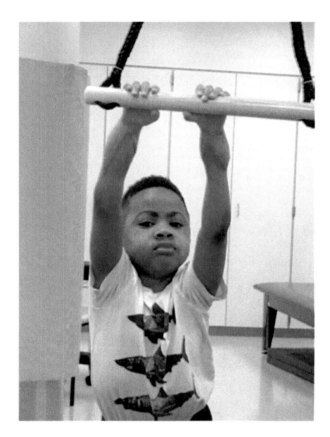

FIGURE 5.2 Eight months following transplantation, Zion achieved bimanual coordination and protective sensation with his transplanted hands. (Reprinted with permission of Elsevier from Amaral S, Kessler SK, Levy TJ, Gaetz W, McAndrew C, Chang B, et al. 18-month outcomes of heterologous bilateral hand transplantation in a child: a case report. *Lancet Child Adolesc Health.* 2017;1(1):35–44.)

cytokine release syndrome. Most recently, in 2019, a composite neck VCA was also successfully performed in Poland involving the tongue, larynx, throat, esophagus, hyoid bone, neck muscles, skin, and laryngeal nerves in a 6-year-old boy. The patient was also infused with allograft donor bone marrow with the hope to withdraw or reduce maintenance immunosuppression. At 9-month follow-up, the child is able to swallow and is learning to speak (9).

CONSIDERATIONS FOR AND MANAGEMENT OF PEDIATRIC VCA RECIPIENTS

ETIOLOGY OF AMPUTATION

Unilateral or bilateral upper limb absence may result from congenital or acquired etiologies. Congenital etiologies include transverse arrest and amniotic band syndrome, while acquired etiologies include trauma, neoplasm, infectious processes, and the associated iatrogenic procedures (10). Infants and children with congenital upper limb differences often adapt very effectively with their compromised limbs (11). For acquired etiologies, the success of physical and psychosocial adaptation depends heavily on the age and level of amputation (12).

FAILED TRIAL OF PROSTHESES

Young children with upper limb absence may initially adapt well during basic motor skill acquisition, but functional independence and social integration become increasingly important and difficult with advancing developmental age (13). Early prosthetic fitting aims to integrate the device into the child's body image and motor development with the aim of early or eventual functional independence (10). Unfortunately, these prostheses are frequently rejected because children perceive that they fail to increase function, are cumbersome to operate, and cause physical discomfort (14, 15). Frequently, children elect for a passive prosthesis for cosmetic reasons (16).

A trial of a functional prosthesis should nevertheless be a requisite for all pediatric VCA candidates to ascertain their functional status and appearance-related concerns with and without an assisting limb. Evaluating the child's integration of the functional prosthesis provides critical information to the therapy team regarding pre- and post-transplant rehabilitation needs. Furthermore, if the functional prosthesis is rejected, a passive prosthesis can be helpful to prepare a prospective patient mentally and physically as a form of preoperative rehabilitation, as a transplanted upper limb will initially be insensate and have limited mobility for many months. Gradually increasing the weight of such a prosthesis may help the child become accustomed to initial weight of the transplanted limb and build stabilizing shoulder girdle strength for support.

ALLOGRAFT SIZE, SELECTION, AND TRANSPORT

Suitable human leukocyte antigen--matched pediatric donor solid organs are scarce, and unlike some solid organs, living donor transplantation is not feasible for VCA. The external, visible nature of VCA introduces further constraints for a suitable donor match, such as organ size, skin tone, hair growth pattern, and skeletal age (17). The need to minimize cold ischemia duration of a metabolically-active limb also diminishes the geographic pool of potential donor organs.

Advancements in ex vivo (extracorporeal) perfusion of solid organs have expanded the acceptability of donor organs by maintaining aerobic metabolism (rather than simply slowing down anaerobic metabolism) and reducing ischemia-reperfusion injury (18). Similar technologies are being tested with composite organs and tissue for replantation or allotransplantation (19, 20). By mitigating the detrimental effects of ischemia time, ex vivo perfusion systems may help overcome the restrictions of geography and enable global transport of age-, size-, and appearance-matched donor pediatric allografts.

ALLOGRAFT GROWTH

Vascular perfusion to the physis is crucial to protect skeletal growth potential after limb revascularization (21). With physeal preservation and minimization of ischemia, replanted limbs grow to near comparable size (92–110%) of the normal limb (22–29).

The difference between replantation and allotransplantation rests in the fact that the donor extremity may have a differential intrinsic growth rate and growth potential compared to the recipient, even in monozygotic twins. In Zuker et al.'s experience with lower extremity transplantation, at 7-year follow-up, there was a 6.5 cm leg length discrepancy despite transplantation of the pelvic ring and entire femur with its proximal and distal physes; however, this limb length discrepancy was more likely to be related to the limb's intrinsically smaller size as opposed to failed physeal growth (5). In Zion's case, having received bilateral forearm allografts with open physes from the same donor, comparable growth and size was observed at 18-month follow-up (7).

PATIENT REHABILITATION

Early presurgical planning alongside the rehabilitation team is essential to evaluate pre-transplant functional status, set patient and family goals, and guide expectations for therapy timeline and expected functional outcomes. Upper extremity rehabilitation after major surgery is rigorous, and children may lack the capacity to appreciate the delayed gratification of repetitive exercises and tests. As such, it is important to ascertain the child and family's needs (e.g., emotional, financial, psychosocial) and offer supports to optimize their long-term commitment to post-transplant rehabilitation.

Preoperatively, evaluation of functional status of the upper limb using standardized tests including performance, patient-reported, and observer-reported (i.e., parental or caregiver) outcome measures should be conducted. Performance outcome on bimanual tasks should be measured with and without the use of a functional prosthetic. Difficult activities such as twisting open a jar, buttoning or zipping up garments, or tying shoelaces should be identified and adaptive strategies noted. It is important to understand how the child wants to use his or her restored hand. Graded evaluation of grasp patterns and in-hand manipulation of the unaffected limb is important as a means of educating the child and family regarding realistic functional outcomes in the transplanted hand; namely, that the transplanted hand may not function to the same level of dexterity as a native hand. Lastly, sensory function and the soft tissue and bony topography of the amputation stump should be evaluated. In addition to functional status measures, baseline patient-reported and observer-reported outcome measure of global health and peer relationships are informative regarding how the child's amputation affects their overall quality of life.

A trial period of rehabilitation may be beneficial prior to or during the time the child is listed for transplantation. First, laterality exercises, motor imagery, and mirror-therapy activities may encourage cortical remodelling prior to transplantation, particularly with respect to prehension and in-hand manipulation as intrinsic function is difficult to achieve post-transplant. As mentioned earlier, fitting a passive prosthetic can help prepare a patient mentally and physically for the potential 6 months of having a transplanted upper limb that is insensate and does not move. Immersive virtual reality activities incorporating visual and sensory feedback may also help with cortical adaptation in preparation for a new limb, including in congenital upper limb amputees (30).

Post-transplantation splinting, stretching, range of motion (ROM) exercises, strength training, motor learning, desensitization, and functional skills training should all be closely guided by the expertise of a dedicated upper extremity rehabilitation team (31, 32). Initial rehabilitation involves protection of the transplanted limb using orthotics, monitoring for acute rejection episodes, and passive ROM exercises to optimize distal joint mobility. As motor and sensory functional reinnervation emerge, rehabilitation goals are modified accordingly to minimize scar and joint contracture, increase strength, facilitate motor learning, and relearn skills for activities of daily living.

FUNCTIONAL REINNERVATION

A successful upper extremity allograft must be functional in both motor and sensory domains, which is predicated on successful reinnervation and cortical integration. Outcomes following peripheral nerve repair in children are generally superior to that of adults with near normal 2-point discrimination, light touch, and Disabilities of Arm Shoulder and Hand (DASH) scores (33–36). This is unsurprising, as the most important prognostic factors following peripheral nerve injury and repair include patient age, mechanism of injury, time from injury to repair, and the distance from site of injury to end organ (33, 37). In children undergoing upper limb VCA, most of these factors are optimized. Children are young, require shorter distances for nerve regeneration, and the site of injury may be controlled with sharp transection and tension-free repair. At 18 months, the motor and sensory outcomes of Zion's bilateral forearm allografts were excellent, although still below age-appropriate normative reference values (7).

Interestingly, FK506 (tacrolimus), the workhorse immunosuppressant of modern solid organ and VCA immunosuppressive protocols, also possesses neuroregenerative properties (38). The early adult upper extremity VCA experience noted unexpectedly rapid end organ reinnervation compared to limb replantation at comparable amputation levels, when FK506 immunosuppression is not administered (39, 40). Nevertheless, even with FK506 therapy, not all adult VCA recipients achieve excellent functional outcomes due to incomplete end organ reinnervation (41). Clinically translatable strategies to promote nerve regeneration offer promise to improve sensorimotor recovery of the allograft. In children, this is most relevant in proximal level (above-elbow or transhumeral) upper extremity transplantation, as well as in older children who have longer limbs and thus larger distances for regeneration. One emerging technique for enhancing nerve regeneration is intraoperative peripheral nerve electrical stimulation at the time of nerve decompression or repair, which has been shown in clinical trials to accelerate target reinnervation and functional outcomes after neuropraxic and neurotmetic injuries (42). Fusion of severed axons with polyethylene glycol (PEG) is another very intriguing technique that has recently been described (43, 44). When applied to a transected nerve, PEG fusion restores direct, albeit mismatched, axon continuity, thereby preventing Wallerian degeneration of the distal axons and enabling much earlier recovery of anterograde and retrograde axonal conduction. Further investigations are certainly warranted.

CORTICAL PLASTICITY

Plasticity refers to the morphological or functional reorganization of the sensorimotor cortex in response to environmental stimulation (30). Compared to adults and adolescents, young children have a greater capacity for cortical remodelling after nerve injury and repair, which facilitates their motor re-education, adaptation with activities, and overall quality of functional recovery (35, 45–47).

Re-establishing cortical control after restoration of a previously present but now amputated composite organ such as a hand should not be a problem. This should also be true in gestational situations where cortical representation for a hand develops normally, but the infant is born without a hand due to disruptive events later in gestation such as amniotic band syndrome or placental embolus. In the adult VCA literature, transplantation of a hand leads to restoration of activity in the primary sensory cortex after chronic denervation (48–50). The confirmation of cortical integration of Zion's transplanted hands clinically and radiographically with magnetoencephalography in the primary motor and sensory cortices, despite absent hands during a period of fine motor acquisition between age 2 and 8 years, underscores the power of cortical neuronal and synaptic plasticity for extremity control (7, 51).

The question that remains incompletely answered is whether sensorimotor cortical integration is possible for a transplanted organ that was never present during early brain development. What can be expected if there was no cortical representation at baseline? This question is relevant to consider if children with congenital upper limb differences without innate cortical representation, such as certain forms of transverse deficiency or phocomelia, are to be considered potential candidates for allotransplantation.

Experience in other reconstructive scenarios may provide some clues by substantiating the potency of cortical reorganization to capture non-innate functions. Individuals with facial paralysis who undergo free functioning muscle transfer neurotized by a masseteric nerve branch of the trigeminal nerve may learn to acquire a spontaneous, emotional smile independent of masseter muscle activation (52). Similarly, after dynamic smile reconstruction with a Labbé temporalis tendon transfer, facial paralysis patients learn to transition from a masticatory smile to a facial expression smile independent of mandibular movements, with functional MRI demonstrating that the smile area increases in size and intensity and migrates to merge with the chewing area (53). In the brachial plexus literature, after intercostal nerve transfer to the biceps nerve, patients gradually learn to flex their elbow at their volition without having to breathe in deeply, implicating synaptic remodelling to enable the biceps cortical center to descend via the peripheral respiratory nerve efferent pathways (54).

In the pediatric transplant literature, the world's first pediatric hand isograft transplant recipient undertaken in Malaysia had congenital transverse arrest at the level of the distal forearm and received an above elbow allograft from her terminal twin sister. At 12-year follow-up, she had excellent wrist motion with median and radial nerve recovery, despite never having somatotopic representation of a wrist joint. In contrast, she did not regain intrinsic hand function (3). In the world's only pediatric lower limb transplant, functional MRI demonstrated reactivation of the appropriate area of the contralateral left primary motor cortex for the right leg, as well as a second patchy area of the right primary motor cortex which may be related to mirror movements (5). The authors hypothesized that transplantation at an early age allowed a cortical rearrangement to "capture" the function of the transplanted leg, implicating that pediatric limb transplantation should not be precluded on the supposition that the cortical infrastructure is not available to control the limb.

IMMUNOSUPPRESSION

The long-term success of VCA is dependent on a maintenance immunosuppression regimen that prevents allograft rejection while minimizing adverse effects. Like solid organ transplantation, induction typically involves monoclonal or polyclonal antibodies with antithymoglobulin, IL-2 receptor antagonists, or alemtuzumab (55). Maintenance immunosuppression includes a conventional combination of corticosteroids, mycophenolate mofetil, tacrolimus, and sirolimus. One advantage of VCA transplants compared to solid organ transplant is their external, visible nature, which enables early detection of rejection episodes with skin punch biopsies or vascular imaging and thus more timely intervention (56).

Strategies to reduce immunosuppression burden include the use of belatacept, a fusion protein for T-cell costimulatory blockade, and the University of Pittsburgh cellular therapy protocol, which involves induction with alemtuzumab and methylprednisolone, bone marrow infusion 2 weeks post-VCA, and maintenance with tacrolimus monotherapy. The most recent pediatric composite neck allotransplantation recipient in Poland also received donor bone marrow infusion 2 weeks post-transplantation with a goal of weaning him from chronic immunosuppression (9). Unlike pediatric solid organ transplantation where some recipients have successfully been weaned off of immunosuppression (57, 58), no VCA recipients have been able to be fully weaned, even with the Pittsburgh protocol of donor bone marrow cellular therapy (59). This may be due to the composite nature of VCA organs, which contain multiple tissue types of variable antigenicity. In spite of this, the rate of chronic rejection appears to be lower in medication-compliant VCA recipients than in solid organ recipients; however, it remains to be defined what exactly characterizes chronic VCA rejection, as vascular intimal hyperplasia, adnexal atrophy, dermal sclerosis, capillary thrombosis, and donor specific antibodies manifest inconsistently between patients (60). Developing a consistent scale for evaluating chronic rejection in skin and/or vessels is an ongoing collaborative objective (2).

Until true allograft immunologic tolerance is achieved with induction of donor specific tolerance or mixed chimerism without graft versus host disease, the life-threatening risks of chronic immunosuppression will continue to dominate the decision-making process for potential VCA candidates for whom an allograft is life-enhancing but not lifesaving. The unfortunate realities of long-term immunosuppression in some VCA patients include renal failure (potentially requiring renal transplant), post-transplant lymphoproliferative disease, metabolic disorders, and death (2). Although the visible nature of VCA transplants facilitates monitoring, there are currently no non-invasive methods of objectively evaluating subacute rejection or chronic graft vasculopathy, such as laboratory values or imaging tests. Nailfold capillaroscopy, a method of assessing upper extremity vascular perfusion in rheumatologic conditions and after digital replantation, requires further investigation for possible use in evaluating microvascular changes in upper extremity VCA (61).

Another exciting direction of research is local immunosuppression, which involves biomaterial-based drug delivery systems that provide sustained medication release at the site of implantation to mitigate the adverse effects of systemic immunosuppression. In animal models of lung, face, and hindlimb transplantation, local drug delivery of FK506 has been shown to prolong allograft survival compared to negative controls and/or decrease the need for systemic immunosuppression (62–66). For local immunosuppression to be clinically translatable, the pharmacodynamics of bioactive drug release must be greatly augmented to enable sustained drug delivery on the order of months to years in human allograft recipients.

OUTCOMES ASSESSMENT TOOLS

Tools such as the DASH, Chen Score for replantation, Comprehensive Functional Score System, and the Carroll Score, while used frequently in adults, were not designed for hand transplantation (41). The Hand Transplant Score System was designed for adults and may not be appropriate or responsive for meaningful factors for children given that they are not validated for children (67). Involving stakeholders such as VCA recipients, psychologists, and occupational therapists will be crucial to design an appropriate scoring system that has excellent construct and content validity, as well as high inter-rater reliability. Such an outcome tool could be used for comparisons between centers and against other treatment modalities such as prostheses and should also be responsive to changes in physical, psychosocial, sexual, and emotional growth of the patient, as well as family dynamics.

PSYCHOSOCIAL ISSUES

Studies of adult VCA have highlighted the importance of addressing psychosocial factors in the assessment phase, as these can significantly impact treatment outcomes (68). In the context of pediatric transplantation, multiple perspectives must be considered: (I) the individual child, (II) the family and caregivers, and (III) the community and wider society (Table 5.2).

TABLE 5.2
Psychosocial Factors to Consider when Assessing Suitability for Pediatric Upper Limb Transplant

Individual Child Factors	Expectations and Functionality		
	Domain	**Rationale**	**Examples**
	Physical and adaptive functioning	Understand current physical and daily functioning skills and limitations, as per age expectations. Assess changes over time	Parent, school and proxy report of adaptive functioning (e.g., ABAS-3)[a], disability scales (e.g., Functional Disability Scale)[b], functional physical skills
	Psychological and mental health	Assess mental health needs and provide intervention (as needed), establish potential risks (e.g., suicidality), and individual capacity to engage in treatment process	Include proxy and caregiver report of trauma (e.g., CRIES)[c], depression (e.g., CDI-2, Columbia Depression Scale)[d,e], anxiety (e.g., MASC-2)[f], treatment adherence, pain (e.g., daily visual analogue scale), behavior (e.g., BASC-3)[g]
	Cognitive status	Evaluate individual level of cognitive functioning, provide guidance regarding consent/assent process, inform treatment interventions and assess ability to adhere to treatment regime	Various cognitive measures to assess intellectual capacity, language, memory, academic and executive functioning skills
	Social functioning	Establish understanding of peer networks and friendships which can impact resiliency and adjustment post-transplant	Interview with child and family, proxy/caregiver report (e.g., Social Skills Improvement System)[h]
	School functioning	Assess educational needs to facilitate social and academic reintegration, advocate for special educational resources	Ongoing consultation with family and school, report cards, prior rehabilitation and psychology assessments
	Self-Image: Integration and Acceptance of Limb		
	Domain	*Rationale*	*Examples*
	Self-image	Highlight individual perception of their body, assess issues such as avoidance of looking/using limb, detachment from self, shame and isolation	Self-reported measures (e.g., Self-Image Profile)[i]
	Treatment Adherence		
	Domain	*Rationale*	*Examples*
	Treatment adherence	Establish history of treatment adherence and develop support strategies for potential barriers	History of medication adherence, medication monitoring systems, formal assessment measures (e.g., Brief Medication Questionnaire, Parental Medication Barriers Scale)[j,k]

(Continued)

TABLE 5.2 (*Continued*)

Psychosocial Factors to Consider when Assessing Suitability for Pediatric Upper Limb Transplant

Family and Caregiver Factors	*Domain*	*Rationale*	*Examples*
	Family stress and mental health	Understand expectations and experiences of having a child with a medical illness/disability. Assess stability of family functioning and mental health risk factors impacting caregiver role	Family Assessment Measure-3[l], Peds QL[m], Pediatric Inventory for Parents[n], Mood questionnaires (e.g., Brief Symptom Inventory)[o]
	Financial/ employment	Establish potential stressors and explore support options for accommodation, finances, employment, medical insurance, etc.	Interview
Community and Societal Factors	*Domain*	*Rationale*	*Examples*
	Extended support network	Establish details of family and friends who can offer practical and emotional support	Interview
	Cultural/ religious	Gain awareness of spiritual, cultural and religious components that need to be integrated into the treatment plan	Interview
	Privacy and the media	Patients have a right to medical confidentiality and a plan should be in place for if, when, and how to handle media and public affairs	Assess family's views about publicity via interview. Liaise with public affairs and media relations department

Table 5.2 References

[a] ABAS-3 – Adaptive Behaviour Assessment System-Third Edition, Harrison, P. and Oakland, T. 2015. WPS Publishers

[b] Functional Disability Scale – Nascimento L.R. (2014) Functional Disability Scales. In: Michalos A.C. (eds), Encyclopedia of Quality of Life and Well-Being Research. Springer, Dordrecht

[c] CRIES – Child Revised Impact of Events Scale, originally developed by Horowtitz et al., 1979. Adapted by Children and War Foundation, 1998 – download for free at https://www.childrenandwar.org/

[d] CDI-2 Children's Depression Inventory Second Edition, Kovacs, M. 2011. MHS Publishers

[e] Columbia DISC Depression Inventory, 2002. DISC Development Group of Columbia University. https://www.mipeds.net/docs/depression.pdf

[f] MASC-2 – Manifest Anxiety Scale for Children-Second Edition. March, J. 2013. MHS Publishers

[g] BASC-3 – Behaviour Assessment System for Children-Third edition. Reynolds, C. and Kamphaus, R. 2015. Pearson Assessments

[h] Social Skills Improvement System Rating Scales (SSIS), Elliott, S and Gresham, F. 2007. Pearson Assessments

[i] Self Image Profiles (SIP), Butler, R. 2001. Pearson Assessments

[j] Brief Medication Questionnaire (BMQ). Svarstad, B., Chewning, B., Sleath, B., and Claesson, C. 1999. *Patient Educ. Counselling*, June, 37 (2): 113–124

[k] Parental Medication Barriers Scale (PMBS). Tackett, A., Peugh, J., Wu, Y and Pai, A. 2014. *Children's Health Care*, 45, 2: 177–191

[l] Family Assessment Measure-III (FAM-III), Skinner, H., Steinhauer, P., and Santa-Barbera, J. 1995. Multi-Health Systems Inc. USA.

[m] Peds QL, Varni, J. 1998 https://www.pedsql.org/about_pedsql.html

[n] Pediatric Inventory for Parents PIP), Streisand, R., Braniecki, S., Tercyak, K., Kazak, A. 2001. *J Pediatric Psychology*; 26 (3): 155–62

[o] Brief Symptom Inventory (BSI), Derogatis L., 1993. Pearson Assessments

INDIVIDUAL CHILD FACTORS

Expectations and Functionality

The child's chronological age and developmental stage, in addition to the mechanism of limb loss and the success of prosthesis use, may impact the individual's hopes and aspirations for a new limb. A careful review of the areas of the child's life that are currently affected by their condition (relating to daily activities, social and emotional functioning), the relative impact of each area, the degree to which they wish each area to improve, and the consequences of not achieving each goal, should be undertaken. If stated goals are unrealistic or unobtainable, these need to be carefully discussed prior to transplantation and should be regularly reviewed across the transplant process. A technique called Patient Generated Index (69) could be utilized with the child and caregiver separately, possibly using an adapted child-friendly version, which would quantify the value of the transplant and cultivate further discussion regarding expectations, risks, and benefits (70).

Self-Image: Integration and Acceptance of Limb

Assessment and treatment of pre-existing psychological issues related to traumatic stress, social stigma or body image should be addressed prior to consideration for transplant (71–73). Various factors may impact acceptance of a new limb, such as external and functional characteristics of the limb, burden of rehabilitation demands and medical complications, understanding of the origin of the limb, individual coping style, cognitive development, family supports, and social acceptance (72), all of which require a cohesive multidisciplinary approach to care. Importantly, intensive post-transplant physical therapy may be particularly challenging for pediatric patients (74) when compared to their adult counterparts, although developmental adaptation may be more rapid due to cortical plasticity (7, 75).

Treatment Adherence

The burden of chronic immunosuppression treatment is seen as one of the greatest primary barriers for limb transplantation (76). This is a significant problem in pediatric kidney transplant recipients, in which approximately 44% of all allograft losses and 23% of late acute rejection episodes are associated with treatment non-adherence (77). These risks are reduced if the child is already taking immunosuppressants for another transplanted organ, or for young children whose caregivers take primary responsibility for providing medications (74). The child's level of cognitive development and mental health status may impact their ability to independently assess longer term outcomes and weigh complex risk-benefits, particularly during adolescence when powerful psychological and social influences are prominent and medication non-adherence is particularly problematic (78, 79). Detailed discussions with the family regarding treatment plans and potential barriers should be integrated into the assessment, with continued review of these issues as the child grows.

FAMILY AND CAREGIVER FACTORS

Family-Centered Care

The value of adopting a family-centered care approach has been well documented across medical populations (80, 81). It allows the team to work in partnership with families to support patient and parent decision-making and acknowledges variations across families in their approach to and understanding of medical treatments. By working in partnership with families, the team is able to build strong and trusting relationships, which are vital during the periods of uncertainty and stress (82).

COMMUNITY AND SOCIETAL FACTORS

The family is part of a wider community (e.g., school, religious and cultural institutions, extended social and recreational networks), and so developing a plan early on regarding continued communication with these agencies will hopefully facilitate post-transplant reintegration. For example, regular contact (e.g., using video platforms) with peers and school may reduce social stigma, and engaging religious or cultural leaders may provide meaningful support for the family. Given potential privacy risks, the medical team should engage the hospital-based Public/Media Affairs group to discuss a collaborative plan with the recipient and donor families regarding sensitive and supportive media coverage.

ETHICAL CONSIDERATIONS

Unlike solid organ transplantation, the objective in limb transplantation is not to be live-saving but to enhance the quality of life; thus, a careful multi-disciplinary examination of the psychosocial and ethical factors specific to each potential recipient is essential (70).

WEIGHING RISKS AND BENEFITS TO THE PATIENT

Evaluating the ethical defensibility of providing an upper limb transplant to a young patient could begin with assessing the patient's current quality of life and the expected future quality of life with and without a transplant (83). This would include a review of psychosocial functioning, reasons for prosthesis abandonment, and the estimated timeline until donor matching. The estimated timeline is important to consider for a child struggling to meet motor developmental milestones.

The risks associated with immunosuppression will also be unique to the specific patient. Children who are already on or about to be on immunosuppression for a solid organ transplant would be favourably considered, although there is the possibility of needing to increase medication doses. Anticipated adverse effects on other organ systems must also be assessed. The longer life expectancy of pediatric recipients mandates greater anticipation of chronic immunosuppression-related complications, notably infection, skin cancer and lymphoproliferative malignancy, diabetes, hypertension, avascular necrosis, and nephrotoxicity (41). Nephrotoxicity has led to renal failure in several adult upper limb transplantees who required renal transplantation, a procedure that comes with its own challenges and major risks to the patient, including immunologic allosensitization from two disparate organ donors. The possibility of a reduced lifespan in exchange for potentially improved quality of life must also be carefully considered.

The possibility of allograft loss must also be discussed upfront. Although pediatric solid organ allograft survival rates have improved over the past years, long-term failure continues to range between 25–35%, and therefore, with time, an increasing number of patients will require a second transplant (84). Approximately 20% of adult upper extremity limb allografts have been lost due to medication non-compliance or chronic rejection, which has important implications for children for whom medication compliance may be a concern and for whom an increased number of expected years of living with the allograft is expected (41, 55).

There is a growing literature appraising the ethical issues associated with upper extremity transplantation, with critics emphasizing important issues such as the incommensurability of values such as length of life and quality of life (70). While experience with VCA has supported a capable person prioritizing quality of life with an upper limb transplant over potentially compromised length of life as a result of immunosuppression therapy, these frameworks cannot be applied in the same manner when health care providers and surrogate decision makers attempt to abstractly weigh these measures for an incapable young person.

CONSENT

Informed consent calls for a fulsome understanding and appreciation of the risks and expected benefits associated with a procedure (67). Much of what can be explained to parents and to patients about expected outcomes is extrapolated from the adult VCA literature, as pediatric VCA is still very much in its infancy. While formally still within pediatric care, consent for an upper limb transplant by a capable 17 year old may offset some of the concerns associated with surrogate decision making (74). In younger children, the decision to embark on the lifelong journey of upper limb functional restoration with VCA falls largely on the parents to make through the lens of best interests of the child. Nonetheless, a decision to transplant could still lead to future resentment from the child if the outcome is less than ideal, or if the outcome is ideal but the patient feels trapped by the burden of perpetual medical treatment and rehabilitation (85). However, consent is a process, not a signature, and in many jurisdictions, the ability to provide consent is linked to capacity rather than a predetermined age. All attempts should be made to explore the pediatric patient's understanding of transplantation, the expected treatment course, the anticipated risks and benefits, and whether the patient would like to proceed. The consent framework applied will also depend in part on whether the transplant is provided as part of research or clinical care, which has implications for costs, oversight, and evaluation of outcomes and the risk-benefit ratio moving forwards (86).

INDICATIONS FOR PEDIATRIC UPPER EXTREMITY ALLOTRANSPLANTATION

The Children's Hospital of Philadelphia (Philadelphia, USA) has listed their pediatric VCA inclusion criteria as children at least 8 years of age with bilateral upper limb amputations, failed trial of prostheses, and able to partake in therapy (67). Boston Children's Hospital (Boston, USA) has also initiated an experimental pediatric hand transplant program, for which their inclusion criteria are individuals 10–25 years of age in good health who live near Boston or are willing to relocate for at least

6 months post-surgery, with either (1) two missing hands, (2) one missing hand and already on immunosuppression for a functioning solid organ transplant, or (3) one missing hand but the other hand is poorly functioning (87).

Our own criteria for developing a pediatric upper limb VCA program at the Hospital for Sick Children (Toronto, Canada) include children who have begun or are about to begin immunosuppression for solid organ allograft, are mature enough to participate in extensive rehabilitation, and have failed prosthesis trials (85). For both acquired or congenital etiologies, bilateral amputees or unilateral amputees with a poorly functioning contralateral upper limb would be considered most favourably.

CONCLUSIONS

For children with debilitating injuries, illnesses, or congenital defects of the upper limb that cannot be rehabilitated with prostheses or reconstructed by even the most complex autologous options, VCA is a compelling option to restore form and function. However, if the goal of VCA is to improve quality of life, then over-medicalization with rejection episodes, burdensome rehabilitation, and medication adverse effects must be minimized. Significant hurdles in reconstructive transplantation have been overcome through multidisciplinary and international collaboration, but many issues remain. The key to progress in VCA is promoting ongoing collaboration, ethical inquiry, research funding, and critical evaluation of the goals and outcomes of surgery. Appropriate patient selection cannot be overstated. For ethically and rigorously screened pediatric patients, upper extremity VCA has a promising future.

COMPLIANCE WITH ETHICAL STANDARDS

CONFLICT OF INTEREST

Kevin Zuo, Anna Gold, Randi Zlotnik Shaul, Emily Ho, Gregory Borshel, and Ronald Zuker declare no conflict of interest.

HUMAN AND ANIMAL RIGHTS AND INFORMED CONSENT

All reported studies/experiments with human or animal subjects performed by the authors have been previously published and complied with all applicable ethical standards (including the Helsinki declaration and its amendments, institutional/national research committee standards, and international/national/institutional guidelines.

REFERENCES

1. Dubernard JM, Owen E, Herzberg G, Lanzetta M, Martin X, Kapila H, et al. Human hand allograft: report on first 6 months. Lancet. 1999;353(9161):1315–20.
2. Kaufman CL, Bhutiani N, Ramirez A, Tien HY, Palazzo MD, Galvis E, et al. Current status of vascularized composite allotransplantation. Am Surg. 2019;85(6):631–7.
3. Pathmanathan V. Arm transplantation for congenital absence of the hand: the 12 year outcome. ANZ J Surg. 2012;82(Suppl. 1):130.

4. Zuker RM, Redett R, Alman B, Coles JG, Timoney N, Ein SH. First successful lower-extremity transplantation: technique and functional result. J Reconstr Microsurg. 2006;22(4):239–44.

5. Fattah A, Cypel T, Donner EJ, Wang F, Alman BA, Zuker RM. The first successful lower extremity transplantation: 6-year follow-up and implications for cortical plasticity. Am J Transplant. 2011;11(12):2762–7.

6. McDiarmid SV. Vascularized composite allotransplantation in children: what we can learn from solid organ transplantation. Curr Opin Organ Transplant. 2018;23(5):605–14.

7. Amaral S, Kessler SK, Levy TJ, Gaetz W, McAndrew C, Chang B, et al. 18-month outcomes of heterologous bilateral hand transplantation in a child: a case report. Lancet Child Adolesc Health. 2017;1(1):35–44.

8. Iglesias M, Leal P, Butron P, Santander-Flores S, Ricano-Enciso D, Gonzalez-Chavez MA, et al. Severe complications after bilateral upper extremity transplantation: a case report. Transplantation. 2014;98(3):e16–7.

9. Jasinka J. Docs reconstruct boy's throat in ground-breaking transplant surgery. Warsaw, Poland, April 11 2019 [Available from: https://www.thefirstnews.com/article/docs-reconstruct-boys-throat-in-ground-breaking-transplant-surgery-5537].

10. Huizing K, Reinders-Messelink H, Maathuis C, Hadders-Algra M, van der Sluis CK. Age at first prosthetic fitting and later functional outcome in children and young adults with unilateral congenital below-elbow deficiency: a cross-sectional study. Prosthet Orthot Int. 2010;34(2):166–74.

11. Michielsen A, Van Wijk I, Ketelaar M. Participation and quality of life in children and adolescents with congenital limb deficiencies: a narrative review. Prosthet Orthot Int. 2010;34(4):351–61.

12. McKechnie PS, John A. Anxiety and depression following traumatic limb amputation: a systematic review. Injury. 2014;45(12):1859–66.

13. de Jong IG, Reinders-Messelink HA, Janssen WG, Poelma MJ, van Wijk I, van der Sluis CK. Mixed feelings of children and adolescents with unilateral congenital below elbow deficiency: an online focus group study. PLOS ONE. 2012;7(6):e37099.

14. Egermann M, Kasten P, Thomsen M. Myoelectric hand prostheses in very young children. Int Orthop. 2009;33(4):1101–5.

15. Wagner LV, Bagley AM, James MA. Reasons for prosthetic rejection by children with unilateral congenital transverse forearm total deficiency. J Prosthet Orthot. 2007;19(2):51–4.

16. Crandall RC, Tomhave W. Pediatric unilateral below-elbow amputees: retrospective analysis of 34 patients given multiple prosthetic options. J Pediatr Orthop. 2002;22(3):380–3.

17. Mendenhall SD, Sawyer JD, West BL, Neumeister MW, Shaked A, Levin LS. Pediatric vascularized composite allotransplantation: what is the landscape for obtaining appropriate donors in the United States? Pediatr Transplant. 2019;23(5):e13466.

18. Cypel M, Yeung JC, Liu M, Anraku M, Chen F, Karolak W, et al. Normothermic ex vivo lung perfusion in clinical lung transplantation. N Engl J Med. 2011;364(15):1431–40.

19. Ozer K, Rojas-Pena A, Mendias CL, Bryner B, Toomasian C, Bartlett RH. Ex situ limb perfusion system to extend vascularized composite tissue allograft survival in swine. Transplantation. 2015;99(10):2095–101.

20. Constantinescu MA, Knall E, Xu X, Kiermeir DM, Jenni H, Gygax E, et al. Preservation of amputated extremities by extracorporeal blood perfusion; a feasibility study in a porcine model. J Surg Res. 2011;171(1):291–9.

21. Bowen CV, Ethridge CP, O'Brien BM, Frykman GK, Gumley GJ. Experimental microvascular growth plate transfers. Part I–Investigation of vascularity. J Bone Joint Surg Br. 1988;70(2):305–10.

22. Beyermann K, Hahn P, Mutsch Y, Lanz U. [Bone growth after finger replantation in childhood]. Handchir Mikrochir Plast Chir. 2000;32(2):88–92.
23. Demiri E, Bakhach J, Tsakoniatis N, Martin D, Baudet J. Bone growth after replantation in children. J Reconstr Microsurg. 1995;11(2):113–22; discussion 22–3.
24. Mc COBB, Franklin JD, Morrison WA, MacLeod AM. Replantation and revascularisation surgery in children. Hand. 1980;12(1):12–24.
25. Kropfl A, Gasperschitz F, Niederwieser B, Primavesi C, Hertz H. [Epiphyseal growth after replantation in childhood]. Handchir Mikrochir Plast Chir. 1994;26(4):194–9.
26. Van Beek AL, Wavak PW, Zook EG. Microvascular surgery in young children. Plast Reconstr Surg. 1979;63(4):457–62.
27. Nunley JA, Spiegl PV, Goldner RD, Urbaniak JR. Longitudinal epiphyseal growth after replantation and transplantation in children. J Hand Surg Am. 1987;12(2):274–9.
28. Messner F, Grahammer J, Hautz T, Brandacher G, Schneeberger S. Ischemia/reperfusion injury in vascularized tissue allotransplantation: tissue damage and clinical relevance. Curr Opin Organ Transplant. 2016;21(5):503–9.
29. Datta N, Devaney SG, Busuttil RW, Azari K, Kupiec-Weglinski JW. Prolonged cold ischemia time results in local and remote organ dysfunction in a murine model of vascularized composite transplantation. Am J Transplant. 2017;17(10):2572–9.
30. Kurzynski M, Jaskolska A, Marusiak J, Wolczowski A, Bierut P, Szumowski L, et al. Computer-aided training sensorimotor cortex functions in humans before the upper limb transplantation using virtual reality and sensory feedback. Comput Biol Med. 2017;87:311–21.
31. Bueno J, Barret JP, Serracanta J, Arno A, Collado JM, Valles C, et al. Logistics and strategy of multiorgan procurement involving total face allograft. Am J Transplant. 2011;11(5):1091–7.
32. Mukesh N, Bramstedt KA. Perspectives of US and Australian hand therapists about pediatric hand transplantation. Prog Transplant. 2017;27(1):73–8.
33. Ruijs AC, Jaquet JB, Kalmijn S, Giele H, Hovius SE. Median and ulnar nerve injuries: a meta-analysis of predictors of motor and sensory recovery after modern microsurgical nerve repair. Plast Reconstr Surg. 2005;116(2):484–94; discussion 95–6.
34. Bolitho DG, Boustred M, Hudson DA, Hodgetts K. Primary epineural repair of the ulnar nerve in children. J Hand Surg Am. 1999;24(1):16–20.
35. Ceynowa M, Mazurek T, Sikora T. Median and ulnar nerve grafting in children. J Pediatr Orthop B. 2012;21(6):525–8.
36. Hudson DA, Bolitho DG, Hodgetts K. Primary epineural repair of the median nerve in children. J Hand Surg Br. 1997;22(1):54–6.
37. Pestronk A, Drachman DB, Griffin JW. Effects of aging on nerve sprouting and regeneration. Exp Neurol. 1980;70(1):65–82.
38. Tung TH. Tacrolimus (FK506): safety and applications in reconstructive surgery. Hand (N Y). 2010;5(1):1–8.
39. Owen ER, Dubernard JM, Lanzetta M, Kapila H, Martin X, Dawahra M, et al. Peripheral nerve regeneration in human hand transplantation. Transplant Proc. 2001;33(1–2):1720–1.
40. Jones JW, Gruber SA, Barker JH, Breidenbach WC. Successful hand transplantation. One-year follow-up. Louisville Hand Transplant Team. N Engl J Med. 2000;343(7):468–73.
41. Shores JT, Brandacher G, Lee WP. Hand and upper extremity transplantation: an update of outcomes in the worldwide experience. Plast Reconstr Surg. 2015;135(2):351e–60e.
42. Chan KM, Curran MW, Gordon T. The use of brief post-surgical low frequency electrical stimulation to enhance nerve regeneration in clinical practice. J Physiol. 2016;594(13):3553–9.

43. Bamba R, Riley DC, Kim JS, Cardwell NL, Pollins AC, Shack RB, et al. Evaluation of a nerve fusion technique with polyethylene glycol in a delayed setting after nerve injury. J Hand Surg Am. 2018;43(1):82.e1–.e7.

44. Paskal AM, Paskal W, Pietruski P, Wlodarski PK. Polyethylene glycol: the future of posttraumatic nerve repair? Systemic review. Int J Mol Sci. 2019;20(6):1478.

45. Chen R, Cohen LG, Hallett M. Nervous system reorganization following injury. Neuroscience. 2002;111(4):761–73.

46. Chemnitz A, Andersson G, Rosen B, Dahlin LB, Bjorkman A. Poor electroneurography but excellent hand function 31 years after nerve repair in childhood. Neuroreport. 2013;24(1):6–9.

47. Duteille F, Petry D, Dautel G, Merle M. A comparison between clinical results and electromyographic analysis after median or ulnar nerve injuries in children's wrists. Ann Plast Surg. 2001;46(4):382–6.

48. Frey SH, Bogdanov S, Smith JC, Watrous S, Breidenbach WC. Chronically deafferented sensory cortex recovers a grossly typical organization after allogenic hand transplantation. Curr Biol. 2008;18(19):1530–4.

49. Giraux P, Sirigu A, Schneider F, Dubernard JM. Cortical reorganization in motor cortex after graft of both hands. Nat Neurosci. 2001;4(7):691–2.

50. Hernandez-Castillo CR, Aguilar-Castaneda E, Iglesias M, Fernandez-Ruiz J. Motor and sensory cortical reorganization after bilateral forearm transplantation: four-year follow-up fMRI case study. Magn Reson Imaging. 2016;34(4):541–4.

51. Gaetz W, Kessler SK, Roberts TPL, Berman JI, Levy TJ, Hsia M, et al. Massive cortical reorganization is reversible following bilateral transplants of the hands: evidence from the first successful bilateral pediatric hand transplant patient. Ann Clin Transl Neurol. 2018;5(1):92–7.

52. Manktelow RT, Tomat LR, Zuker RM, Chang M. Smile reconstruction in adults with free muscle transfer innervated by the masseter motor nerve: effectiveness and cerebral adaptation. Plast Reconstr Surg. 2006;118(4):885–99.

53. Garmi R, Labbe D, Coskun O, Compere JF, Benateau H. Lengthening temporalis myoplasty and brain plasticity: a functional magnetic resonance imaging study. Ann Chir Plast Esthet. 2013;58(4):271–6.

54. Chen R, Anastakis DJ, Haywood CT, Mikulis DJ, Manktelow RT. Plasticity of the human motor system following muscle reconstruction: a magnetic stimulation and functional magnetic resonance imaging study. Clin Neurophysiol. 2003;114(12):2434–46.

55. Kollar B, Tasigiorgos S, Dorante MI, Carty MJ, Talbot SG, Pomahac B. Innovations in reconstructive microsurgery: reconstructive transplantation. J Surg Oncol. 2018;118(5):800–6.

56. Kaufman CL, Ouseph R, Blair B, Kutz JE, Tsai TM, Scheker LR, et al. Graft vasculopathy in clinical hand transplantation. Am J Transplant. 2012;12(4):1004–16.

57. Takatsuki M, Uemoto S, Inomata Y, Egawa H, Kiuchi T, Fujita S, et al. Weaning of immunosuppression in living donor liver transplant recipients. Transplantation. 2001;72(3):449–54.

58. Leventhal J, Abecassis M, Miller J, Gallon L, Ravindra K, Tollerud DJ, et al. Chimerism and tolerance without GVHD or engraftment syndrome in HLA-mismatched combined kidney and hematopoietic stem cell transplantation. Sci Transl Med. 2012;4(124):124ra28.

59. Schneeberger S, Gorantla VS, Brandacher G, Zeevi A, Demetris AJ, Lunz JG, et al. Upper-extremity transplantation using a cell-based protocol to minimize immunosuppression. Ann Surg. 2013;257(2):345–51.

60. Kollar B, Pomahac B, Riella LV. Novel immunological and clinical insights in vascularized composite allotransplantation. Curr Opin Organ Transplant. 2019;24(1):42–8.

61. Roy M, Haykal S, Zuo, KJ, Ghazarian D, McCabe SJ.Nailfold capillaroscopy: potential use in vascularized composite allotransplantation of the hand. 6th Biennial Meeting of the American Society for Reconstructive Transplantation; Nov 15–17, 2018; Chicago, IL, USA.

62. Gharb BB, Rampazzo A, Altuntas SH, Madajka M, Cwykiel J, Stratton J, et al. Effectiveness of topical immunosuppressants in prevention and treatment of rejection in face allotransplantation. Transplantation. 2013;95(10):1197–203.

63. Solari MG, Washington KM, Sacks JM, Hautz T, Unadkat JV, Horibe EK, et al. Daily topical tacrolimus therapy prevents skin rejection in a rodent hind limb allograft model. Plast Reconstr Surg. 2009;123(Suppl. 2):17s–25s.

64. Olariu R, Denoyelle J, Leclere FM, Dzhonova DV, Gajanayake T, Banz Y, et al. Intra-graft injection of tacrolimus promotes survival of vascularized composite allotrans-plantation. J Surg Res. 2017;218:49–57.

65. Dzhonova DV, Olariu R, Leckenby J, Banz Y, Prost JC, Dhayani A, et al. Local injections of tacrolimus-loaded hydrogel reduce systemic immunosuppression-related toxicity in vascularized composite allotransplantation. Transplantation. 2018;102(10):1684–94.

66. Deuse T, Blankenberg F, Haddad M, Reichenspurner H, Phillips N, Robbins RC, et al. Mechanisms behind local immunosuppression using inhaled tacrolimus in preclinical models of lung transplantation. Am J Respir Cell Mol Biol. 2010;43(4):403–12.

67. Amaral S, Levin LS. Pediatric and congenital hand transplantation. Curr Opin Organ Transplant. 2017;22(5):477–83.

68. Kumnig M, Jowsey-Gregoire SG. Key psychosocial challenges in vascularized com-positc allotransplantation. World J Transplant. 2016;6(1):91–102.

69. Ruta DA, Garratt AM, Leng M, Russell IT, MacDonald LM. A new approach to the measurement of quality of life. The Patient-Generated Index. Med Care. 1994;32(11):1109–26.

70. Caplan A, Purves D. A quiet revolution in organ transplant ethics. J Med Ethics. 2017;43(11):797–800.

71. Chang G, Pomahac B. Psychosocial changes six months after face transplantation. Psychosomatics. 2013;54(4):367–71.

72. Bramstedt KA. A lifesaving view of vascularized composite allotransplantation: patient experience of social death before and after face, hand, and larynx transplant. J Patient Exp. 2018;5(2):92–100.

73. Rumsey N, Harcourt D. Body image and disfigurement: issues and interventions. Body Image. 2004;1(1):83–97.

74. Hedges CE, Rosoff PM. Transplants for non-lethal conditions: a case against hand transplantation in minors. J Med Ethics. 2018;44(10):661–5.

75. Colen DL, Bank J, McAndrew C, Levin LS. Reconstruction for all: the case for pediat-ric hand transplantation. Vascularized Composite Allotransplantation. 2015;2(3):47–52.

76. Bertrand AA, Sen S, Otake LR, Lee GK. Changing attitudes toward hand allotransplan-tation among North American hand surgeons. Ann Plast Surg. 2014;72(Suppl. 1):S56–60.

77. Dobbels F, Ruppar T, De Geest S, Decorte A, Van Damme-Lombaerts R, Fine RN. Adherence to the immunosuppressive regimen in pediatric kidney transplant recipi-ents: a systematic review. Pediatr Transplant. 2010;14(5):603–13.

78. Dharnidharka VR, Lamb KE, Zheng J, Schechtman KB, Meier-Kriesche HU. Across all solid organs, adolescent age recipients have worse transplant organ sur-vival than younger age children: A US national registry analysis. Pediatr Transplant. 2015;19(5):471–6.

79. Meaux JB, Green A, Nelson MK, Huett A, Boateng B, Pye S, et al. Transition to self-management after pediatric heart transplant. Prog Transplant. 2014;24(3):226–33.

80. Visser-Meily A, Post M, Gorter JW, Berlekom SB, Van Den Bos T, Lindeman E. Rehabilitation of stroke patients needs a family-centred approach. Disabil Rehabil. 2006;28(24):1557–61.
81. Kokorelias KM, Gignac MAM, Naglie G, Cameron JI. Towards a universal model of family centered care: a scoping review. BMC Health Serv Res. 2019;19(1):564.
82. Brown K, Mace SE, Dietrich AM, Knazik S, Schamban NE. Patient and family-centred care for pediatric patients in the emergency department. CJEM. 2008;10(1):38–43.
83. Flynn J, Shaul RZ, Hanson MD, Borschel GH, Zuker R. Pediatric facial transplantation: ethical considerations. Plast Surg (Oakv). 2014;22(2):67–9.
84. Doumit G, Gharb BB, Rampazzo A, Papay F, Siemionow MZ, Zins JE. Pediatric vascularized composite allotransplantation. Ann Plast Surg. 2014;73(4):445–50.
85. Haykal SZ, Zucker RM. Chapter 65. Vascularized composite allotransplantation in the pediatric population. In: Bentz MLB, Bauer S, Zuker RM, editors. Principles and practice of pediatric plastic surgery. Second ed. CRC Press; 2016. p. 1893–912.
86. Shaul RZ, Borschel G, Flynn J, Hanson MD, Wright L, Zuker RM. Ethical issues in pediatric vascularized composite allotransplantation. In: Greenberg RA, Goldberg A, Rodriguez-Arias D, editors. Ethical issues in pediatric organ transplantation. Switzerland: Springer International; 2016. p. 169–91.
87. Hospital BCs. Boston Children's Hospital Hand Transplant Program Eligibility 2020 [Available from: http://www.childrenshospital.org/centers-and-services/programs/f-_-n/hand-transplant-program/eligibility].

Section III

Graft Monitoring in Reconstructive Transplantation

6 Targeted Imaging and Therapeutic Technologies in Neuroregeneration

Jelena M. Janjic, Mihály Balogh,
Sandeep Kumar Reddy Adena,
Amanda Fitzpatrick, John A. Pollock,
Vijay Gorantla, and Andrew J. Shepherd

CONTENTS

Introduction 101
Cellular Targets in Neuroregeneration 102
Cell Therapy in Neuroregeneration.. 104
Nanoparticles for Imaging and Support of Neuoregeneration 105
Immunomodulation and Imaging Immune Cells with Nanoparticles.................. 106
Macrophage-Targeted Nanosystems 107
Targeting to Neurons in Neuroregeneration.. 110
    Carbon Nanotubes, Nanohorns, and Nanoparticles 110
    Quantum Dots 111
    Metal NPs.. 111
Nanosystems as Mechanistic Tools In Vivo... 112
Conclusions and Future Directions.. 113
References 113

INTRODUCTION

More than 1.4 million Americans experience peripheral nerve injuries (PNIs) each year, and close to a million of those injuries require a surgical intervention.[1–3] Estimates of the incidence of PNI after accidental trauma secondary to motor vehicle accidents, sharp lacerations, penetrating trauma, stretching or crushing trauma and fractures, and gunshot wounds have ranged from 3% to 87%. Iatrogenic injuries are thought to account for 12% of cases of PNI worldwide, although this is likely a gross underestimate.[3,4] PNI can result in motor or sensory deficits, intractable acute or chronic neuropathic pain with significant treatment costs, and morbidity and loss of function that impact the quality of life.[4] Distal axonal degeneration and loss of target fidelity are unavoidable consequences of PNI. The key is to maintain or maximize the pro-regenerative capacity of the de-axonized distal nerve to support recipient axonal regeneration to distal sensory/motor targets and to achieve functional neuro-integration.

Neuroregeneration is defined as the progressive structural and functional recovery of the damaged nervous system. It is a complex process including the generation of new neurons, glia, myelin, and synapses, as well as the regaining of motor and sensory functions and also cognitive and emotional abilities. Unfortunately, neuroregeneration is very slow compared to the regeneration of other body systems. Various approaches can induce the regrowth of nerve fibers. Usually, nerve regeneration is promoted by administering drugs[5], electrical stimulation,[6,7] or physical factors (magnetic field).[8,9] In recent years, nerve surgery, bioartificial structures (such as conduits) and the microsurgical suture technique have demonstrated remarkable progress.[10] Transection or crushing injuries and Wallerian degeneration (WD) occur at a distance from the site of the injury. Axonal regeneration occurs within hours of nerve injury, and regrowth of nerve fibers takes place from the proximal nerve segment. Traumatic neuroma formation can occur at the site of the lesion due to obstruction of axonal guidance. Degenerative processes can also result in poor reinnervation of the target tissue or organ. All these challenges highlight the necessity for the innovation of new targeted and cell-based therapeutic strategies for stimulation and control of neuroregeneration. Furthermore, there is a need to noninvasively image molecular and cellular processes of neuroregeneration in order to optimize therapeutic development and open the doors to treatment personalization. The focus of this chapter is on noninvasive diagnostic and therapeutic interventions with nanotechnology.

CELLULAR TARGETS IN NEUROREGENERATION

Distal axonal degeneration and loss of target fidelity is an unavoidable consequence of PNI. The goals of neuroregenerative therapies are: 1) maintain or maximize the pro-regenerative capacity of the de-axonized distal nerve, 2) support recipient axonal regeneration to distal sensory/motor targets, and 3) achieve functional neuro-integration. Any approach to such goals must be comprehensive and multifaceted. It must simultaneously facilitate natural host reparative processes—involving Schwann cells (SCs) and macrophages—to promote expeditious and targeted axonal outgrowth, as well as to provide neurotrophic support of the distal neuromuscular junction and end-plates for functional reinnervation and recovery. The treatment paradigm must include selective neurotrophic agents, which when delivered in a targeted fashion, act via multiple, non-redundant cellular/molecular mechanisms or pathways. This will have a global, complementary impact on intracellular and extracellular processes involving differentiation, migration, or signaling in the neuroinflammation, neurodegeneration, and neuroregeneration phases following PNI.[11]

Following PNI, neuro-immune interactions are fundamental to the process of WD. An early phase of neuroinflammation involves macrophage recruitment and rapid clearance of myelin debris, improving blood-nerve barrier permeability and activation of nearby SCs to produce new myelin, facilitating nerve regeneration. Nerve transection/injury triggers a massive transformation of myelinating and non-myelinating (Remak) SCs to form the reparative (Büngner) SCs of injured nerves.[12–15] A major component of SC reprogramming during WD is autophagocytosis (myelinophagy) by SCs, as myelin is inhibitory to axonal regeneration. SCs break down 40–50% of the myelin in the vicinity of the injury during the first 5–7 days after PNI.[16,17] The neural-immune interactions in WD after PNI involve leukocyte trafficking and infiltration of the lesion site after SC de-differentiation, and then spread to the entire distal stump beginning at day 4.[18,19] Both hematogenous (infiltrating) monocyte-derived macrophages (55% of cells) and resident endoneurial macrophages (45% of cells) play a role in WD.[20] WD is an important antecedent phase for successful repair in the complex mechanism of proper neuronal regeneration. If the efficient innate-immune response of WD is hampered (e.g., by diabetes), the process of functional recovery can be highly damaged as well.[21] In line with these findings, Cui and co-workers showed that macrophages are also capable of promoting a neurotrophic environment, thereby facilitating regrowth of the damaged nerve.[22]

Based on the injury and the cellular and molecular milieu, macrophages can assume two well-studied phenotypes, pro-inflammatory (M1) and anti-inflammatory/pro-healing (M2),[23] though it is likely these represent two extremes along a continuum of potential phenotypes. Classically activated M1 macrophages accumulate in the area of inflammation in the early stage and participate in the pro-inflammatory phase where debris clearance is facilitated. They produce numerous pro-inflammatory mediators (e.g., chemokines, cytokines).[24] These macrophages later polarize into alternatively activated M2 macrophages, relieving inflammation and improving repair by playing a neuroprotective role.[25] The exact role and importance of each cell type (SCs, macrophages, dendritic cells, neutrophils, B-cells, helper T-cells, cytotoxic T-cells) and arm of the immune response (innate, adaptive, complement), and how these components interact and compensate for the other in the time course of WD and axonal regeneration after PNI, is just emerging. It is an established notion that an efficient innate immune response with an orchestrated interplay of SCs and resident and hematogenous M1 macrophages is important for myelin clearance during WD after PNI.[26,27]

The key macrophage receptor regulating M1-M2 conversion is CD163. CD163 scavenges hemoglobin:haptoglobin (Hb:Hp) complexes, which leads to the nuclear translocation of the transcription factor Nrf2 (NF-E2-related factor 2), upregulation of heme oxygenase (HO)-1 cytoprotective protein, and release of the anti-inflammatory cytokine interleukin (IL)-10.[28] There is literature data showing that a range of natural and synthetic antioxidants may drive M1 to M2 switching through Nrf2/HO-1, leading to improved kidney function in diabetes.[28–30] Therefore, Nrf2, which is the transcriptional regulator upstream of HO-1, could be a potential novel target in neuroregeneration support and management. Several studies also confirm the immunomodulatory role of SCs in suppressing inflammatory gene expression after PNI and promoting M2 polarization.[31,32] However, recent rodent PNI studies challenge this assumption by showing that SCs are capable of substantial myelin degradation in the absence of M1 macrophages and are the pivotal, primary cells in WD.[23–25,33–36] Experimental PNI models confirm that myelin lipid degradation products accumulate in SCs beginning at 4 days after injury, peak around 9 days after injury, and subside significantly by 2 weeks after injury.[37] Indeed, early myelin debris clearance after PNI is mediated by multiple, independent, and redundant mechanisms, with SCs being key drivers as compared to M1 resident macrophages.[18,19,37–39] These findings are also supported by other research in adaptive immunodeficiencies involving immunoglobulin or functional T-cell defects, where normal or increased myelin debris clearance is observed 1 week after denervation due to compensatory SC myelinophagy.[40] The development, maturation, differentiation, and de-differentiation of SCs relies on key intracellular transcription or signaling pathways that include but are not limited to protein-kinase A, C, Akt, Erk/MAPK, Hippo, mTOR, c-jun, and the immunophilin, FKBP52.[41]

CELL THERAPY IN NEUROREGENERATION

Cell therapy is a potentially promising approach for the management of nerve regeneration, through which trophic and growth factors are provided by SCs.[42,43] Following PNI, engrafted cells such as SCs form the myelin sheath and promote nerve repair by producing various growth factors. In the past decade, cell therapy for nerve defects has evolved to the use of mesenchymal stem cells (MSCs), embryonic stem cells, olfactory cells, stem cells of hair follicles, and other stem cells since the production of viable SCs in the required quantity occasionally fails.[44–46] Commonly used cells in cell therapy for nerve regeneration are MSCs, neural stem cells, and induced pluripotent stem cells (IPSCs). MSCs show immunosuppressive activity and have the capacity to modulate immune responses.[47,48] They are generally derived from bone marrow, umbilical cord stroma, adipose tissue, or amniotic fluid.[49–51] One of the main advantages of choosing bone marrow or adipose tissue is that they provide an easily accessible and autologous source of stem cells for transplantation therapies. The interaction between MSCs and immune cells leads to the suppression of T and B lymphocyte activity, thereby inhibiting dendritic cell maturation.[52] Neural stem cells exhibit a wide range of therapeutic actions following nerve injury. They have the significant properties of self-renewal and multi-potency to generate neurons, astrocytes, and oligodendrocytes appropriately throughout life. To make neural stem cells viable for transplantation, these cells must be effectively cultured and expanded ex vivo. Neural stem cells can be extracted directly from neural tissue, such as the neuroectoderm in developing fetuses, or the subgerminal or subventricular zone in adults (since neurogenesis occurs throughout life in these regions).[53] In recent times, the development of IPSCs expands the sources of cells for such therapies and represents a significant development in the progress of neuroregeneration.[54,55] Undifferentiated IPSCs can differentiate to SCs or neural crest stem cells with myelinating abilities.[56] They significantly boost axonal growth and recovery of neurosensory functions.[57] They can also enhance axonal regeneration and myelination without inducing teratomas.[58] IPSC-based nerve conduits in combination with basic fibroblast growth factor show improved regenerative effects.[59] For nerve injury application, cells are often collectively used with synthetic or natural materials to form artificial nerve tissue and are classified as biological drugs. Stem cell usage in clinical trials for PNI therefore needs proper regulatory approval to ensure that such cell therapies meet safety and efficacy standards.

Despite the exceptional prospects, there still exist some concerns regarding the safety and efficiency of stem cell therapy. For example, cell therapy requires a large population of cells to be collected, cultured, expanded, and cryopreserved before transplantation. Tumorigenicity of stem cells is also a justifiable concern; however, malignancy does not usually occur after administration.[60] To preserve phenotypic stability, stem cell homogeneity must also be taken into consideration since the in vitro culture, and expansion of cells introduce significant heterogeneity in cell phenotype and treatment outcomes. Since a severe and prolonged nerve injury often leads to muscle atrophy, stem cells can also be targeted to muscles by injecting them to the injured nerve sites.[61,62] Considering the complexity of cellular interactions in neuroregeneration following nerve injury, noninvasive nanoimaging is a promising solution. The role of nanoimaging in monitoring neuroregeneration has been discussed earlier in depth.[63] Here, we will focus on utilizing nanoimaging in support of new therapeutic strategies development and novel nanotechnology-based treatments in support of neuroregeneration.

NANOPARTICLES FOR IMAGING AND SUPPORT OF NEUOREGENERATION

Currently, a variety of nanomaterials and nanoparticle formations are applied for imaging methodologies and drug delivery to sites of injury. Current approaches take advantage of the composition of the nanomaterial, such as the ability to follow carbon nanoparticles (NPs) with cellular imaging techniques or the antioxidant properties of silver nanoparticles (SNPs) and gold nanoparticles (GNPs). In this section, we survey select examples of nanoparticle designs as tools for diagnostic and therapeutic delivery and offer direction on their application in immunomodulation in neuroregeneration.

NPs are an incredibly diverse class of materials with a typical size range of 10–500 nm. Their varied functions are due in part to their diversity of form (e.g., nanosized rods, cubes, shells, cones, and tubes).[64] Based on their chemical composition, they can be broadly classified into organic materials (liposomes, nanoemulsions, carbon nanotubes, dendrimers, and other polymers) and inorganic materials (e.g., metals).[65] NPs have been used extensively in biomedical applications, especially in diagnostics and drug/gene delivery.[66] They enable precise drug targeting, enhancement of therapeutic moiety bioavailability, and are uniquely multifunctional: combining diagnostics, therapeutics, and biosensing.[67] Here, we focus on their potential as direct immunomodulation agents for manipulating the innate immune system for therapeutic purposes. Delivering appropriate cargo, they can "re-train" the immune system to detect and eliminate foreign entities, and the key to these therapeutic strategies is their ability to induce immune stimulation or suppression.[68] As drug carrier systems for therapeutic molecules, NPs aim to improve drug/gene delivery and therapeutic effects and decrease their associated side effects.[69] In recent times, numerous efforts have been made to study the impact of various types of NPs on neurons, and there are several reports suggesting that NPs can promote neuroprotection and neuronal differentiation.[70–72] Further, particular NPs can be inherently immunomodulatory. For example, Fullerene produces immunosuppressive effects,

TABLE 6.1

Summary of Commonly Used Nanoparticles in Neuroregeneration

Class	Size	Applicability
Quantum dots	2–10 nm	Biocompatibility, good optical properties, long photo-stability and useful for immune cell tracking.
Lipid NPs	20 nm–2.5 μm	Can carry both hydrophobic and hydrophilic drugs, controlled drug release kinetics.
• Liposomes	5–100 nm	
• Micelles	30–100 nm	
• Exosomes		
Polymeric NPs	1–200 nm	Sustained drug release, biocompatible, many synthesis strategies.
• Polylactic acid NPs		
• Poly (lactic-co-glycolic acid)		
Metallic NPs	1–50 nm	Biocompatible, readily cross blood-brain barrier, can reduce oxidative stress, and can be easily encapsulated.
• Gold	3–200 nm	
• Silver	10–150 nm	
• Metal oxide		

and SNPs and GNPs produce anti-inflammatory effects. Several types of NPs showed improved therapeutic results in neurons, and among them, carbon-based,[73] gold and silver NPs[74,75] were predominant. A brief summary of common classes of NPs with their potential uses and their applicability in neuroregeneration imaging and therapeutics is shown in Table 6.1.

IMMUNOMODULATION AND IMAGING IMMUNE CELLS WITH NANOPARTICLES

The immune system acts in concert with the nervous and endocrine systems to constitute an interactive and communicative network. The presence of receptors for neurotransmitters on immune cells and innervation of key sites of immunomodulation such as lymph nodes makes neuroimmunomodulation possible.[76] By a variety of signal transduction events, neuroimmune interactions are modulated. It involves cytokines, cyclic nucleotides, neurohormones, neuropeptides, neurosteroids, neurotransmitters, and calcium-dependent protein kinases. Crucially, NPs can be utilized in neuroimmunomodulation through their uptake by monocyte-derived macrophages.[77] This nonspecific uptake by phagocytic cells can lead to selective homing to lymphoid organs and the production of immunomodulatory effects dependent on the therapeutic moiety carried by the nanosystem.[78] Two basic strategies exist for targeting pro-inflammatory M1 macrophages: 1) macrophage depletion by NP-loaded cytotoxic drugs and 2) immunomodulation by NPs carrying specific agents to the injury microenvironment to repolarize macrophages from M1 to M2 phenotype.[79] Furthermore, the effects of neuroimmunomodulation can be monitored in living subjects using macrophage-targeted nanoimaging.[63] Systemic macrophage depletion is not desirable due to the resultant suppression of the innate immune response to infection. A more precision-targeted strategy has been established in our recent studies where theranostic (therapeutic and diagnostic) nanosystems were used to both modulate the immune response to nerve injury and monitor noninvasively the effects of macrophage-targeted immunomodulation.[80–84]

MACROPHAGE-TARGETED NANOSYSTEMS

Macrophages emerged as the most accessible cellular targets for NP-based therapies, due to their ability to take up NPs injected in the blood stream, which allows for their in vivo tracking using near-infrared fluorescence (NIRF) and magnetic resonance imaging (MRI).[85–89] Passive targeting of circulating inflammatory cells by complex colloidal nanosystems known as perfluorocarbon nanoemulsions (PFC-NEs) has been extensively investigated for the purposes of 19F MRI of inflammation.[89–92] PFCs are chemically and biologically inert 19F MRI agents, which allow for quantitative and qualitative assessment of inflammation in vivo without apparent background. PFC-NEs have been successfully used to measure the spatial and temporal distribution of infiltrating macrophages in transplant models (kidney, heart), and such PFC-NE-labeled macrophage infiltration correlates well with histopathologic findings of rejection.[86] In a related study, PFC-NEs were also used to quantify macrophage infiltration as a surrogate measure of inflammation in pig hearts in a myocardial infarction model.[93] PFC-NEs have been broadly applied to specifically and selectively quantify macrophage trafficking changes following transplantation,[86] abscess,[94] and inflammatory bowel disease.[95] We have demonstrated the utility of macrophage-targeted PFC-NEs for imaging neuroinflammation in rodent models, as summarized in Figure 6.1.[96,97] The severity of nerve injury correlated with numbers of infiltrating macrophages, which increased signal at the site of injury as measured by both NIRF imaging and 19F MRI.

Over the past decade, efforts to expand our macrophage-targeted nanosystem technologies led to the design and development of macrophage-targeted PFC-NEs, which are "triphasic," composed of three immiscible liquids: PFC (fluorous phase), hydrocarbon (organic phase), and water (aqueous phase). The advantage of such triphasic PFC-NEs lies in their increased capacity to incorporate lipophilic drugs[98] and/or NIRF dyes due to the higher organic volume fraction compared to that of other reported PFC-NEs, with no significant change in droplet size.[99–103] These NIRF-labeled PFC-NEs show an excellent correlation between NIRF signal and 19F nuclear magnetic resonance (NMR) signal in cells and tissues ex vivo at experimental end-points (Figure 6.1a–b).[91] Consequently, 19F NMR can be used to quantify the presence of macrophages in excised tissues at the end-point. Furthermore, immunofluorescence studies show that NIRF-labeled PFC-NEs show selectivity for macrophages over neutrophils (Figure 6.1c). NIRF-labeled PFC-NEs have therefore been shown to provide in vivo and ex vivo NIRF and 19F MRI signatures. These imaging studies demonstrate the feasibility of tracking and quantification of macrophage infiltration and trafficking patterns in neuroregeneration.

Using a chronic constriction injury (CCI) model of nerve injury in rats, we established that macrophage-targeted nano-emulsions (PFC-NEs) can serve as effective imaging agents to monitor changes in macrophage infiltration in live animals and as real-time surrogate biomarkers for changes in neuroinflammation following nanomedicine-based treatment.[80–84] Observed changes in pain behavior in response

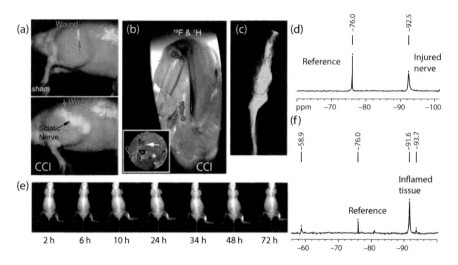

FIGURE 6.1 NIRF-labeled PFC-NE macrophage detection in live animals and at end-point in rodent models of nerve injury and inflammation. (a) NIRF imaging of macrophage infiltration patterns in sham and chronic constriction injury (CCI) of sciatic nerve in rats. (b) End-point 19F MRI of PFC-NE-labeled macrophage accumulation at CCI. (c) End-point NIRF imaging of excised CCI nerve. (d) 19F NMR spectrum of excised CCI nerve populated with PFC-NE-labeled macrophages. (e) Live sequential NIRF imaging in complete Freund's adjuvant (CFA)-treated mice. Increasing NIRF signal correlates with PFC-NE-labeled macrophage accumulation at the site of CFA injection. (f) 19F NMR spectrum of excised CFA-treated paw tissue infiltrated with PFC-NE-labeled macrophages. (Data reproduced from Patel, S. K., Beaino, W., Anderson, C. J. & Janjic, J. M. Theranostic nanoemulsions for macrophage COX-2 inhibition in a murine inflammation model. *Clin Immunol* 160, 59–70, doi:10.1016/j.clim.2015.04.019 [2015]; Vasudeva, K. et al. Imaging neuroinflammation in vivo in a neuropathic pain rat model with near-infrared fluorescence and 19F magnetic resonance. PLOS ONE 9, e90589, doi:10.1371/journal.pone.0090589 [2014].)

to macrophage-targeted nanomedicines were achieved at extremely low drug doses of the COX-2 inhibitor celecoxib (0.24 mg/kg, 100-fold lower than a typical systemic dose in animals) (Figure 6.2). This change coincided with an intriguing trend of decreased macrophage-specific nanoimaging signal in nanomedicine treated animals vs. control, as measured by 19F MRI and NIRF imaging. Briefly, the experiment was performed as follows: on day 8, rats were injected intravenously with either drug-free nanomedicine, drug-loaded nanomedicine (celecoxib-loaded macrophage-targeted nanoemulsion, CXB-NE), or free drug (CXB) control. Pain hypersensitivity developed in both CCI animal groups but not in the sham group (n = 3 per condition). After CXB-NE injection, pain hypersensitivity was restored to baseline levels in ~2 days, whereas the CCI animals with free drug continued to exhibit pain hypersensitivity, as did animals injected with drug-free NE. Histological data suggest that the number of CD68+ cells (macrophages) decreased in excised tissues, which corresponded to a decrease in macrophage infiltration observed in complete Freund's adjuvant (CFA)-injected mice. Therefore, there is a strong indication that the number of macrophages infiltrating an injured nerve is reduced by NE-based delivery of CXB to these cells.

These compelling results provide key evidence that neuroimmunomodulation in nerve injury can lead to new therapeutic and diagnostic strategies. Furthermore, we

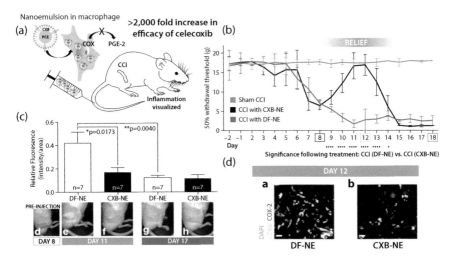

FIGURE 6.2 (a) Macrophage-targeted COX-2 inhibition with CXB-NE in CCI rat model. (b) Macrophage-targeted CXB-NE provides extended (5d) pain relief compared to drug-free nanoemulsion (DF-NE) controls, when injected intravenously in CCI rats. Pain sensitivity was measured by von Frey hindpaw stimulation. (c) NIRF imaging decrease in macrophage infiltration in CXB-NE-treated animals that sustains up to day 17, when both groups lack signal. This cofirms that pain relief is corresponding to CXB-NE-induced macrophage supression. (d) COX-2-expressing macrophages targeted by CXB-NE are reduced in CCI injury as compared to DF-NE controls. (Data adapted from Janjic, J. M. et al. Low-dose NSAIDs reduce pain via macrophage targeted nanoemulsion delivery to neuroinflammation of the sciatic nerve in rat. *J Neuroimmunol* 318, 72–79, doi:10.1016/j.jneuroim.2018.02.010 [2018]; Saleem, M., Deal, B., Nehl, E., Janjic, J. M. & Pollock, J. A. Nanomedicine-driven neuropathic pain relief in a rat model is associated with macrophage polarity and mast cell activation. *Acta Neuropathol Commun* 7, 108, doi:10.1186/s40478-019-0762-y [2019]; Saleem, M. et al. A new best practice for validating tail vein injections in rat with nearinfrared-labeled agents. *J Vis Exp* 146, e59295, doi:10.3791/59295 [2019]; Stevens, A. M., Liu, L., Bertovich, D., Janjic, J. M. & Pollock, J. A. Differential expression of neuroinflammatory mRNAs in the rat sciatic nerve following chronic constriction injury and pain-relieving nanoemulsion NSAID delivery to infiltrating macrophages. *Int J Mol Sci* 20, doi:10.3390/ijms20215269 [2019]; Stevens, A. M., Saleem, M., Deal, B., Janjic, J. & Pollock, J. A. Targeted cyclooxygenase-2 inhibiting nanomedicine results in pain-relief and differential expression of the RNA transcriptome in the dorsal root ganglia of injured male rats. *Mol Pain* 16, doi:10.1177/1744806920943309 [2020].)

also found that targeted immunomodulation using CXB-NE led to a phenotype shift from pro-inflammatory (M1) to pro-regeneration (M2) macrophage phenotype[81] and an increase in the expression of neuroregeneration-associated genes.[83,84] Figure 6.2 summarizes key findings from these studies. Further studies are underway to establish these neuroregeneration supportive effects in large animal models.

Biomimetic NPs are emerging as an appealing choice due to their integration of the functions of biological materials with the flexibility of synthetic materials typically utilized in NP construction. In a recent study, melatonin-stimulated MSC-derived exosomes (MT-Exo) inhibited the inflammatory phase of diabetic wound healing by regulating M1 and M2 macrophage polarization and accelerated the transition from the inflammatory to tissue regeneration phase.[104] This suggests that MT-Exo is a promising approach for the healing of diabetic wounds. MT pretreatment could endow MSC-derived exosomes with better biological effects, increasing the ratio of M2 polarization to M1 polarization, thereby inhibiting inflammation and promoting tissue repair.[104] Rather than targeting macrophages through pathway inhibition, biomimetic drug delivery systems can also be derived directly from macrophage membranes. Another recent study utilized the macrophage membrane to coat reactive oxygen species (ROS)-responsive NPs as an experimental treatment for atherosclerosis.[105] Because these NPs are derived from macrophage membranes, the NPs were able to avoid clearance while leading the NPs to the inflammatory tissues and sequestering proinflammatory cytokines to suppress local inflammation.[105]

TARGETING TO NEURONS IN NEUROREGENERATION

CARBON NANOTUBES, NANOHORNS, AND NANOPARTICLES

Carbon nanotubes (CNTs) are potentially useful in neuroregeneration support due to their physical and mechanical properties. CNTs have a large specific surface area and high aspect ratio to penetrate cell membranes for direct translocation into cells. Their specific mechanical properties also offer the potential to support and promote the regeneration of neural tissue in conjunction with existing nerve repair conduits.[106] These characteristics make CNTs an attractive choice as a drug delivery vehicle. CNTs can act independently or by incorporation to other types of complex structures (e.g., polymer networks). As a soluble standalone formulation, CNTs added directly to neuronal cell culture medium have the potential to control neural cell functions. Alternatively, through surface modification, CNTs can be attached to substrates such as scaffolds.[107] As a scaffold, CNTs act as a reservoir of adsorbed proteins and play a role in boosting neuronal electrical performance. In a recent study, direct electrical coupling was hypothesized due to the observation of discontinuous and tight contacts between multi-walled carbon nanotubes (MWCNT) and single-wall carbon nanotubes (SWCNT) bundles and neuronal membranes.[107] While mechanical strength and lack of electrical conductivity limit the applications of materials such as hydrogels, CNT-hydrogel hybrid systems can overcome these challenges and increase biocompatibility.[107,108] In another study, a series of Chitin/carbon nanotubes (Ch/CNT) composite hydrogels exhibited nanofibrillar network structure, excellent mechanical properties, and biodegradability in vitro. They allowed for the potential to enhance the proliferation of neurons and SCs in vitro, and promotion of cell adhesion, proliferation, and neurite outgrowth (with no cytotoxic or neurotoxic effects).[109]

While CNTs are similar in atomic arrangement and physiochemical features to single-walled carbon-nanohorns (SNH), they differ in their structural characteristics and morphology. Differences in their geometry contribute to different uptake by cellular targets. Using macrophages as the cell model, SNH demonstrated greater nanosafety for future clinical applications in biomedicine as well as greater biocompatibility with macrophages as the target.[110]

Carbon NPs are attractive bioimaging agents in neuroregeneration due to their ability to follow drug distribution and monitor its effects through luminescent or fluorescent signals.[111] In a recent study, soluble fullerol NPs were utilized to treat neuroinflammation in a mouse model of low back pain by suppressing the inflammatory responses of dorsal root ganglia (DRG) neurons in addition to cellular apoptosis by decreasing the level of ROS as well as potentially enhancing anti-oxidative enzyme gene expression.[112] These therapeutic features are attractive for neuroregeneration as they offer better control of neuroinflammation combined with diagnostic monitoring of treatment efficacy.

QUANTUM DOTS

Quantum dots (QDs) are fluorescent semiconductor nanocrystals which emit fluorescent wavelengths correlated with their size. QDs usually range from 1 to 100 nm in diameter and are chemically stable under physiological conditions. QDs have long-term photostability,[113] and to increase their physiologic function, they are often bioconjugated with a ligand.[114,115] They usually consist of a metalloid crystalline core which is generally made of cadmium selenide, cadmium sulfide, cadmium telluride, indium arsenide, or indium phosphide, and is surrounded by a shell which is usually made of zinc sulfide to enhance aqueous solubility.[116] They are fully biocompatible and are widely used in biological and biomedical applications. They are used extensively in image quantification of disease diagnosis and progression, monitoring of dopaminergic neurotoxicity, and in vivo tracking of transplanted cell activities and movement inside the body.[117–119]

METAL NPs

Metal NPs possess unique and improved physicochemical properties and quantum size effect due to their substantial reactive surface area and explicit electronic structures. They also possess unique electrical and optical properties that make them distinctive and more relevant than large-size materials. The shape and size of the metal NPs influence their electrical, optical, magnetic, and catalytic properties. The extensive applications of metal NPs in the field of biomedicine to deliver the drugs are attributable to their theranostic approaches. Due to their very small size, they can cross the blood-brain barrier and enhance imaging of the brain. For drug delivery into the central nervous system, they can be conjugated with various ligands like antibodies or proteins. As NPs have a large surface area, their surfaces are accessible to further alteration with hydrophilic, hydrophobic, anionic, cationic, or any neutral moieties to the surrounding environment so that their applications can be further refined and optimized.

When compared to other metal NPs, GNPs exhibit exceptional advantages due to their distinctive properties, very small size, inert nature, biocompatibility, high dispersity, non-cytotoxicity, stability, larger surface area and tunable physical, chemical, optical, and electronic properties. They have been widely used as drug carriers, imaging probes, photo-thermal converters, radiosensitizers, and in targeted drug delivery systems. Biocompatible polymers are being utilized for the surface modification of GNPs in order to enhance the stability and payloads of the NPs and promote prolonged systemic circulation followed by cellular uptake. The plasmonic properties of the gold core, specifically surface plasmon resonance (SPR), make it an ideal candidate for imaging applications. The striking of the particle with light creates an oscillating electromagnetic wave, which subsequently induces the resonation of surface conduction electrons. The generated resonance leads to the formation of an ionic core as an oscillatory dipole along the axis of light radiation.[120,121] The shape, composition, structure, and environment of GNPs influence the SPR.[122] The light which is absorbed by the GNPs by using SPR is either emitted, scattered, released as heat, or used to quench the nearby fluorescence.[123] GNPs can efficiently convert the absorbed energy to heat, which has been used for photothermal drug delivery. All these optical properties of GNPs owing to the localized SPR, together with their excellent photostability, make them a powerful contrast agent in in vivo imaging through computed tomography (CT) and X-ray imaging.[124–126] When compared to traditional CT contrast agents like iodine, GNPs absorb and reduce X-rays more effectively, thereby increasing the precision and enhancing the contrast in the visualization of nanoparticle location.[127,128] The tunable absorption and scattering properties of GNPs make them useful as imaging probes in various optical imaging techniques like MRI, photoacoustic tomography (PAT), positron emission tomography (PET) and single photon emission computed tomography (SPECT).[129–132] All these imaging techniques are useful for diagnostic purposes and enable them for noninvasive assessment of anatomical, molecular, and functional information with image-guided drug delivery.[133,134] GNPs serve as efficient drug carriers and are capable of carrying a large amount of drugs owing to their tremendous surface area. The targeted drug delivery of GNPs improves the cellular uptake of the drug at the intended site, reducing the distribution of the drug to off-target tissues and organs, thereby increasing the drug's therapeutic window.

SNPs naturally possess antibacterial characteristics and have the ability to cross the blood-brain barrier. When they are injected through the intraperitoneal route, they can reach the hippocampus and can induce an immune response in the brain.[135] In some cases, they induce inflammatory and neurodegenerative gene expression responses.[136] However, this immune response improves the ability of microglia to reduce their toxicity toward dopaminergic neurons and also express the enzymes that produce an overall anti-inflammatory effect.[137] One of the main disadvantages of SNPs is that they cause neurotoxicity due to their accumulation in the brain over a period of time and its nonspecific delivery to the brain.[138] To reduce their cytotoxicity and make them effective, they must be conjugated with ligands and targeted specifically to individual neural cell types. Nonetheless, SNPs should not be dismissed, as their enhanced ability to cross the blood-brain barrier could lead to exciting options for drug delivery or immunotherapy.

NANOSYSTEMS AS MECHANISTIC TOOLS IN VIVO

The many rodent PNI models create a variety of opportunities to study nerve injuries and outcomes of neuroregeneration by assessing behavioral hypersensitivity, retrograde labeling of neurons with corresponding assessment of their levels of protein expression immunohistochemically in both the pain and pain-relieved state, as well as the correlation of changes in RNA expression.[83] However, the pain and chronic pain phenomena does not rely on just the neurons, rather on three main cell types that influence the development of neuroinflammation caused from PNI, including the neurons, glia, and infiltrating immune cells and their expression of inflammatory mediators such as COX-2 and cytokines with the activation of the inflammasome. To date, there remain large gaps in our knowledge of the interplay and signaling between these three cell types and the changes in gene expression that lead to pain hypersensitivity and neuroregeneration. Even less is known about the transcriptome response to targeted drug therapy that relieves pain. To address this, we have used a qPCR 84-gene array to assess mRNA expression associated with the neuroinflammatory response.[83] When a macrophage-targeted immunomodulating nanoparticle (CXB-NE) is present, we observed mRNA changes consistent with the reduced recruitment of macrophages, evident by a reduction in chemokine and cytokine expression. Furthermore, genes associated with the adhesion of macrophages, as well as changes in the neuronal and glial mRNAs were observed. Moreover, genes associated with neuropathic pain, including Maob, NMDA-Receptor2b, TrpV3, IL-6, Calcium channel Cacna1b/Cav2.2, Integrin Itgam/Cd11b, Sodium channel Scn9a/Nav1.7, and Tac1, which produces substance P and neurokinin A, were all found to respond to the CXB-NE during pain relief as compared to those animals that received drug-free vehicle. These results demonstrate that by targeting macrophage production of inflammatory mediators at the site of injury, pain relief includes a partial reversal of the gene expression profiles associated with chronic pain. To expand this approach further, we have carried out sequencing of total RNA from DRG of naïve, drug-free nanomedicine-treated and drug-loaded nanomedicine-treated CCI rats, identifying about 15,000 genes, of which over 100 exhibit differential expression between the drug-treated and drug-free conditions. In combination, these approaches allow us to characterize the gene expression profile of nerve regeneration and injury recovery. With the use of targeted nanosystems, we are able to determine with high specificity the changes brought on by the targeted introduction of drug therapy on the gene expression profile while neuroimmunomodulation is achieved in support of neuroregeneration.

CONCLUSIONS AND FUTURE DIRECTIONS

Nanomedicine is very much an emerging field in neuroregeneration. In the above examples, we hope to have demonstrated the potential of nanotechnology in cell targeted imaging and drug delivery strategies. We also discussed briefly select examples of successful immunomodulation with NPs in nerve injury models. These findings open new avenues for both therapeutic and mechanistic strategies with strong potential for precise and personalized neuroimmunomodulation in neuroregeneration in patients who suffer PNI, from car accidents to major surgeries and trauma.

REFERENCES

1. Tubbs RS et al. *Nerves and Nerve Injuries*. 673 (Elsevier Ltd, 2015).
2. Taylor, C. A., Braza, D., Rice, J. B. & Dillingham, T. The incidence of peripheral nerve injury in extremity trauma. *Am J Phys Med Rehabil* **87**, 381–385, doi:10.1097/PHM.0b013e31815e6370 (2008).

3. Robinson, L. R. Traumatic injury to peripheral nerves. *Suppl Clin Neurophysiol* **57**, 173–186 (2004).

4. Scholz, T. et al. Peripheral nerve injuries: an international survey of current treatments and future perspectives. *J Reconstr Microsurg* **25**, 339–344, doi:10.1055/s-0029-1215529 (2009).

5. Mohammadi, R., Azad-Tirgan, M. & Amini, K. Dexamethasone topically accelerates peripheral nerve repair and target organ reinnervation: a transected sciatic nerve model in rat. *Injury* **44**, 565–569 (2013).

6. Maciel, F. O., Viterbo, F., Chinaque, L. d. F. C. & Souza, B. M. Effect of electrical stimulation of the cranial tibial muscle after end-to-side neurorrhaphy of the peroneal nerve in rats. *Acta Cirurgica Brasileira* **28**, 39–47 (2013).

7. Cavalcante Miranda de Assis, D. et al. The parameters of transcutaneous electrical nerve stimulation are critical to its regenerative effects when applied just after a sciatic crush lesion in mice. *BioMed Res Int* **2014**, 572949 (2014).

8. Das, S., Kumar, S., Jain, S., Avelev, V.D. and Mathur, R. Exposure to ELF-magnetic field promotes restoration of sensori-motor functions in adult rats with hemisection of thoracic spinal cord. *Electromagn Biol Med* **31**, 180–194 (2012).

9. Beck-Broichsitter, B. E. et al. Does pulsed magnetic field therapy influence nerve regeneration in the median nerve model of the rat? *BioMed Res Int* **2014**, 401760 (2014).

10. Bersnev, V., Khamzaev, R. & Boroda, I. Results of using an epineural suture of the sciatic nerve. *Vestnik khirurgii imeni II Grekova* **168**, 61–63 (2009).

11. Chan, K. M., Gordon, T., Zochodne, D. W. & Power, H. A. Improving peripheral nerve regeneration: from molecular mechanisms to potential therapeutic targets. *Exp Neurol* **261**, 826–835, doi:10.1016/j.expneurol.2014.09.006 (2014).

12. Gomez-Sanchez, J. A. et al. Schwann cell autophagy, myelinophagy, initiates myelin clearance from injured nerves. *J Cell Biol* **210**, 153–168, doi:10.1083/jcb.201503019 (2015).

13. Jessen, K. R. & Mirsky, R. The repair Schwann cell and its function in regenerating nerves. *J Physiol* **594**, 3521–3531, doi:10.1113/JP270874 (2016).

14. Jessen, K. R., Mirsky, R. & Lloyd, A. C. Schwann cells: development and role in nerve repair. *Cold Spring Harb Perspect Biol* **7**, a020487, doi:10.1101/cshperspect.a020487 (2015).

15. Lutz, A. B. Purification of Schwann cells from the neonatal and injured adult mouse peripheral nerve. *Cold Spring Harb Protoc* **2014**, 1312–1319, doi:10.1101/pdb.prot074989 (2014).

16. Stoll, G., Griffin, J. W., Li, C. Y. & Trapp, B. D. Wallerian degeneration in the peripheral nervous system: participation of both Schwann cells and macrophages in myelin degradation. *J Neurocytol* **18**, 671–683 (1989).

17. Hirata, K. & Kawabuchi, M. Myelin phagocytosis by macrophages and nonmacrophages during Wallerian degeneration. *Microsc Res Tech* **57**, 541–547, doi:10.1002/jemt.10108 (2002).

18. Perry, V. H. & Brown, M. C. Role of macrophages in peripheral nerve degeneration and repair. *Bioessays* **14**, 401–406, doi:10.1002/bies.950140610 (1992).

19. Bruck, W. The role of macrophages in Wallerian degeneration. *Brain Pathol* **7**, 741–752 (1997).

20. Mueller, M. et al. Macrophage response to peripheral nerve injury: the quantitative contribution of resident and hematogenous macrophages. *Lab Invest* **83**, 175–185, doi:10.1097/01.lab.0000056993.28149.bf (2003).

21. Rotshenker, S. Vol. 8 1–14 (BioMed Central, 2011).

22. Cui, Q., Yin, Y. & Benowitz, L. I. The role of macrophages in optic nerve regeneration. *Neuroscience* **158**, 1039–1048, doi:10.1016/j.neuroscience.2008.07.036 (2009).

23. Sica, A. & Mantovani, A. Macrophage plasticity and polarization: in vivo veritas. *J Clin Invest* **122**, 787–795 (2012).
24. Pollard, J. W. Trophic macrophages in development and disease. *Nat Rev Immunol* **9**, 259–270, doi:10.1038/nri2528 (2009).
25. Chen, P., Piao, X. & Bonaldo, P. Role of macrophages in Wallerian degeneration and axonal regeneration after peripheral nerve injury. *Acta Neuropathol* **130**, 605–618, doi:10.1007/s00401-015-1482-4 (2015).
26. Rotshenker, S. Wallerian degeneration: the innate-immune response to traumatic nerve injury. *J Neuroinflammation* **8**, 109, doi:10.1186/1742-2094-8-109 (2011).
27. Gaudet, A. D., Popovich, P. G. & Ramer, M. S. Wallerian degeneration: gaining perspective on inflammatory events after peripheral nerve injury. *J Neuroinflammation* **8**, 110, doi:10.1186/1742-2094-8-110 (2011).
28. Landis, R. C., Quimby, K. R. & Greenidge, A. R. M1/M2 macrophages in diabetic nephropathy: Nrf2/HO-1 as therapeutic targets. *Curr Pharm Des* **24**, 2241–2249, doi:10.2174/1381612824666180716163845 (2018).
29. Jiménez-Osorio, A. S., González-Reyes, S. & Pedraza-Chaverri, J. Vol. 448 182–192 (Elsevier B.V., 2015).
30. Naito, Y., Takagi, T. & Higashimura, Y. Vol. 564 83–88 (Academic Press Inc., 2014).
31. Stratton, *J. A.* et al. The immunomodulatory properties of adult skin-derived precursor Schwann cells: implications for peripheral nerve injury therapy. *Eur J Neurosci* **43**, 365–375, doi:10.1111/ejn.13006 (2016).
32. Jha, A. K. et al. Network integration of parallel metabolic and transcriptional data reveals metabolic modules that regulate macrophage polarization. *Immunity* **42**, 419–430, doi:10.1016/j.immuni.2015.02.005 (2015).
33. Fernandez-Valle, C., Bunge, R. P. & Bunge, M. B. Schwann cells degrade myelin and proliferate in the absence of macrophages: evidence from in vitro studies of Wallerian degeneration. *J Neurocytol* **24**, 667–679 (1995).
34. Gaudet, A. D., Popovich, P. G. & Ramer, M. S. Wallerian degeneration: gaining perspective on inflammatory events after peripheral nerve injury. *J Neuroinflammation* **8**, 110, doi:10.1186/1742-2094-8-110 (2011).
35. Taskinen, H. S. & Roytta, M. The dynamics of macrophage recruitment after nerve transection. *Acta Neuropathol* **93**, 252–259 (1997).
36. Ydens, E. et al. Acute injury in the peripheral nervous system triggers an alternative macrophage response. *J Neuroinflammation* **9**, 176, doi:10.1186/1742-2094-9-176 (2012).
37. Brosius Lutz, A. et al. Schwann cells use TAM receptor-mediated phagocytosis in addition to autophagy to clear myelin in a mouse model of nerve injury. *Proc Natl Acad Sci U S A* **114**, E8072–E8080, doi:10.1073/pnas.1710566114 (2017).
38. Hirata, K., Mitoma, H., Ueno, N., He, J. W. & Kawabuchi, M. Differential response of macrophage subpopulations to myelin degradation in the injured rat sciatic nerve. *J Neurocytol* **28**, 685–695 (1999).
39. Shen, Z. L. et al. Cellular activity of resident macrophages during Wallerian degeneration. *Microsurgery* **20**, 255–261 (2000).
40. Cashman, C. R. & Hoke, A. Deficiency of adaptive immunity does not interfere with Wallerian degeneration. *PLOS ONE* **12**, e0177070, doi:10.1371/journal.pone.0177070 (2017).
41. Castelnovo, L. F. et al. Schwann cell development, maturation and regeneration: a focus on classic and emerging intracellular signaling pathways. *Neural Regen Res* **12**, 1013–1023, doi:10.4103/1673-5374.211172 (2017).
42. Gordon, T. The role of neurotrophic factors in nerve regeneration. *Neurosurg Focus* **26**, E3 (2009).
43. Lutz, A. B. & Barres, B. A. Contrasting the glial response to axon injury in the central and peripheral nervous systems. *Dev Cell* **28**, 7–17 (2014).

44. Martinez, A. M. B., de Oliveira Goulart, C., dos Santos Ramalho, B., Oliveira, J. T. & Almeida, F. M. Neurotrauma and mesenchymal stem cells treatment: from experimental studies to clinical trials. *World J Stem Cells* **6**, 179 (2014).
45. Widgerow, A. D. et al. "Strategic sequences" in adipose-derived stem cell nerve regeneration. *Microsurgery* **34**, 324–330 (2014).
46. Zack-Williams, S. D., Butler, P. E. & Kalaskar, D. M. Current progress in use of adipose derived stem cells in peripheral nerve regeneration. *World J Stem Cells* **7**, 51 (2015).
47. Stagg, J. & Galipeau, J. Mechanisms of immune modulation by mesenchymal stromal cells and clinical translation. *Curr Mol Med* **13**, 856–867 (2013).
48. Hsueh, Y.-Y. et al. Functional recoveries of sciatic nerve regeneration by combining chitosan-coated conduit and neurosphere cells induced from adipose-derived stem cells. *Biomaterials* **35**, 2234–2244 (2014).
49. Daly, W., Yao, L., Zeugolis, D., Windebank, A. & Pandit, A. A biomaterials approach to peripheral nerve regeneration: bridging the peripheral nerve gap and enhancing functional recovery. *J R Soc Interface* **9**, 202–221 (2012).
50. Li, Y., Guo, L., Ahn, H. S., Kim, M. H. & Kim, S. W. Amniotic mesenchymal stem cells display neurovascular tropism and aid in the recovery of injured peripheral nerves. *J Cell Mol Med* **18**, 1028–1034 (2014).
51. Pereira, T. et al. Promoting nerve regeneration in a neurotmesis rat model using poly (DL-lactide–caprolactone) membranes and mesenchymal stem cells from the Wharton's jelly: in vitro and in vivo analysis. *BioMed Res Int* **2014**, 302659 (2014).
52. Rubtsov, Y. P. et al. Regulation of immunity via multipotent mesenchymal stromal cells. *Acta Naturae (англоязычная версия)* **4**, 23–31 (2012).
53. Lee, J. P., McKercher, S., Muller, F. J. & Snyder, E. Y. Neural stem cell transplantation in mouse brain. *Curr Protoc Neurosci* **42**, doi:10.1002/0471142301.ns0310s42 (2008).
54. Okita, K., Ichisaka, T. & Yamanaka, S. Generation of germline-competent induced pluripotent stem cells. *Nature* **448**, 313–317 (2007).
55. Takahashi, K., Okita, K., Nakagawa, M. & Yamanaka, S. Induction of pluripotent stem cells from fibroblast cultures. *Nat Protoc* **2**, 3081 (2007).
56. Wang, A. et al. Induced pluripotent stem cells for neural tissue engineering. *Biomaterials* **32**, 5023–5032 (2011).
57. Uemura, T. et al. Transplantation of induced pluripotent stem cell-derived neurospheres for peripheral nerve repair. *Biochem Biophys Res Commun* **419**, 130–135 (2012).
58. Uemura, T. et al. Long-term efficacy and safety outcomes of transplantation of induced pluripotent stem cell-derived neurospheres with bioabsorbable nerve conduits for peripheral nerve regeneration in mice. *Cells Tissues Organs* **200**, 78–91 (2014).
59. Ikeda, M. et al. Acceleration of peripheral nerve regeneration using nerve conduits in combination with induced pluripotent stem cell technology and a basic fibroblast growth factor drug delivery system. *J Biomed Mater Res A* **102**, 1370–1378 (2014).
60. Sullivan, R., Dailey, T., Duncan, K., Abel, N. & Borlongan, C. V. Peripheral nerve injury: stem cell therapy and peripheral nerve transfer. *Int J Mol Sci* **17**, 2101 (2016).
61. Kubo, T., Randolph, M. A., Gröger, A. & Winograd, J. M. Embryonic stem cell–derived motor neurons form neuromuscular junctions in vitro and enhance motor functional recovery in vivo. *Plast Reconstr Surg* **123**, 139S–148S (2009).
62. Schaakxs, D., Kalbermatten, D. F., Raffoul, W., Wiberg, M. & Kingham, P. J. Regenerative cell injection in denervated muscle reduces atrophy and enhances recovery following nerve repair. *Muscle Nerve* **47**, 691–701 (2013).
63. Janjic, J. M. & Gorantla, V. S. Peripheral nerve nanoimaging: monitoring treatment and regeneration. *AAPS J* **19**, 1304–1316, doi:10.1208/s12248-017-0129-x (2017).
64. Balasubramanian, B. et al. Synthesis of monodisperse TiO2– paraffin core– shell nanoparticles for improved dielectric properties. *ACS Nano* **4**, 1893–1900 (2010).

65. Karim, E., Rosli, R. & Chowdhury, E. H. Systemic delivery of nanoformulations of anti-cancer drugs with therapeutic potency in animal models of cancer. *Curr Cancer Ther Rev* **12**, 204–220 (2016).

66. Saha, A., Mohanta, S. C., Deka, K., Deb, P. & Devi, P. S. Surface-engineered multifunctional Eu: Gd2O3 nanoplates for targeted and pH-responsive drug delivery and imaging applications. *ACS Appl Mater Interfaces* **9**, 4126–4141 (2017).

67. Aftab, S. et al. Nanomedicine: an effective tool in cancer therapy. *Int J Pharm* **540**, 132–149 (2018).

68. Gomes, A. C., Mohsen, M. & Bachmann, M. F. Harnessing nanoparticles for immunomodulation and vaccines. *Vaccines* **5**, 6 (2017).

69. Xing, R., Liu, G., Zhu, J., Hou, Y. & Chen, X. Functional magnetic nanoparticles for non-viral gene delivery and MR imaging. *Pharm Res* **31**, 1377–1389 (2014).

70. Sun, B. et al. Nerve growth factor-conjugated mesoporous silica nanoparticles promote neuron-like PC12 cell proliferation and neurite growth. *J Nanosci Nanotechnol* **16**, 2390–2393 (2016).

71. Dante, S. et al. Selective targeting of neurons with inorganic nanoparticles: revealing the crucial role of nanoparticle surface charge. *ACS Nano* **11**, 6630–6640 (2017).

72. Guerzoni, L. P., Nicolas, V. & Angelova, A. In vitro modulation of TrkB receptor signaling upon sequential delivery of curcumin-DHA loaded carriers towards promoting neuronal survival. *Pharm Res* **34**, 492–505 (2017).

73. Singh, N. et al. Chitin and carbon nanotube composites as biocompatible scaffolds for neuron growth. *Nanoscale* **8**, 8288–8299 (2016).

74. Lin, *R.* et al. Improving sensitivity and specificity of capturing and detecting targeted cancer cells with anti-biofouling polymer coated magnetic iron oxide nanoparticles. *Colloids Surface B: Biointerfaces* **150**, 261–270 (2017).

75. Wei, M., Li, S., Yang, Z., Zheng, W. & Le, W. Gold nanoparticles enhance the differentiation of embryonic stem cells into dopaminergic neurons via mTOR/p70S6K pathway. *Nanomedicine* **12**, 1305–1317 (2017).

76. Felten, D. L. et al. Sympathetic innervation of lymph nodes in mice. *Brain Res Bull* **13**, 693–699 (1984).

77. Garash, R., Bajpai, A., Marcinkiewicz, B. M. & Spiller, K. L. Drug delivery strategies to control macrophages for tissue repair and regeneration. *Exp Biol Med (Maywood)* **241**, 1054–1063, doi:10.1177/1535370216649444 (2016).

78. Liu, Z., Jiang, W., Nam, J., Moon, J. J. & Kim, B. Y. S. Immunomodulating nanomedicine for cancer therapy. *Nano Lett* **18**, 6655–6659, doi:10.1021/acs.nanolett.8b02340 (2018).

79. Hu, G. et al. Nanoparticles targeting macrophages as potential clinical therapeutic agents against cancer and inflammation. *Front Immunol* **10**, 1998, doi:10.3389/fimmu.2019.01998 (2019).

80. Janjic, J. M. et al. Low-dose NSAIDs reduce pain via macrophage targeted nanoemulsion delivery to neuroinflammation of the sciatic nerve in rat. *J Neuroimmunol* **318**, 72–79, doi:10.1016/j.jneuroim.2018.02.010 (2018).

81. Saleem, M., Deal, B., Nehl, E., Janjic, J. M. & Pollock, J. A. Nanomedicine-driven neuropathic pain relief in a rat model is associated with macrophage polarity and mast cell activation. *Acta Neuropathol Commun* **7**, 108, doi:10.1186/s40478-019-0762-y (2019).

82. Saleem, *M.* et al. A new best practice for validating tail vein injections in rat with near-infrared-labeled agents. *J Vis Exp* **146**, e59295, doi:10.3791/59295 (2019).

83. Stevens, A. M., Liu, L., Bertovich, D., Janjic, J. M. & Pollock, J. A. Differential expression of neuroinflammatory mRNAs in the rat sciatic nerve following chronic constriction injury and pain-relieving nanoemulsion NSAID delivery to infiltrating macrophages. *Int J Mol Sci* **20**, doi:10.3390/ijms20215269 (2019).

84. Stevens, A. M., Saleem, M., Deal, B., Janjic, J. & Pollock, J. A. Targeted cyclooxygenase-2 inhibiting nanomedicine results in pain-relief and differential expression of the RNA transcriptome in the dorsal root ganglia of injured male rats. *Mol Pain* **16**, doi:10.1177/1744806920943309 (2020).

85. Gustafsson, B., Youens, S. & Louie, A. Y. Development of contrast agents targeted to macrophage scavenger receptors for MRI of vascular inflammation. *Bioconjug Chem* **17**, 538–547, doi:10.1021/bc060018k (2006).

86. Hitchens, T. K. et al. 19F MRI detection of acute allograft rejection with in vivo perfluorocarbon labeling of immune cells. *Magn Reson Med* **65**, 1144–1153, doi:10.1002/mrm.22702 (2011).

87. Rausch, M., Hiestand, P., Baumann, D., Cannet, C. & Rudin, M. MRI-based monitoring of inflammation and tissue damage in acute and chronic relapsing EAE. *Magn Reson Med* **50**, 309–314, doi:10.1002/mrm.10541 (2003).

88. Riou, A. et al. MRI assessment of the intra-carotid route for macrophage delivery after transient cerebral ischemia. *NMR Biomed* **26**, 115–123, doi:10.1002/nbm.2826 (2013).

89. Weise, G., Basse-Luesebrink, T. C., Wessig, C., Jakob, P. M. & Stoll, G. In vivo imaging of inflammation in the peripheral nervous system by (19)F MRI. *Exp Neurol* **229**, 494–501, doi:10.1016/j.expneurol.2011.03.020 (2011).

90. Stoll, G., Basse-Lusebrink, T., Weise, G. & Jakob, P. Visualization of inflammation using (19) F-magnetic resonance imaging and perfluorocarbons. *Wiley Interdiscip Rev Nanomed Nanobiotechnol* **4**, 438–447, doi:10.1002/wnan.1168 (2012).

91. Balducci, A. et al. A novel probe for the non-invasive detection of tumor-associated inflammation. *Oncoimmunology* **2**, e23034, doi:10.4161/onci.23034 (2013).

92. Kadayakkara, D. K. et al. Inflammation driven by overexpression of the hypoglycosylated abnormal mucin 1 (MUC1) links inflammatory bowel disease and pancreatitis. *Pancreas* **39**, 510–515, doi:10.1097/MPA.0b013e3181bd6501 (2010).

93. Bonner, F. et al. Monocyte imaging after myocardial infarction with 19F MRI at 3 T: a pilot study in explanted porcine hearts. *Eur Heart J Cardiovasc Imaging* **16**, 612–620, doi:10.1093/ehjci/jev008 (2015).

94. Hertlein, T. et al. Visualization of abscess formation in a murine thigh infection model of *Staphylococcus aureus* by 19F-magnetic resonance imaging (MRI). *PLOS ONE* **6**, e18246, doi:10.1371/journal.pone.0018246 (2011).

95. Kadayakkara, D. K., Ranganathan, S., Young, W. B. & Ahrens, E. T. Assaying macrophage activity in a murine model of inflammatory bowel disease using fluorine-19 MRI. *Lab Invest* **92**, 636–645, doi:10.1038/labinvest.2012.7 (2012).

96. Patel, S. K., Beaino, W., Anderson, C. J. & Janjic, J. M. Theranostic nanoemulsions for macrophage COX-2 inhibition in a murine inflammation model. *Clin Immunol* **160**, 59–70, doi:10.1016/j.clim.2015.04.019 (2015).

97. Vasudeva, K. et al. Imaging neuroinflammation in vivo in a neuropathic pain rat model with near-infrared fluorescence and (1)(9)F magnetic resonance. *PLOS ONE* **9**, e90589, doi:10.1371/journal.pone.0090589 (2014).

98. Patel, S. K., Zhang, Y., Pollock, J. A. & Janjic, J. M. Cyclooxgenase-2 inhibiting perfluoropoly (ethylene glycol) ether theranostic nanoemulsions-in vitro study. *PLOS ONE* **8**, e55802, doi:10.1371/journal.pone.0055802 (2013).

99. Pan, H., Soman, N. R., Schlesinger, P. H., Lanza, G. M. & Wickline, S. A. Cytolytic peptide nanoparticles ('NanoBees') for cancer therapy. *Wiley Interdiscip Rev Nanomed Nanobiotechnol* **3**, 318–327, doi:10.1002/wnan.126 (2011).

100. Lee, S. J., Schlesinger, P. H., Wickline, S. A., Lanza, G. M. & Baker, N. A. Interaction of melittin peptides with perfluorocarbon nanoemulsion particles. *J Phys Chem B* **115**, 15271–15279, doi:10.1021/jp209543c (2011).

101. Akers, W. J. et al. Targeting of alpha(nu)beta(3)-integrins expressed on tumor tissue and neovasculature using fluorescent small molecules and nanoparticles. *Nanomedicine* **5**, 715–726, doi:10.2217/nnm.10.38 (2010).

102. Caruthers, S. D., Cyrus, T., Winter, P. M., Wickline, S. A. & Lanza, G. M. Anti-angiogenic perfluorocarbon nanoparticles for diagnosis and treatment of atherosclerosis. *Wiley Interdiscip Rev Nanomed Nanobiotechnol* **1**, 311–323, doi:10.1002/wnan.9 (2009).

103. Soman, N. R., Lanza, G. M., Heuser, J. M., Schlesinger, P. H. & Wickline, S. A. Synthesis and characterization of stable fluorocarbon nanostructures as drug delivery vehicles for cytolytic peptides. *Nano Lett* **8**, 1131–1136, doi:10.1021/nl073290r (2008).

104. Liu, W. et al. Melatonin-stimulated MSC-derived exosomes improve diabetic wound healing through regulating macrophage M1 and M2 polarization by targeting the PTEN/AKT pathway. *Stem Cell Res Ther* **11**, 259, doi:10.1186/s13287-020-01756-x (2020).

105. Gao, C. et al. Treatment of atherosclerosis by macrophage-biomimetic nanoparticles via targeted pharmacotherapy and sequestration of proinflammatory cytokines. *Nat Commun* **11**, 2622, doi:10.1038/s41467-020-16439-7 (2020).

106. Oprych, K. M., Whitby, R. L., Mikhalovsky, S. V., Tomlins, P. & Adu, J. Repairing peripheral nerves: is there a role for carbon nanotubes? *Adv Healthc Mater* **5**, 1253–1271, doi:10.1002/adhm.201500864 (2016).

107. Redondo-Gómez, C. et al. Recent advances in carbon nanotubes for nervous tissue regeneration. *Adv Polym Technol* **2020**, 1–16, doi:10.1155/2020/6861205 (2020).

108. Vashist, A. et al. Advances in carbon nanotubes-hydrogel hybrids in nanomedicine for therapeutics. *Adv Healthc Mater* **7**, e1701213, doi:10.1002/adhm.201701213 (2018).

109. Wu, S. et al. Biocompatible chitin/carbon nanotubes composite hydrogels as neuronal growth substrates. *Carbohydr Polym* **174**, 830–840, doi:10.1016/j.carbpol.2017.06.101 (2017).

110. He, B. et al. Single-walled carbon-nanohorns improve biocompatibility over nanotubes by triggering less protein-initiated pyroptosis and apoptosis in macrophages. *Nat Commun* **9**, 2393, doi:10.1038/s41467-018-04700-z (2018).

111. Maiti, D., Tong, X., Mou, X. & Yang, K. Carbon-based nanomaterials for biomedical applications: a recent study. *Front Pharmacol* **9**, 1401, doi:10.3389/fphar.2018.01401 (2018).

112. Liu, Q. et al. Novel treatment of neuroinflammation against low back pain by soluble fullerol nanoparticles. *Spine (Phila Pa 1976)* **38**, 1443–1451, doi:10.1097/BRS.0b013e31828fc6b7 (2013).

113. Dubertret, B. et al. In vivo imaging of quantum dots encapsulated in phospholipid micelles. *Science* **298**, 1759–1762 (2002).

114. Yang, W. et al. Facile synthesis of Gd–Cu–In–S/ZnS bimodal quantum dots with optimized properties for tumor targeted fluorescence/MR in vivo imaging. *ACS Appl Mater Interfaces* **7**, 18759–18768 (2015).

115. Zhang, B. et al. Nanomaterials in neural-stem-cell-mediated regenerative medicine: imaging and treatment of neurological diseases. *Adv Mater* **30**, 1705694 (2018).

116. Cupaioli, F. A., Zucca, F. A., Boraschi, D. & Zecca, L. Engineered nanoparticles. how brain friendly is this new guest? *Prog Neurobiol* **119**, 20–38 (2014).

117. Tokuraku, K., Marquardt, M. & Ikezu, T. Real-time imaging and quantification of amyloid-β peptide aggregates by novel quantum-dot nanoprobes. *PLOS ONE* **4**, e8492 (2009).

118. Agarwal, R. et al. Delivery and tracking of quantum dot peptide bioconjugates in an intact developing avian brain. *ACS Chem Neurosci* **6**, 494–504 (2015).

119. Ma, W., Liu, H.-T. & Long, Y.-T. Monitoring dopamine quinone-induced dopaminergic neurotoxicity using dopamine functionalized quantum dots. *ACS Appl Mater Interfaces* **7**, 14352–14358 (2015).

120. González-Díaz, J. B. et al. Plasmonic Au/Co/Au nanosandwiches with enhanced magneto-optical activity. *Small* **4**, 202–205 (2008).

121. Male, D., Gromnicova, R. & Mcquaid, C. Gold Nanoparticles for Imaging and Drug Transport to the CNS. *Int Rev Neurobiol* **130**, 155–198 (Elsevier, 2016).

122. Huang, X., Jain, P. K., El-Sayed, I. H. & El-Sayed, M. A. Gold nanoparticles: interesting optical properties and recent applications in cancer diagnostics and therapy. *Nanomedicine* **5**, 681–693 (2007).

123. Swierczewska, M., Lee, S. & Chen, X. The design and application of fluorophore–gold nanoparticle activatable probes. *Phys Chem Chem Phys* **13**, 9929–9941 (2011).

124. El-Sayed, I. H., Huang, X. & El-Sayed, M. A. Selective laser photo-thermal therapy of epithelial carcinoma using anti-EGFR antibody conjugated gold nanoparticles. *Cancer Lett* **239**, 129–135 (2006).

125. Au, L. et al. A quantitative study on the photothermal effect of immuno gold nanocages targeted to breast cancer cells. *ACS Nano* **2**, 1645–1652 (2008).

126. Stewart, M. E. et al. Nanostructured plasmonic sensors. *Chem Rev* **108**, 494–521 (2008).

127. Curry, T., Kopelman, R., Shilo, M. & Popovtzer, R. Multifunctional theranostic gold nanoparticles for targeted CT imaging and photothermal therapy. *Contrast Media Mol Imaging* **9**, 53–61 (2014).

128. Shilo, M., Motiei, M., Hana, P. & Popovtzer, R. Transport of nanoparticles through the blood–brain barrier for imaging and therapeutic applications. *Nanoscale* **6**, 2146–2152 (2014).

129. Hainfeld, J., Slatkin, D., Focella, T. & Smilowitz, H. Gold nanoparticles: a new X-ray contrast agent. *Br J Radiol* **79**, 248–253 (2006).

130. Murph, S. E. H. et al. Manganese–gold nanoparticles as an MRI positive contrast agent in mesenchymal stem cell labeling. *J Nanopart Res* **14**, 658 (2012).

131. Jang, B. et al. Gold nanorods for target selective SPECT/CT imaging and photothermal therapy in vivo. *Quant Imaging Med Surg* **2**, 1 (2012).

132. Wang, L. V. & Hu, S. Photoacoustic tomography: in vivo imaging from organelles to organs. *Science* **335**, 1458–1462 (2012).

133. Willmann, J. K., Van Bruggen, N., Dinkelborg, L. M. & Gambhir, S. S. Molecular imaging in drug development. *Nat Rev Drug Discov* **7**, 591–607 (2008).

134. Janib, S. M., Moses, A. S. & MacKay, J. A. Imaging and drug delivery using theranostic nanoparticles. *Adv Drug Deliv Rev* **62**, 1052–1063 (2010).

135. Aliev, G. et al. Nanoparticles as alternative strategies for drug delivery to the Alzheimer brain: electron microscopy ultrastructural analysis. *CNS & Neurological Disorders-Drug Targets* **14**, 1235–1242 (2015).

136. Huang, C.-L. et al. Silver nanoparticles affect on gene expression of inflammatory and neurodegenerative responses in mouse brain neural cells. *Environ Res* **136**, 253–263 (2015).

137. Gonzalez-Carter, D. A. et al. Silver nanoparticles reduce brain inflammation and related neurotoxicity through induction of H 2 S-synthesizing enzymes. *Sci Rep* **7**, 42871 (2017).

138. Tang, J. et al. Distribution, translocation and accumulation of silver nanoparticles in rats. *J Nanosci Nanotechnol* **9**, 4924–4932 (2009).

7 Biomarkers and Surrogates of Acute Rejection in Vascularized Composite Allograft Transplantation

Calum Honeyman, Helen Stark,
Hayson Chenyu Wang, Joanna Hester,
Henk Giele, and Fadi Issa

CONTENTS

Introduction 122
Defining Serum and Tissue Biomarkers and Surrogates of Rejection
in VCA 122
Clinical and Histopathological Assessment 123
Cell Phenotypes Within Peripheral Blood 124
Cell Phenotypes Within Tissue 125
Gene Expression Profiling 126
    Rejection-Related Genes 126
    Adhesion Molecules 128
Donor-Derived Cell-Free DNA 128
Microrna Profiling 129
Proteomics 129
Imaging 130
Sentinel Skin Flaps to Monitor VCA 131
Future Directions and Challenges 136
    The Microbiome 136
    Future Techniques of Immune Phenotyping 137
    Challenges 137
Conclusions 138
Acknowledgements 138
References 138

DOI: 10.1201/9780429260179-10

INTRODUCTION

The past two decades has seen vascularized composite allograft (VCA) transplantation become an established treatment option for select civilian and military patients with devastating tissue loss (Honeyman and Fries 2019). Over 200 VCAs have now been performed, including face, hand, abdominal wall, uterus, penis, lower limb, and neck organ transplants (Tasigiorgos et al. 2019; Shores, Brandacher, and Lee 2015; Giele et al. 2016; Brännström et al. 2015; Grajek et al. 2017; Diefenbeck et al. 2011; Cetrulo et al. 2017). Despite encouraging clinical outcomes, the toxic side-effects of life-long immunosuppression (malignancy, infection, and renal failure) and inability to safely control acute and chronic rejection are slowing progress in the field of VCA (Siemionow 2017; Shores et al. 2017; Krezdorn et al. 2019).

Even in compliant patients, rates of acute rejection (AR) in the first year after VCA are high (88% for upper extremity and 73% for face transplantation). This is significant when compared to rates of 10–30% reported for deceased donor solid organ transplant (SOT) recipients (Dhaliwal and Thohan 2006; Niederhaus et al. 2013; Lund et al. 2015; Petruzzo et al. 2017). The increased susceptibility of VCAs to AR was thought to be related to the increased antigenicity of the skin relative to other transplanted tissue components (Lee et al. 1991). However, this theory is incompletely understood and the reliability of skin as a primary monitor of deeper tissues in VCA transplants has recently been questioned (Robbins et al. 2019). Evidence suggests that repeated episodes of AR contribute to chronic rejection (CR) and associated graft vasculopathy (GV) (Unadkat et al. 2010; Ng et al. 2019). Problematically, current immunosuppression protocols and rescue therapies fail to prevent or reverse the development of GV after it has been confirmed histologically. In this situation, graft loss is inevitable (Ng et al. 2019).

Currently, no serum or tissue biomarkers or surrogates exist in the fields of VCA or SOT that can predict rejection before it is established and damage has taken place. As such, there is a significant need for research directed towards the discovery, validation, and clinical study of minimally invasive and quantifiable immune signatures that are predictive of impending rejection. These markers must be reliable, reproducible, and easily translatable to a clinical laboratory.

The aim of this chapter is to summarize progress in the development of non-invasive skin or serum biomarkers for the recognition or prediction of AR in the field of VCA transplantation. The early detection and treatment of AR will ensure the risk of CR is reduced.

DEFINING SERUM AND TISSUE BIOMARKERS AND SURROGATES OF REJECTION IN VCA

This chapter concerns biomarkers and surrogates of immune responses specific to VCA. Surrogates are a subset of biomarkers that, according to the Biomarkers Definitions Working Group, have a "characteristic that is objectively measured and evaluated as an indicator of normal biological processes, pathogenic processes, or pharmacologic responses to a therapeutic intervention". A surrogate endpoint is defined as "a biomarker that is intended to substitute for a clinical endpoint.

A surrogate endpoint is expected to predict clinical benefit (or harm or lack of benefit or harm) based on epidemiological, therapeutic, pathophysiological, or other scientific evidence" (Biomarkers Definitions Working Group 2001). Examples of surrogate endpoints used in SOT include serum markers (liver function tests and creatinine for monitoring liver and renal transplants, respectively) and tissue markers (histopathology changes from diagnostic or protocol biopsy specimens).

CLINICAL AND HISTOPATHOLOGICAL ASSESSMENT

Current monitoring of VCAs for AR is focussed on a combination of clinical and histopathological assessment. The ability of clinicians and patients to monitor the visible skin component of most VCAs for signs of rejection (demonstrable as a rash, erythema, or oedema) is unique in the field of transplantation. As the majority of VCA recipients will experience at least one episode of AR in the first post-transplant year, continuous monitoring of the VCA skin allows early detection and successful reversal of AR in almost all cases (Petruzzo et al. 2017).

The gold standard for diagnosing rejection is a tissue biopsy, performed as part of routine surveillance or in response to clinical signs of rejection visualized on the allograft skin. Histopathology is reported in accordance with the Banff 2007 working classification of skin-containing composite tissue allograft pathology (Cendales et al. 2008). Clinicopathological and cellular features of AR present in a similar way between VCA types, including hand, face, and abdominal wall transplantation (Kanitakis et al. 2003; Cendales et al. 2006; Levi et al. 2003).

In 2007, the Ninth Banff Conference on Allograft Pathology was held to unify the four pre-existing VCA pathological scoring systems, leading to standardized international pathology reporting and research outcomes (Zdichavsky et al. 1999; Bejarano et al. 2004; Kanitakis et al. 2005; Cendales et al. 2006). This initial Banff classification was based on pathology from 28 hand transplants, nine abdominal wall transplants, and one vascularized knee joint transplant with a sentinel skin flap (SSF) (Schneider et al. 2016). In 2013, the classification was updated to include C4d-negative antibody-mediated rejection, recognizing the clinical cases of antibody-mediated rejection (AMR) reported (Haas et al. 2014; Weissenbacher et al. 2014). The Banff scoring system grades the histopathological features of AR on a scale from 0 (no features) to 4 (frank necrosis of the epidermis).

A number of relevant limitations of the current system exist. Firstly, no histopathological feature on a VCA skin biopsy is 100% specific for a given diagnosis (Sarhane et al. 2013). Visible skin changes vary in accordance with the severity of rejection on biopsy, but these changes are not specific to VCA, and common skin conditions including dermatitis and rosacea can mimic rejection in VCA recipients (Kanitakis 2008; Pomahac et al. 2011). Currently, there is limited correlation between grade of VCA biopsy and recommended treatment or outcomes. In a study of six face transplant recipients, approximately 80% of grade 3 rejection episodes resolved with topical immunosuppression or adjustment of oral maintenance immunosuppression alone, with no requirement for additional rescue boluses as might be expected from experience in SOT (Kollar et al. 2018). This has also been reported in the management of AR for hand transplant recipients (Chen et al. 2020). Atypical clinical presentations of AR can occur, making the diagnosis more challenging and include hand transplant rejection confined to the palmar skin and nail beds (Schneeberger et al. 2008).

Secondly, a significant degree of subjectivity and intra- or inter-observer error is inherent when reporting skin-containing VCA pathology specimen (Sarhane et al. 2013). This is a common issue faced in all areas of transplantation, particularly when comparing borderline and AR samples (Furness and Taub 2006; Veríssimo Veronese et al. 2005).

Finally, and perhaps the most significant limitation currently faced, is that by the time clinical signs of rejection are apparent and biopsied, irreversible damage has already occurred (Whitehouse and Sanchez-Fueyo 2014). Current methods to detect rejection employ static tools to try and capture a dynamic and evolving process that is poorly understood. Without the ability to accurately detect signs of impending rejection, clinicians are unable to prevent the repeated cycle of damage that ultimately leads to GV and allograft loss (Sarhane et al. 2014).

There remains a clear unmet need for an objective, non-invasive, quantifiable method of detecting and reporting VCA rejection at an early immunological stage. In the next sections, we will examine the different modalities which are being developed with this purpose in mind.

CELL PHENOTYPES WITHIN PERIPHERAL BLOOD

Analysis of peripheral blood lymphocyte subsets by multi-parameter flow cytometry is a valuable way of monitoring changes in the immune cell compartments following VCA and a potential source of future biomarkers. It has been shown that an increased number of circulating memory T cells is associated with a higher risk for rejection in kidney and heart transplantation (Heidt et al. 2011). Recipient T cells play a major role in skin allograft rejection. Borges and colleagues characterized the immune responses of six full face transplant recipients, showing that effector memory T cells (T_{EM}) were the commonest subset after transplantation and that these cells were mostly of a Th2 phenotype. Within $CD4^+$ T cells, T_{EM}s ($CD45RA^-CCR7^-$) were the most common subset, whilst $CD8^+$ T cells contained both T_{EM}s and effector memory RA T cells (T_{EMRA}). However, they found that the number of total circulating $CD4^+$ and $CD8^+$ cells were not significantly different between pre-rejection and post-rejection time points. A nonsignificant reduction in T_{EM}s ($CD45RA^-CCR7^-$) and an increase in both $CD4^+$ and $CD8^+$ T_{EMRA}s ($CD45RA^+CCR7^-$) was observed, compared with pre-rejection time points. Meanwhile, regulatory T cells (Tregs; $CD4^+Foxp3^+$) significantly accumulated in the graft during rejection, leading to decreased numbers of Tregs in circulating blood at rejection compared with pre-rejection timepoints (Borges et al. 2016).

In another study, Win et al. analyzed the peripheral blood of a presensitized face transplant recipient before and after transplantation to capture the immunological features of AMR or T cell-mediated rejection (TCMR) (Win et al. 2017). They observed an increased T effector population in the $CD8^+$ population during TCMR episodes, but with preservation of the regulatory T cell population. Both circulating T follicular helper (Tfh) cell ($CD4^+PD1^+CXCR5^+$) and memory B cell ($CD19^+CD27^+$)

populations increased one week after transplantation, concurrent with suspected episodes of AMR, but not during TCMR episodes. There is some limited evidence that immune phenotypes after transplantation differ between SOT and VCA transplantation. Kamińska et al. compared immune cell subsets in peripheral blood of five stable hand transplant recipients and 30 stable kidney transplant recipients (Kamińska et al. 2017). Unlike the four-fold depletion of B cells in stable kidney transplant recipients, the population of B cells in five stable hand transplant recipients showed little change compared with healthy people. The Treg population size ($CD4^+$ $CD25^+CD127^{low}$) in hand transplant recipients was similar to that in healthy controls, whereas kidney transplant recipients showed a reduced Treg population size. Hand transplant recipients also had an increase in both total $CD8^+$ T cell numbers, as well as $CD8^+CD28^-$ numbers. More $CD8^+CD28^-$ cells were observed in hand transplant recipients with an eightfold increase in absolute cell counts compared to healthy controls. However, whilst these studies provide useful information on baseline characteristics in VCA immune cell composition, they have not yet led a clinically useful biomarker that can predict or detect rejection in the peripheral blood.

CELL PHENOTYPES WITHIN TISSUE

A significantly higher number of T cells reside in the skin than in the peripheral circulation (Etra, Raimondi, and Brandacher 2018). There is also a greater representation of T cells with an effector memory phenotype in the skin, which bear a diverse T-cell receptor repertoire and have a characteristic Th1 phenotype. An abundance of $CD8^+$ memory T cells in the skin of VCAs, which may be recruited from the circulation, has also been detected (Iske et al. 2019). Baran et al. have characterized the morphological and histological features of skin rejection in hand transplant recipients (Baran et al. 2015). Transplanted skin, when compared to the patient's own skin, revealed higher numbers of $CD8^+$ lymphocytes and $CD68^+$ macrophages, but not $CD4^+$ T cells. $CD20^+$ B cells were found in allograft skin in all cases, but not in the patient's own skin. However, dendritic cells in allograft dermal infiltrate and epidermis both increased. An increased number of CD1a cells were also present in the dermis in allograft skin of a patient with Banff grade 1 rejection. Furthermore, donor cells in the epidermal compartment proved to be exclusively dendritic-appearing $CD8^+$ T cells in a series of 113 sequential biopsies of full facial transplants, with a mixture of donor and recipient $CD8^+$ and $CD4^+$ T cells in the pilosebaceous and perivascular compartments. Unlike central memory T cells that circulate in the peripheral blood, donor T cells in rejecting allografts were predominantly (>90%) of the Trm phenotype ($CD69^+$, $CD103^+$, CLA^+) (Lian et al. 2014).

Mild skin rejection is a common observation in VCA transplants, presenting with a T cell-dominated dermal cell infiltrate. Hautz et al. found the infiltrate was mainly comprised of $CD3^+$ T lymphocytes, and $CD8^+$ cells were more prominent than $CD4^+$ cells. The percentage of $CD3^+$ T lymphocytes and the CD4/CD8-ratio increased with time, and $CD20^+$ B lymphocytes were sparse (Hautz et al. 2012). Although recipient T cells are thought to play a major role in skin graft rejection, unexpectedly, clinical face transplant biopsies during AR episodes showed most lymphocytes to be $CD8^+$ memory T cells of donor origin, suggesting the possibility that donor T cells have a role in the pathogenesis of VCA rejection (Lian et al. 2014). Rejection episodes of full face transplant recipients were characterized by a significant accumulation of CD4+ and CD8+ T cells as well as all CD14+ cells in the allograft (Borges et al. 2016). Again, whilst the information from these studies contributes to our knowledge of the immune composition in VCA skin biopsies, more work is needed to provide a clinically relevant biomarker profile that can be used to improve patient outcomes.

GENE EXPRESSION PROFILING

Microarrays and more recently RNA-seq technologies allow evaluation of the patterns of gene expression, alternate splicing events, as well as novel transcriptome modifiers providing new information regarding diagnosis, prognosis, and potential therapy. Transcriptomic studies have significantly contributed to our understanding of the molecular mechanisms and biological complexity of VCA immunology.

REJECTION-RELATED GENES

Win et al. compared the gene expression profiles of rejection allograft biopsies with non-rejection biopsies in a highly sensitized face transplant recipient (Win et al. 2017). They observed activation of the interferon gamma (IFN-γ) signalling pathway (including IRF1 and STAT1), overexpression of genes responsible for the recruitment of cytotoxic cells through production of chemokine ligands (primarily through the CXCR3/CCR5 pathway, including CXCL9 and CCL5), and genes with immune effector function (genes expressed by CD8+ cytotoxic T cells and natural killer cells upon activation, including GZMB [granzyme B]). IFN-γ is considered a critical cytokine in sustaining inflammation during allograft rejection, synergistically functioning with tumour necrosis factor-α (TNF-α) to induce the expression of CXCR3 ligands (CXCL9, CXCL10, CXCL11) and CCR5 ligands (CCL3, CCL4, CCL5). CXCR3 and CCR5 ligands are the most frequently upregulated chemokines during acute allograft rejection. These chemokines secreted by dendritic cells, activated macrophages and T cells, endothelial cells, and NK cells, in turn, lead to increased production of IFN-γ, with a resultant amplification of the inflammatory stimuli and further release of chemoattractant molecules (Spivey et al. 2011). Expression of interleukin (IL)-1b, IL-6, IL-10, IFN-γ, TGFβ, CCL2, CCL3, CCL4, CCL5, CXCL1, and CXCL2 is significantly increased in both syngeneic and allogeneic grafts compared to normal skin in rat models, indicating their involvement in damage-related inflammation, rather than rejection per se (Win et al. 2017; Spivey et al. 2011; Friedman et al. 2017; Kollar, Pomahac, and Riella 2019).

Win et al. also analyzed 31 genes contributing most to the variability between the AMR and TCMR episode. They found AMR was associated with an overexpression of endothelial genes such as ICAM1, VCAM1, and SELE, whereas TCMR was characterized by up-regulated expression of GZMB, a cytotoxicity-associated gene

(Win et al. 2017). In a published abstract from 2019, Win et al. used NanoString technology to analyze and compare unique gene expression profiles of face transplant and SOT recipients. They showed that 82% of upregulated genes were shared between face and SOT recipients. However, face transplant rejection was associated with the upregulation of 36 unique genes, including the immunomodulatory genes SOCS1, and induction of lipid antigen-presenting CD1 proteins, that may represent future therapeutic targets to manage AR in face transplant patients going forward ("Comparison with Solid Organ Transplants Reveals Distinct Face Transplant Rejection Gene Signature That Reflects the Unique Immunobiology of Skin"; American Transplant Congress. n.d.).

Wolfram et al. analyzed a panel of 17 inflammatory cytokine genes to compare inflammatory skin disease models (contact hypersensitivity) with acute skin rejection (Wolfram et al. 2015). They found that the gene expression profiles of CCL7, IL-1b, IL-18, and TNF in the skin was highly indicative of rejection rather than inflammatory diseases. Furthermore, IL-12b, IL-17a, and IL-1b gene expression levels significantly differed between the rejection and inflammatory disease models with only moderate interaction and were independent from skin types.

Kamińska et al. assessed the expression of a set of genes related to the T cell populations in peripheral blood mononuclear cells to elucidate the difference of the immune status between stable hand transplant recipients and stable kidney transplant recipients (Kamińska et al. 2017). In the hand transplant group, rejection-related genes (CD8, IL-10, NOTCH1, PDCD1, TNF) were upregulated compared to that in healthy individuals. In the kidney transplant group, no gene expression differed from that in healthy individuals. Also, the rejection-related genes (CD8, NOTCH, TNF) were expressed at a higher level in the hand transplant group compared to those in the kidney transplant group.

Forkhead box protein 3 (FOXP3) is an essential molecular marker of Treg development and function in the thymus and peripheral lymphoid organs. A number of studies have explored the association between FOXP3, the master transcription factor for Tregs, and AR. Tregs are involved in inflammatory processes where they act to prevent the overshoot of normal immune responses. Hautz et al. found FOXP3 along with indoleamine 2,3-dioxygenase expression correlated well with the severity of rejection of human hand allografts (Hautz et al. 2009). FOXP3 expression was mainly found in samples undergoing severe rejection, and its levels increased with time (Hautz et al. 2009; Hautz et al. 2012; Eljaafari et al. 2006). Jindal et al. took skin biopsies from a rat hind-limb model at the first clinical signs of AR in hIL-2/Fc (a long-lasting human IL-2 fusion protein) recipient rats and compared the expression of FOXP3 to effector genes (GZMB, IFN-γ, and perforin [Prf1]). These respective gene expression profiles correlated with the long-term outcome of the allograft, with higher regulatory:effector ratios in the reversible rejectors that went on long-term survival (Jindal et al. 2015).

Glucocorticoid-induced tumour necrosis factor receptor (GITR) is a surface receptor molecule involved in inhibiting the suppressive activity of Tregs and extending the survival of effector T cells. GITR has been shown to be upregulated in stable hand transplant recipients compared to stable kidney transplant recipients and healthy controls (Kamińska et al. 2017). Moreover, IL-18, TNFα, CCL7, CCL17, CX3CL1, CXCL9, CXCL10, and CXCL11 are significantly upregulated in rat allogeneic grafts compared to normal skin or syngeneic grafts, indicating their involvement in the adaptive alloresponse (Friedman et al. 2017).

ADHESION MOLECULES

ICAM-1, an adhesion molecule gene, is expressed by the vascular endothelium, macrophages, and lymphocytes. The expression of ICAM-1 can be induced by cytokines such as IL-1 and TNF. ICAM-1 ligation produces proinflammatory effects recruitment by signalling through cascades involving a number of kinases (Smith 1993). E-selectin, P-selectin and L-selectin function as a lectin, recognising carbohydrate structures on the leukocyte or endothelial cell surface. Hautz et al. found that adhesion molecules LFA-1, ICAM-1, E-selectin, P-selectin, and VE-cadherin were upregulated in human hand allografts with mild rejection (grade I), and for P-selectin, expression increased with time after transplant (Hautz et al. 2012). Win et al. also found a large increase of ICAM1 in a face transplant recipient undergoing AMR (Win et al. 2017).

DONOR-DERIVED CELL-FREE DNA

The majority of DNA is intracellular and contained within the nucleus or mitochondria. A small proportion of DNA is extracellular or "cell-free" (cfDNA) and rises in response to pathological states, including malignancy, myocardial infarction, and autoimmune diseases (Salvi et al. 2016; Duvvuri and Lood 2019; Chang et al. 2003). cfDNA acts as a marker of apoptosis and cell-death and can be measured in serum or urine using shotgun sequencing or droplet digital PCR (Schütz et al. 2017). An interesting point to note, highlighted in a recent article by Dholakia et al., is the possibility that donor-derived (dd)-cfDNA may also have a role to play in stimulating the immune system, potentially adding "insult on injury" (Dholakia, De Vlaminck, and Khush 2020).

Lo et al. were the first to describe the presence of dd-cfDNA in kidney and liver transplant recipients and highlighted the potential utility of measuring the dd-cfDNA concentration as a non-invasive marker of AR (Lo et al. 1998). A recent systematic review by Knight et al. concluded that there was evidence in the literature to support dd-cfDNA as a biomarker of rejection in organ transplantation (Knight, Thorne, and Lo Faro 2019). They noted that the majority of studies (including kidney, liver, lung, and heart transplants) reported a relationship between dd-cfDNA and biopsy-proven ACR. Furthermore, following treatment for AR, dd-cfDNA levels, in most cases, returned to baseline. More recently, Yang et al. have demonstrated the utility of urinary cfDNA, in combination with five other markers, to monitor for AR in kidney transplant patients (Yang et al. 2020).

Only one study has investigated the utility of dd-cfDNA in VCA recipients. In this study, dd-cfDNA levels were prospectively measured in a single face and bilateral arm transplant recipient. In this small pilot study, they were unable to detect dd-cfDNA in the recipients' plasma during stable graft function or episodes of rejection (Haug et al. 2019).

MICRORNA PROFILING

MicroRNAs (miRNAs) are small noncoding single-stranded RNA molecules that are involved in the post-translational regulation of gene expression (Anglicheau, Muthukumar, and Suthanthiran 2010). They have been recognized to play an important role in the development of immune cells and the modulation of innate and adaptive immune responses. Mas et al. highlighted the multiple potential roles of miRNAs in organ transplant monitoring, including the early recognition of rejection, as markers of graft quality and in monitoring for tolerance and chronic rejection (Mas et al. 2013).

Oda et al. investigated the role of miRNAs in a rat hindlimb VCA model (Oda et al. 2016). They found elevated levels of miRNA146a and miRNA155 associated with AR episodes, appearing before clinical or histological rejection was apparent (Oda et al. 2016) Both of these miRNAs are known to have multiple immune system functions, and the authors suggested they could have potential as biomarkers for AR. They followed up this work in 2017 using the same rat model (Oda et al. 2017). They went on to investigate miRNA in allogeneic and syngeneic hindlimb transplants in an effort to remove the potential confounding effects of transplantation. In this model, they found three miRNAs associated with AR, miRNA-146a and miRNA-155, as in their previous work, and miRNA-182. Whilst miRNA-182 had the highest specificity and sensitivity, the cut-off level was close to normal baseline, limiting its usefulness. Therefore, of the three, they felt miRNA-155 was the best potential biomarker for AR. Although this study provides some interesting insights into miRNA in the field of VCA, the authors themselves note a number of limitations, not least the fact that this work is all in rats and the crossover to humans needs further investigation.

Further work in this area has been undertaken in a rat model of VCA transplantation ("Mechanistic Insights by RNA Profiling on Rejecting Vascularized Composite Allotransplants"; American Transplant Congress n.d.). In this study, peripheral blood samples were taken pre-transplantation, then blood and skin samples were taken at rejection time points to identify mRNAs and miRNAs that were differentially expressed. This generated a huge number of potential targets, many of them involved in immune signalling pathways. Once again, this work requires further validation in human samples.

PROTEOMICS

High output proteomic assays enable the identification of large sets of protein and peptide expression profiles that can be extracted from blood, urine, tissue, or breath samples (Christians, Klawitter, and Klawitter 2016). There has been significant interest in the use of protein signatures as non-invasive biomarkers of rejection across all fields of transplantation, with a number of novel biomarker targets identified

(Mischak et al. 2015). To date, proteomic profiling has been used exclusively for early discovery and proof-of-concept studies.

Kollar et al. used the SOMAscan proteomics platform to look for non-invasive protein biomarkers in 24 serum samples obtained from six face transplant recipients (Kollar et al. 2018). They analyzed 1310 proteins and detected a five protein signature (MMP3, ACY1, IL1R2, SERPINA4, CPB2) capable of differentiating severe rejection from no rejection and non-severe rejection episodes. After technical validation using ELISA, MMP3 appeared the most promising biomarker, increasing significantly during episodes of severe rejection episodes. MMP3 is a proteolytic enzyme, implicated in wound repair and remodelling, previously investigated as a potential biomarker target in both lung and renal transplantation (Gill and Parks 2008; Liu et al. 2016; Rodrigo et al. 2000). In a subsequent multi-centre validation study of MMP3 as a non-invasive biomarker of rejection in skin-bearing VCAs, data was examined from 19 VCA recipients (nine face transplants and 10 upper extremity transplants), 14 healthy controls and 38 patients with auto-immune skin diseases (Kollar et al. 2019). Serum MMP3 concentrations were measured using the ELISA that had previously been validated (Kollar et al. 2018). In this study, MMP3 levels increased significantly between pre- and post-transplantation, and additionally during severe rejection. However, there was no association between biopsy grades and MMP3 levels, although severe rejection was associated with at least a five-time increase in MMP3 from pre-transplant levels. Importantly, auto-immune skin conditions were associated with low levels of MMP3. Overall, using a non-invasive serum marker, identified from proteomics, AR in VCA could be predicted with 76% sensitivity and 81% specificity. Despite showing early promise, the study was limited by the relatively small numbers of patients examined. Additionally, due to the retrospective nature of the study, there were challenges related to missing data (pre-transplant serum samples for select patients), non-standardized serum sample measurements, and significant variations in AR episodes and their management. This study is the first of its kind in the field of VCA, and a significant step towards the validation of a clinically applicable biomarkers in VCA. The next stage will be to build toward a prospective, randomized study.

IMAGING

Advanced imaging technology plays an essential role in the pre-operative assessment of VCA patients, with the creation of custom 3D cutting guides to optimize surgery and as part of postoperative monitoring strategies, predominantly employed to identify early signs of GV (Caterson and McCarty 2018; Soga et al. 2010; Kumamaru et al. 2014). The opportunity to use non-invasive imaging strategies to detect impending VCA rejection, prior to clinical or histological changes, is very appealing and applicable to all fields of transplantation and VCA.

In 1988, Hovius et al. were the first to investigate the utility of a laser Doppler flowmeter in an allogeneic rat limb transplant model, but were unable to demonstrate preclinical signs of rejection. The authors thought this may be due to an inability to perform continuous measurements over time, and may have been related to the inadequate sensitivity of the imaging modality employed at that time (Hovius et al. 1988). Over 30 years later, high-resolution ultrasound biomicroscopy (UBM) had shown some early promise in the field of VCA. UBM is a powerful, non-invasive vascular imaging modality that has been extensively studied in pre-clinical and clinical settings (Myredal et al. 2010; Rowinska et al. 2012). In one study, UBM was used to monitor six upper extremity transplants, showing early intimal changes associated with GV, not reliably identified with previous imaging, including brachial indices and computed tomography (CT)/magnetic resonance (MR) angiography (Kaufman et al. 2012). The authors hypothesized that another useful advantage of UBM may be a decreased requirement for potentially morbid deep tissue biopsies. However, the use of UBM in hand transplantation has seen little progress and has not been validated after this initial publication. In a 2013 review, Kaufman et al. did go on to highlight that vessel intimal thickness increases with age, and that only large changes in vessel wall thickness should be considered significant (Kaufman et al. 2013). Perhaps this finding limited the use of this technique in clinical practice.

UBM has subsequently been used as a non-invasive strategy for facial allograft monitoring (Kueckelhaus, Imanzadeh, et al. 2015). Kueckelhaus et al. were unable to show a statistical difference in the donor facial artery-to-recipient radial artery ratio, and no intimal proliferation in the facial arteries of patients, ranging from 8 months to 4½ years after transplant. However, they have gone on to validate the sensitivity of this technique for the early detection of CR in facial allotransplantation.

Outside the field of VCA, other imaging modalities are showing promise in the detection of AR. This includes the pre-clinical and clinical use of magnetic resonance imaging (MRI) and positron emission tomography (PET)-CT for surveillance after cardiac and renal transplantation (Dolan et al. 2019; Chen et al. 2017). However, prospective, longitudinal studies and cost analysis are required to further validate the utility of both modalities going forward, compared to traditional gold standard of tissue biopsy. Both MRI and PET may have a role in VCA monitoring, particularly the assessment of deeper tissues for early signs of rejection, currently an under investigated and controversial area (Robbins et al. 2019).

At present, no imaging modalities exist that can detect changes associated with AR in pre-clinical or clinical VCA studies. However, better defining the role of multiparametric MRI or PET-CT in the detection of VCA AR in pre-clinical and clinical settings is essential, particularly how they might be employed to monitor deeper tissue components of a VCA over time. In reality, the role of advanced imaging is likely to form one part of a non-invasive VCA follow-up protocol that attempts to predict AR based on quantifiable anatomical changes. However, this is far from a clinical reality, limited by cost, small patient numbers, and limited collaboration between centres at present.

SENTINEL SKIN FLAPS TO MONITOR VCA

SSFs are donor-derived skin *flaps* (axial pattern fasciocutaneous free flaps with their own blood supply) or donor-derived skin *grafts* (full-thickness or split-thickness, secondarily vascularized after transfer), inset into a distant site of a VCA recipient. Thus far, SSFs have most commonly been used for the purpose of immune monitoring in face transplantation and as a convenient biopsy site that minimises morbidity from repeated facial allograft biopsies. Kueckelhaus et al. used donor SSFs to reconstruct unmet soft tissue defects from additional injuries in face transplant recipients (e.g., radial forearm flap to reconstruct a web space contracture) and also found SSFs to be useful in differentiating episodes of rejection, infection and dermatological conditions affecting facial allograft skin (Kueckelhaus, Fischer, et al. 2015). To date, SSFs or grafts have been used in approximately 5% (11/205) of VCAs performed worldwide. This includes eight primarily vascularized flaps to monitor facial allografts, an allogenic knee transplant, and three secondarily vascularized full-thickness skin grafts to monitor hand transplants, summarized in Table 7.1.

The first published report of an SSF as a remote monitor for a VCA was in Germany in 2002 (Diefenbeck et al. 2007). Diefenbeck et al. employed a primarily vascularized SSF to monitor the last of six allogeneic knee transplants they performed (M. Diefenbeck et al. 2006). Twenty-eight months after the transplant, the patient experienced an episode of acute skin rejection (pain, redness, and itching), confirmed as AR by SSF biopsy. Following treatment with high-dose methylprednisolone, arthroscopic biopsy confirmed concordant rejection in the knee allograft. At 36 months, a section of the SSF became necrotic, with pathological changes indicating chronic rejection of the SSF. These changes were also observed in the articular cartilage and bone of the knee allograft. Ultimately a deep infection developed that could not be salvaged, leading to an above-knee amputation, but the premise of SSF as a reliable monitor in the field of VCA was established.

In 2004, Lanzetta et al. described their outcomes from a series of three Italian hand transplant recipients that received donor-derived full thickness skin grafts, inset into the left hip for monitoring purposes (Lanzetta et al. 2004). Despite initially concordant rejection between the SSF and hand transplants, over time the monitoring capacity of the SSF was lost in a process referred to as "creeping substitution", where recipient skin replaced donor skin and therefore the SSF lost its monitoring value (Lanzetta and Rovati 2007).

When considering the utility of SSFs, it is important to consider whether the transplanted skin is primarily vascularized (e.g., radial forearm flap) or secondarily vascularized (e.g., full-thickness or split-thickness skin grafts). When compared to conventional skin grafts, primarily vascularized flaps show significant differences in immune cell trafficking and in mechanisms of antigen presentation (Horner et al. 2010). Furthermore ischaemia-reperfusion injury is greater in skin grafts, potentially provoking an immune response, unlike in the primarily vascularized skin flap (Issa 2016). Hence, studies relating the use of skin grafts must be interpreted differently from those that use vascularized skin flaps, the latter being more analogous to the limb or face VCA. It should be noted that the terms SSF and sentinel skin graft are used interchangeably in published literature and do not always reflect the method of vascularization employed. Where primarily vascularized SSFs have been used, there appears to be a high level of concordance between VCA allograft and SSF. In a dataset of 46 events of simultaneous SSF and facial allografts, Kueckelhaus et al. showed concordant rejection for Banff grades 0,1,2,3 rejection of 83.3%, 53.85%, 66.67%, and 100% respectively (Kueckelhaus, Fischer, et al. 2015).

TABLE 7.1

International Summary of SSFs Used to Monitor VCAs

Relevant publications	From	Country	No. of Patients	VCA Type	SSF Type	SSF Inset Location	Maximum Recorded Follow-up	Time from VCA to Rejection Episode	SSF Findings	VCA Findings	AR Treatment	Maintenance Immuno-Suppression
Devauchelle et al. 2006	2005	France	1	Partial face	RFFF	Sub-mammary	10 years	*Patient 1*				
								Day 20	G1	G2 (om)	Increased steroid	Tac, MMF, steroid
Dubernard et al. 2007											Steroid boluses / Steroid & Tac (top)	steroid
Kanitakis et al. 2006								Day 214	G2	G3	Steroid boluses / Steroid & Tac (top)	Tac, MMF, steroid
Morelon et al. 2017								Month 94	G3	G3, G3 (om)	Increased steroid / Steroid boluses	Steroid, MMF, sirolimus
Petruzzo et al. 2015								Month 102	Signs of necrosis (C4d neg) AMR	G3 (C4d pos)	Steroid boluses / IVIG	Steroid, MMF, Tac
								Month 107	Removed N/A	Removed	Plasmapheresis, Eculizumab	
	2009	France	1	Partial face	RFFF	Abdomen	4 years	*Patient 2*				
								Day 41	G3	G2-3 (om)	Steroid boluses	Tac, MMF, steroid
								Day 103	G3	G1 (om)	Increased PO steroid	Tac, MMF, steroid
								Day 186	G3	G2, G3 (om)	Steroid boluses / Increased PO steroid	Tac, steroids
								Day 239	G1	G1	Increased PO steroid	Tac, steroids
								Day 474	NR	G2	Steroid boluses	Steroids
								Day 527	NR	G3	Campath-1	Steroids
								Day 540	NR	G3	Campath-1	Tac, steroids
								Day 931	NR	NR	IV steroids	Tac, steroids, everolimus

(Continued)

TABLE 7.1 (Continued)
International Summary of SSFs Used to Monitor VCAs

Relevant publications	From	Country	No. of Patients	VCA Type	SSF Type	SSF Inset Location	Maximum Recorded Follow-up	Time from VCA to Rejection Episode	SSF Findings	VCA Findings	AR Treatment	Maintenance Immuno-Suppression
Kueckelhaus, Fischer, et al. 2015	2009	USA	4	Face	RFFF	First web space, dorsum of hand, axilla, and inguinal region	5 years	*Patient 1*				
								3 months	Low grade	G1-2	Steroid boluses	Tac, MMF
								4 months	G0	G1-2	Rosacea	Tac, MMF
								34 months	G3	G3	Increased Tac	Tac, MMF
								54 months	G3	G3	Increased maintenance and PO steroids for 4 weeks	Tac, MMF
								Patient 2				
								23 months	G3	G3	Steroid boluses, steroid taper, increased maintenance	Tac, MMF
								Patient 3				
								3 weeks	G2	G2	Steroid boluses	Tac, MMF
								17 months	G3	G3	Steroid boluses, steroid taper, increased maintenance	Tac, MMF
								Patient 4				
								1 month	SSF lost due to vascular insufficiency	Facial allograft unaffected	N/A	Tac, MMF
Michael Diefenbeck et al. 2007; 2011	2000	Germany	1	Knee allograft	NR	Lateral thigh	4.7 years	28 months	Bx confirmed AR*	Concordant knee VCA AR*	Steroid boluses	Tac, MMF, steroid
								36 months	SSF CR	Concordant knee VCA CR and necrosis on arthroscopic bx	NR	Tac, MMF, steroid
								56 months	Deep infection and loss of SSF	Deep infection and loss of VCA	N/A	Tac only due to surgical site infection

Reference	Year	Country	n	VCA	Flap	Sentinel site	Follow-up	Timepoint	Grade 1	G2	Treatment	Immunosuppression
Amer et al. 2018 "American Society for Reconstructive Transplantation Conference Abstracts 2018"	2016	USA	1	Face	PTAF	Inguinal area	1 year	Day 57	NR	NR	Steroid boluses	Tac, MMF, steroid
Volokh et al. 2019	2015	Russia	1	Partial face	RFFF	Forearm	1 year	NR	NR	NR	NR	MMF, cyclosporine, steroid
Lanzetta et al. 2004 "Rationale for Additional Monitoring of the Hand" n.d.	2000	Italy	3	Bilateral hand transplant	FTSG	Hip	NR	*Patient 1* Day 76	Mild AR*	Normal	No change	Tac, MMF, steroid
								Day 83	Mild AR*	Mild AR*	Increased Tac, steroid boluses, Tac & steroid (top)	Tac, MMF, steroid
								Patient 2 Day 60	Mild AR*	Normal*	Increased Tac, steroid boluses, Tac & steroid (top)	Tac, MMF, steroid
								Patient 3	None	None	None	Tac, MMF, steroid

Abbreviations: AR = acute rejection; FTSG = full-thickness skin graft; IVIG = intravenous immunoglobulin; Tac = tacrolimus; top = topical; MMF = mycophenolate mofetil; OM = oral mucosa; PTAF = posterior tibial artery flap; PO = per oral; RFFF = radial forearm flap; SSFs = sentinel skin flaps; NR = not recorded; VCA = vascularized composite allograft. NB: *Grade not specified

The longest documented follow-up for a combined SSF and VCA recipient came after the first successful partial face transplant performed in France in 2005. Devauchelle et al. inset a donor radial forearm flap into the recipient's submammary area for monitoring and biopsy purposes (Devauchelle et al. 2006). The patient experienced two episodes of AR in the first post-transplant year, concordant between the SSF and facial allograft skin (Dubernard et al. 2007). Four years after the face transplant, protocol biopsies highlighted subclinical grade 2 rejection in the SSF only, but the decision was made not to treat this based on the normal clinical appearance of facial allograft and submammary skin flap (Petruzzo et al. 2012). Despite no further rejection episodes, the patient developed donor specific antibodies (DSAs) seven years after her transplant. At 94 months post-transplant, the skin, SSF, and mucosal biopsies all showed concordance for grade 3 rejection. Nine months later, the patient developed GV in the facial allograft and SSF, leading to necrosis. The SSF and facial allograft showed similar macroscopic and pathological changes, thought to be due to AMR-associated GV (Morelon et al. 2017).

Currently, SSFs serve as a useful adjunct to traditional monitoring and biopsy protocols, predominantly in facial transplantation. A number of pertinent research questions related to SSF in VCA monitoring remain: (1) What is the long-term monitoring concordance of SSFs in facial allograft monitoring? (2) What is the effect and role of SSFs in the setting of AMR and CR? (3) What are the specific immune cell pathways linking SSF and VCA rejection, and can they be utilized as part of a non-invasive monitoring protocol to detected impending ACR? (4) Could there be a potential protective effect of combining SSF and VCA?

The role of SSF for immune monitoring in SOT is under active investigation by researchers at the University of Oxford, including a clinical trial of SSF in pancreas transplantation. Published data from Oxford has highlighted the immune monitoring benefits of the abdominal wall transplants during small bowel transplantation (Barnes et al. 2016; Weissenbacher et al. 2018).

FUTURE DIRECTIONS AND CHALLENGES

THE MICROBIOME

There has been an increasing interest in the immunogenic role of the microbiome, secondary to improvements in the techniques for analysis (metagenomic methods such as 16S rRNA). There is a growing body of evidence that the symbiotic relationship between our microbiome and immune system extends to modulatory effects which when dysregulated can lead to disease (Tabibian and Kenderian 2017).

Oh et al. demonstrated significant differences in ileal microbiota after small bowel transplantation between rejection and no rejection episodes (Oh et al. 2012). They noted decreases in Firmicutes and Lactobacillales and increases in Proteobacteria phylae. It was unclear whether this was as a result of rejection or a causative factor, but demonstrates that monitoring the composition of microbiome has the potential to indicate a rejection episode. Further evidence, from a rat model of liver transplantation, of the potential of gut microbiome to indicate rejection was reported by Ren et al. 2014 (Ren et al. 2014).

Although the gut is perhaps what first comes to mind when thinking about the microbiome, there are significant populations in the lung and on skin. Evidence reported by Charlson et al. highlights that lung transplant recipients have significantly different populations of bacteria compared to healthy controls (Charlson et al. 2012).

A recent review by Dery et al. considers both the immunological and therapeutic possibilities of the microbiome in transplantation (Dery et al. 2020). Focussing on VCA, they hypothesize that the skin microbiome, which is "densely populated by highly diverse microbiota" may play an important role in modulating rejection. Furthermore, there is existing evidence that the gut microbiome has an important role in skin allograft survival. Whilst there is limited evidence at present that the microbiome may be used to monitor for rejection, this is certainly an area that warrants further research.

FUTURE TECHNIQUES OF IMMUNE PHENOTYPING

Peyster et al. report on the use of in situ immune profiling of heart transplant biopsies using quantitative multiplex immunofluorescence techniques (Peyster et al. 2020). They were able to define a profile both associated with AR and future rejection episodes. In addition to these multiplex immunofluorescence techniques, there are an increasing number of spatial genomic techniques being developed which in the future will likely contribute new biomarkers for detection of AR. Multiplexed gene detection platforms are continuously improving, with probe-based assays that allow for easy detection of hundreds of genes in peripheral blood or in tissues. Transplantation-specific panels are becoming increasingly available, with genes incorporated based on previous studies of transcriptomic profiling, such as work from Halloran et al. (Halloran, Famulski, and Reeve 2016).

CHALLENGES

A key challenge faced by researchers in this field is how to obtain appropriate samples that either precede or closely relate to the onset of rejection. One approach is to take protocol samples throughout the follow up period. SSFs offer the intriguing alternative not only of alerting researchers to early rejection, but also allowing relevant samples to be taken in a timely and safe fashion. At present, most biomarker research relies on using hypotheses based on what is already known about immune responses in transplantation. This inevitably leads to bias in the results gained. Whilst newer genomic techniques have the power to give more unbiased results, they produce large amounts of data. This data output requires expert bioinformatic support to analyze findings. Due to the restricted indications for VCA, there is a small pool of patients and therefore samples for research. This has limited the ability of researchers to translate interesting findings into a clinically validated and relevant test. Collaboration between centres will be key in achieving this goal.

CONCLUSIONS

Despite the challenges of biomarker research, it is an area of active research, with a clear clinical need. There have been significant advances in recent years, in part due to development of improved techniques and technology, many of which are becoming more easily accessible, less expensive, and increasingly incorporated into clinical analysis laboratories. It is likely that a combination of strategies may be used to profile rejection more accurately in these patients in the future.

ACKNOWLEDGEMENTS

Calum Honeyman would like to thank the William Rooney Plastic Surgery and Burns Research Trust and the J.P. Moulton Charitable Foundation for their generous support during his period of research in Oxford.

REFERENCES

Amer, Hatem, Sheila J Jowsey-Gregoire, Charles B Rosen, Manish Gandhi, Brooks S Edwards, Lori E Ewoldt, and Samir Mardini. 2018. "Mayo Clinic's First Face Transplant." *Transplantation* 102 (July): S433. https://doi.org/10.1097/01.tp.0000543215.07156.0a.
"American Society for Reconstructive Transplantation Conference Abstracts 2018." 2018. *SAGE Open Medicine* 6 (January): 205031211880866. https://doi.org/10.1177/2050312118808661.
American Transplant Congress. n.d. "Mechanistic Insights by RNA Profiling on Rejecting Vascularized Composite Allotransplants. Accessed April 9, 2020. https://atcmeetingabstracts.com/abstract/mechanistic-insights-by-rna-profiling-on-rejecting-vascularized-composite-allotransplants/.
American Transplant Congress. n.d. "Comparison with Solid Organ Transplants Reveals Distinct Face Transplant Rejection Gene Signature That Reflects the Unique Immunobiology of Skin." Accessed April 22, 2020. https://atcmeetingabstracts.com/ abstract/comparison-with-solid-organ-transplants-reveals-distinct-face-transplantrejection-gene-signature-that-reflects-the-unique-immunobiology-of-skin/.
Anglicheau, Dany, Thangamani Muthukumar, and Manikkam Suthanthiran. 2010. "MicroRNAs: Small RNAs with Big Effects." *Transplantation Journal* 90 (2): 105–12. https://doi.org/10.1097/TP.0b013e3181e913c2.
Baran, Wojciech, Maria Koziol, Zdzisław Woźniak, Mirosław Banasik, Maria Boratyńska, Anja Kunze, and Knut Schakel. 2015. "Increased Numbers of 6-Sulfo LacNAc (Slan) Dendritic Cells in Hand Transplant Recipients." *Annals of Transplantation* 20 (October): 649–54. https://doi.org/10.12659/aot.894828.
Barnes J, Issa F, Vrakas G, Friend P, Giele H. 2016. "The Abdominal Wall Transplant as a Sentinel Skin Graft. *Current Opinion in Organ Transplantation* 21 (5): 536–40. doi:10.1097/MOT.0000000000000352.
Bejarano, Pablo A, David Levi, Mehdi Nassiri, Vladimir Vincek, Monica Garcia, Deborah Weppler, Gennaro Selvaggi, Tamoaki Kato, and Andreas Tzakis. 2004. "The Pathology of Full-Thickness Cadaver Skin Transplant for Large Abdominal Defects: A Proposed Grading System for Skin Allograft Acute Rejection." *American Journal of Surgical Pathology* 28 (5): 670–75. https://doi.org/10.1097/00000478-200405000-00016.
Biomarkers Definitions Working Group. 2001. "Biomarkers and Surrogate Endpoints: Preferred Definitions and Conceptual Framework." *Clinical Pharmacology & Therapeutics* 69 (3): 89–95. https://doi.org/10.1067/mcp.2001.113989.

Borges, T J, J T O'Malley, L Wo, N Murakami, B Smith, J Azzi, S Tripathi, et al. 2016. "Codominant Role of Interferon-γ- and Interleukin-17-Producing T Cells During Rejection in Full Facial Transplant Recipients." *American Journal of Transplantation* 16 (7): 2158–71. https://doi.org/10.1111/ajt.13705.

Brännström, Mats, Liza Johannesson, Hans Bokström, Niclas Kvarnström, Johan Mölne, Pernilla Dahm-Kähler, Anders Enskog, et al. 2015. "Livebirth after Uterus Transplantation." *Lancet* 385 (9968): 607–16. https://doi.org/10.1016/S0140-6736(14)61728-1.

Caterson, Edward J, and Justin C McCarty. 2018. "Face Transplant: Status of Current Supporting Technology to Plan and Perform the Operation and Monitor the Graft in the Postoperative Period." *Journal of Craniofacial Surgery* 29 (4): 1. https://doi.org/10.1097/SCS.0000000000004605.

Cendales, L C, J Kanitakis, S Schneeberger, C Burns, P Ruiz, L Landin, M Remmelink, et al. 2008. "The Banff 2007 Working Classification of Skin-Containing Composite Tissue Allograft Pathology." *American Journal of Transplantation* 8 (7): 1396–1400. https://doi.org/10.1111/j.1600-6143.2008.02243.x.

Cendales, Linda C, Allan D Kirk, J Margaret Moresi, Phillip Ruiz, and David E Kleiner. 2006. "Composite Tissue Allotransplantation: Classification of Clinical Acute Skin Rejection." *Transplantation* 81 (3): 418–22. https://doi.org/10.1097/01.tp.0000185304.49987.d8.

Cetrulo, Curtis L, Kai Li, Harry M Salinas, Matthew D Treiser, Ilse Schol, Glen W Barrisford, Francis J McGovern, et al. 2018. "Penis Transplantation: First US Experience." *Annals of Surgery* 267 (5): 983–88. https://doi.org/10.1097/SLA.0000000000002241.

Chang, Christine P-Y, Rhu-Hsin Chia, Tsu-Lan Wu, Kuo-Chien Tsao, Chien-Feng Sun, and James T Wu. 2003. "Elevated Cell-Free Serum DNA Detected in Patients with Myocardial Infarction." *Clinica Chimica Acta; International Journal of Clinical Chemistry* 327 (1–2): 95–101. https://doi.org/10.1016/s0009-8981(02)00337-6.

Charlson, Emily S, Joshua M Diamond, Kyle Bittinger, Ayannah S Fitzgerald, Anjana Yadav, Andrew R Haas, Frederic D Bushman, and Ronald G Collman. 2012. "Lung-Enriched Organisms and Aberrant Bacterial and Fungal Respiratory Microbiota after Lung Transplant." *American Journal of Respiratory and Critical Care Medicine* 186 (6): 536–45. https://doi.org/10.1164/rccm.201204-0693OC.

Chen, Yi Ting, Shun Chen Huang, Chien Chang Chen, Lee Moay Lim, Po Liang Lu, Ya Ping Hou, Yin Chih Fu, Chia Hsin Chen, and Yur Ren Kuo. 2020. "Topical Tacrolimus and Steroids Modulate T Cells in Acute Rejection of Hand Allotransplantation: Two Case Reports." *Microsurgery* 40 (2): 217–23. https://doi.org/10.1002/micr.30439.

Chen, Yihan, Li Zhang, Jinfeng Liu, Pingyu Zhang, Xiaoyuan Chen, and Mingxing Xie. 2017. "Molecular Imaging of Acute Cardiac Transplant Rejection: Animal Experiments and Prospects." *Transplantation* 101 (9): 1977–86. https://doi.org/10.1097/TP.0000000000001780.

Christians, Uwe, Jelena Klawitter, and Jost Klawitter. 2016. "Biomarkers in Transplantation-Proteomics and Metabolomics." *Therapeutic Drug Monitoring* 38 (Suppl 1): S70–74. https://doi.org/10.1097/FTD.0000000000000243.

Dery, Kenneth J, Kentaro Kadono, Hirofumi Hirao, Andrzej Górski, and Jerzy W Kupiec-Weglinski. 2020. "Microbiota in Organ Transplantation: An Immunological and Therapeutic Conundrum?" *Cellular Immunology* 351:104080. doi: 10.1016/j.cellimm.2020.104080.

Devauchelle, Bernard, Lionel Badet, Benoit Lengelé, Emmanuel Morelon, Sylvie Testelin, Mauricette Michallet, Cédric D'Hauthuille, and Jean-Michel Dubernard. 2006. "First Human Face Allograft: Early Report." *Lancet* 368 (9531): 203–9. https://doi.org/10.1016/S0140-6736(06)68935-6.

Dhaliwal, Amandeep, and Vinay Thohan. 2006. "Cardiac Allograft Vasculopathy: The Achilles' Heel of Long-Term Survival after Cardiac Transplantation." *Current Atherosclerosis Reports* 8 (2): 119–30. http://www.ncbi.nlm.nih.gov/pubmed/16510046.

Dholakia, Shamik, Iwijn De Vlaminck, and Kiran K Khush. 2020. "Adding Insult on Injury." *Transplantation* 104(11): 2266–71.doi: 10.1097/TP.0000000000003240

Diefenbeck, M, F Wagner, M H Kirschner, A Nerlich, T Muckley, and G O Hofmann. 2006. "Management of Acute Rejection 2 Years after Allogeneic Vascularized Knee Joint Transplantation." *Transplant International* 19 (7): 604–6. https://doi.org/10.1111/j.1432-2277.2006.00327.x.

Diefenbeck, Michael, Andreas Nerlich, Stefan Schneeberger, Frithjof Wagner, and Gunther O Hofmann. 2011. "Allograft Vasculopathy after Allogeneic Vascularized Knee Transplantation." *Transplant International* 24 (1): e1–5. https://doi.org/10.1111/j.1432-2277.2010.01178.x.

Diefenbeck, Michael, Frithjof Wagner, Martin H Kirschner, Andreas Nerlich, Thomas Mückley, and Gunther O Hofmann. 2007. "Outcome of Allogeneic Vascularized Knee Transplants." *Transplant International* 20 (5): 410–18. https://doi.org/10.1111/j.1432-2277.2007.00453.x.

Dolan, Ryan S, Amir A Rahsepar, J Blaisdell, Kenichiro Suwa, Kambiz Ghafourian, Jane E Wilcox, Sadiya S Khan, et al. 2019. "Multiparametric Cardiac Magnetic Resonance Imaging Can Detect Acute Cardiac Allograft Rejection After Heart Transplantation." *JACC: Cardiovascular Imaging* 12 (8P2): 1632–41. https://doi.org/10.1016/j.jcmg.2019.01.026.

Dubernard, Jean-Michel, Benoit Lengelé, Emmanuel Morelon, Sylvie Testelin, Lionel Badet, Christophe Moure, Jean-Luc Beziat, et al. 2007. "Outcomes 18 Months after the First Human Partial Face Transplantation." *New England Journal of Medicine* 357 (24): 2451–60. https://doi.org/10.1056/NEJMoa072828.

Duvvuri, Bhargavi, and Christian Lood. 2019. "Cell-Free DNA as a Biomarker in Autoimmune Rheumatic Diseases." *Frontiers in Immunology* 10 (March): 502. https://doi.org/10.3389/fimmu.2019.00502.

Eljaafari, Assia, Lionel Badet, Jean Kanitakis, Christophe Ferrand, Annie Farre, Palmina Petruzzo, Emmanuel Morelon, et al. 2006. "Isolation of Regulatory T Cells in the Skin of a Human Hand-Allograft, up to Six Years Posttransplantation." *Transplantation* 82 (12): 1764–68. https://doi.org/10.1097/01.tp.0000250937.46187.ca.

Etra, Joanna W, Giorgio Raimondi, and Gerald Brandacher. 2018. "Mechanisms of Rejection in Vascular Composite Allotransplantation." *Current Opinion in Organ Transplantation* 23 (1): 28–33. https://doi.org/10.1097/MOT.0000000000000490.

Friedman, Or, Narin Carmel, Meirav Sela, Ameen Abu Jabal, Amir Inbal, Moshe Ben Hamou, Yakov Krelin, Eyal Gur, and Nir Shani. 2017. "Immunological and Inflammatory Mapping of Vascularized Composite Allograft Rejection Processes in a Rat Model." *PLOS ONE* 12 (7): e0181507. https://doi.org/10.1371/journal.pone.0181507.

Furness, Peter N, and Nick Taub. 2006. "Interobserver Reproducibility and Application of the ISN/RPS Classification of Lupus Nephritis - A UK-Wide Study." *American Journal of Surgical Pathology* 30 (8): 1030–35. https://doi.org/10.1097/00000478-200608000-00015.

Giele, Henk, Anil Vaidya, Srikanth Reddy, Giorgios Vrakas, and Peter Friend. 2016. "Current State of Abdominal Wall Transplantation." *Current Opinion in Organ Transplantation* 21 (2): 159–64. https://doi.org/10.1097/MOT.0000000000000276.

Gill, Sean E, and William C Parks. 2008. "Metalloproteinases and Their Inhibitors: Regulators of Wound Healing." *International Journal of Biochemistry and Cell Biology* 40 (6–7): 1334–47. https://doi.org/10.1016/j.biocel.2007.10.024.

Grajek, Maciej, Adam Maciejewski, Sebastian Giebel, Łukasz Krakowczyk, Rafał Ulczok, Cezary Szymczyk, Janusz Wierzgon, et al. 2017. "First Complex Allotransplantation of Neck Organs." *Annals of Surgery* 266 (2): e19–24. https://doi.org/10.1097/SLA.0000000000002262.

Haas, M, B Sis, L C Racusen, K Solez, D Glotz, R B Colvin, M C R Castro, et al. 2014. "Banff 2013 Meeting Report: Inclusion of C4d-Negative Antibody-Mediated Rejection and Antibody-Associated Arterial Lesions." *American Journal of Transplantation* 14:272–83. https://doi.org/10.1111/ajt.12590.

Halloran, Philip F, Konrad S Famulski, and Jeff Reeve. 2016. "Molecular Assessment of Disease States in Kidney Transplant Biopsy Samples." *Nature Reviews Nephrology.* 12(9):534–48.https://doi.org/10.1038/nrneph.2016.85.

Haug, Valentin, Yanan Kuang, Sotirios Tasigiorgos, Branislav Kollar, Abhishek Mogili, Pasi A Jänne, Simon Talbot, Cloud P Paweletz, and Bohdan Pomahac. 2020. "Circulating Donor-Derived Cell-Free DNA as a Biomarker in Vascularized Composite Allotransplantation?" *Transplantation* 104 (3): e79–80. https://doi.org/10.1097/TP.0000000000003000.

Hautz, T, G Brandacher, B Zelger, H G Müller, A W P Lee, D Fuchs, R Margreiter, and S Schneeberger. 2009. "Indoleamine 2,3-Dioxygenase and Foxp3 Expression in Skin Rejection of Human Hand Allografts." *Transplantation Proceedings* 41 (2): 509–12. https://doi.org/10.1016/j.transproceed.2009.01.008.

Hautz, Theresa, Bettina Zelger, Gerald Brandacher, Hansgeorg Mueller, Johanna Grahammer, Bernhard Zelger, Wp Andrew Lee, et al. 2012. "Histopathologic Characterization of Mild Rejection (Grade I) in Skin Biopsies of Human Hand Allografts." *Transplant International* 25 (1): 56–63. https://doi.org/10.1111/j.1432-2277.2011.01369.x.

Heidt, Sebastiaan, David San Segundo, Sushma Shankar, Shruti Mittal, Anand S R Muthusamy, Peter J Friend, Susan V Fuggle, and Kathryn J Wood. 2011. "Peripheral Blood Sampling for the Detection of Allograft Rejection: Biomarker Identification and Validation." *Transplantation* 92 (1): 1–9. https://doi.org/10.1097/TP.0b013e318218e978.

Honeyman, Calum, and Charles Anton Fries. 2019. "Vascularised Composite Allotransplantation – Basic Science and Clinical Applications." *International Journal of Orthoplastic Surgery* 2 (1): 13–22. https://doi.org/10.29337/ijops.28.

Horner, Benjamin M, Kelly K Ferguson, Mark A Randolph, Joel A Spencer, Alicia L Carlson, Erica L Hirsh, Charles P Lin, and Peter E M Butler. 2010. "In Vivo Observations of Cell Trafficking in Allotransplanted Vascularized Skin Flaps and Conventional Skin Grafts." *Journal of Plastic, Reconstructive & Aesthetic Surgery* 63 (4): 711–19. https://doi.org/10.1016/j.bjps.2009.01.036.

Hovius, Steven E R, L N A van Adrichem, P M A van der Heijden, V D Vuzevski, R van Strik, and J C van der Meulen. 1988. "Postoperative Monitoring of Allogeneic Limb Transplantation in Rats."*Annals of Plastic Surgery* 21 (6): 559–65. https://doi.org/10.1097/00000637-198812000-00012.

Iske, Jasper, Yeqi Nian, Ryoichi Maenosono, Max Maurer, Igor M Sauer, and Stefan G Tullius. 2019. "Composite Tissue Allotransplantation: Opportunities and Challenges."*Cellular and Molecular Immunology* 16: 343–49. https://doi.org/10.1038/s41423-019-0215-3.

Issa, Fadi. 2016. "Vascularized Composite Allograft-Specific Characteristics of Immune Responses." *Transplant International* 29 (6): 672–81. https://doi.org/10.1111/tri.12765.

Jindal, R, J Unadkat, W Zhang, D Zhang, T W Ng, Y Wang, J Jiang, et al. 2015. "Spontaneous Resolution of Acute Rejection and Tolerance Induction with IL-2 Fusion Protein in Vascularized Composite Allotransplantation." *American Journal of Transplantation* 15 (5): 1231–40. https://doi.org/10.1111/ajt.13118.

Kamińska, Dorota, Katarzyna Kościelska-Kasprzak, Magdalena Krajewska, Adam Chełmoński, Jerzy Jabłecki, Marcelina Żabińska, Marta Myszka, et al. 2017. "Immune Activation- and Regulation-Related Patterns in Stable Hand Transplant Recipients." *Transplant International* 30 (2): 144–52. https://doi.org/10.1111/tri.12883.

Kanitakis, Jean. 2008. "The Challenge of Dermatopathological Diagnosis of Composite Tissue Allograft Rejection: A Review." *Journal of Cutaneous Pathology* 35 (8): 738–44. https://doi.org/10.1111/j.1600-0560.2007.00889.x.

Kanitakis, Jean, Lionel Badet, Palmina Petruzzo, Jean Luc Béziat, Emmanuel Morelon, Nicole Lefrançois, Camille Françès, et al. 2006. "Clinicopathologic Monitoring of the Skin and Oral Mucosa of the First Human Face Allograft: Report on the First Eight Months." *Transplantation* 82 (12): 1610–15. https://doi.org/10.1097/01.tp.0000248780.55263.33.

Kanitakis, Jean, Denis Jullien, Palmina Petruzzo, Nadey Hakim, Alain Claudy, Jean-Pierre Revillard, Earl Owen, and Jean-Michel Dubernard. 2003. "Clinicopathologic Features of Graft Rejection of the First Human Hand Allograft." *Transplantation* 76 (4): 688–93. https://doi.org/10.1097/01.TP.0000079458.81970.9A.

Kanitakis, Jean, Palmina Petruzzo, Denis Jullien, Lionel Badet, Maria Clara Dezza, Alain Claudy, Marco Lanzetta, Nadey Hakim, Earl Owen, and Jean-Michel Dubernard. 2005. "Pathological Score for the Evaluation of Allograft Rejection in Human Hand (Composite Tissue) Allotransplantation." *European Journal of Dermatology* 15 (4): 235–38. http://www.ncbi.nlm.nih.gov/pubmed/16048749.

Kaufman, C L, R Ouseph, B Blair, J E Kutz, T M Tsai, L R Scheker, H Y Tien, et al. 2012. "Graft Vasculopathy in Clinical Hand Transplantation." *American Journal of Transplantation* 12 (4): 1004–16. https://doi.org/10.1111/j.1600-6143.2011.03915.x.

Kaufman, Christina L, Rosemary Ouseph, Michael R Marvin, Yorell Manon-Matos, Brenda Blair, and Joseph E Kutz. 2013. "Monitoring and Long-Term Outcomes in Vascularized Composite Allotransplantation." *Current Opinion in Organ Transplantation* 18(6): 652–8. https://doi.org/10.1097/MOT.0000000000000025.

Knight, Simon Robert, Adam Thorne, and Maria Letizia Lo Faro. 2019. "Donor-Specific Cell-Free DNA as a Biomarker in Solid Organ Transplantation. A Systematic Review." *Transplantation* 103 (2): 273–83. https://doi.org/10.1097/TP.0000000000002482.

Kollar, Branislav, Bohdan Pomahac, and Leonardo V Riella. 2019. "Novel Immunological and Clinical Insights in Vascularized Composite Allotransplantation."*Current Opinion in Organ Transplantation* 24 (1): 42–48. https://doi.org/10.1097/MOT.0000000000000592.

Kollar, Branislav, Andrey Shubin, Thiago J Borges, Sotirios Tasigiorgos, Thet Su Win, Christine G Lian, Simon T Dillon, et al. 2018. "Increased Levels of Circulating MMP3 Correlate with Severe Rejection in Face Transplantation." *Scientific Reports* 8 (1): 14915. https://doi.org/10.1038/s41598-018-33272-7.

Kollar, Branislav, Audrey Uffing, Thiago J Borges, Andrey V Shubin, Bruno T Aoyama, Céline Dagot, Valentin Haug, et al. 2019. "MMP3 Is a Non-Invasive Biomarker of Rejection in Skin-Bearing Vascularized Composite Allotransplantation: A Multicenter Validation Study." *Frontiers in Immunology* 10 (November): 2771. https://doi.org/10.3389/fimmu.2019.02771.

Krezdorn, Nicco, Christine G Lian, Michael Wells, Luccie Wo, Sotirios Tasigiorgos, Shuyun Xu, Thiago J Borges, et al. 2019. "Chronic Rejection of Human Face Allografts." *American Journal of Transplantation* 19 (4): 1168–77. https://doi.org/10.1111/ajt.15143.

Kueckelhaus, Maximilian, Sebastian Fischer, Christine G Lian, Ericka M Bueno, Francisco M Marty, Stefan G Tullius, Julian J Pribaz, George J Murphy, and Bohdan Pomahac. 2015. "Utility of Sentinel Flaps in Assessing Facial Allograft Rejection." *Plastic and Reconstructive Surgery* 135 (1): 250–58. https://doi.org/10.1097/PRS.0000000000000797.

Kueckelhaus, Maximilian, Amir Imanzadeh, Sebastian Fischer, Kanako Kumamaru, Muayyad Alhefzi, Ericka Bueno, Nicole Wake, Marie D Gerhard-Herman, Frank J Rybicki, and Bohdan Pomahac. 2015. "Noninvasive Monitoring of Immune Rejection in Face Transplant Recipients." *Plastic and Reconstructive Surgery* 136 (5): 1082–89. https://doi.org/10.1097/PRS.0000000000001703.

Kumamaru, K K, G C Sisk, D Mitsouras, K Schultz, M L. Steigner, E George, D S Enterline, E M Bueno, B Pomahac, and F J Rybicki. 2014. "Vascular Communications between Donor and Recipient Tissues after Successful Full Face Transplantation." *American Journal of Transplantation* 14 (3): 711–19. https://doi.org/10.1111/ajt.12608.

Lanzetta, M, P Petruzzo, G Vitale, S Lucchina, E R Owen, J M Dubernard, N Hakim, and H Kapila. 2004. "Human Hand Transplantation: What Have We Learned?" *Transplantation Proceedings* 36 (3): 664–68. https://doi.org/10.1016/j.transproceed.2004.03.006.

Lanzetta, Marco, and Luca Rovati. 2007. "Monitoring Rejection with a Distant Sentinel Skin Graft." *Hand Transplantation*, 263–68. https://doi.org/10.1007/978-88-470-0374-3_34.

Lee, W P, M J Yaremchuk, Y C Pan, M A Randolph, C M Tan, and A J Weiland. 1991. "Relative Antigenicity of Components of a Vascularized Limb Allograft." *Plastic and Reconstructive Surgery* 87 (3): 401–11. http://www.ncbi.nlm.nih.gov/pubmed/1998012.

Levi, David M, Andreas G Tzakis, Tomoaki Kato, Juan Madariaga, Naveen K Mittal, Jose Nery, Seigo Nishida, and Phillip Ruiz. 2003. "Transplantation of the Abdominal Wall." *Lancet* 361 (9376): 2173–76. https://doi.org/10.1016/S0140-6736(03)13769-5.

Lian, Christine Guo, Ericka M Bueno, Scott R Granter, Alvaro C Laga, Arturo P Saavedra, William M Lin, Joseph S Susa, et al. 2014. "Biomarker Evaluation of Face Transplant Rejection: Association of Donor T Cells with Target Cell Injury." *Modern Pathology* 27 (6): 788–99. https://doi.org/10.1038/modpathol.2013.249.

Liu, X, Z Yue, J Yu, E Daguindau, K Kushekhar, Q Zhang, Y Ogata, et al. 2016. "Proteomic Characterization Reveals that MMP-3 Correlates with Bronchiolitis Obliterans Syndrome Following Allogeneic Hematopoietic Cell and Lung Transplantation." *American Journal of Transplantation* 16 (8): 2342–51. https://doi.org/10.1111/ajt.13750.

Lo, Y M Dennis, Mark SC Tein, Calvin CP Pang, Chung K Yeung, Kwok-Lung Tong, and N Magnus Hjelm. 1998. "Presence of Donor-Specific DNA in Plasma of Kidney and Liver-Transplant Recipients." *Lancet* 351 (9112): 1329–30. https://doi.org/10.1016/S0140-6736(05)79055-3.

Lund, Lars H, Leah B Edwards, Anna Y Kucheryavaya, Christian Benden, Anne I Dipchand, Samuel Goldfarb, Bronwyn J Levvey, et al. 2015. "The Registry of the International Society for Heart and Lung Transplantation: Thirty-Second Official Adult Heart Transplantation Report—2015; Focus Theme: Early Graft Failure." *The Journal of Heart and Lung Transplantation* 34 (10): 1244–54. https://doi.org/10.1016/j.healun.2015.08.003.

Mas, V R, C I Dumur, M J Scian, R C Gehrau, and D G Maluf. 2013. "MicroRNAs as Biomarkers in Solid Organ Transplantation." *American Journal of Transplantation* 13(1):11–19. https://doi.org/10.1111/j.1600-6143.2012.04313.x.

Mischak, Harald, Raymond Vanholder, Christian Delles, and Antonia Vlahou. 2015. "Proteomic Biomarkers in Kidney Disease: Issues in Development and Implementation." *Nature Reviews Nephrology* 11: 221–32. https://doi.org/10.1038/nrneph.2014.247.

Morelon, E, P Petruzzo, J Kanitakis, S Dakpé, O Thaunat, V Dubois, G Choukroun, et al. 2017. "Face Transplantation: Partial Graft Loss of the First Case 10 Years Later." *American Journal of Transplantation* 17 (7): 1935–40. https://doi.org/10.1111/ajt.14218.

Myredal, Anna, Li Ming Gan, Walter Osika, Peter Friberg, and Mats Johansson. 2010. "Increased Intima Thickness of the Radial Artery in Individuals with Prehypertension and Hypertension." *Atherosclerosis* 209 (1): 147–51. https://doi.org/10.1016/j.atherosclerosis.2009.09.017.

Ng, Zhi Yang, Alexandre G Lellouch, Ivy A Rosales, Luke Geoghegan, Amon-Ra Gama, Robert B Colvin, Laurent A Lantieri, Mark A Randolph, and Curtis L Cetrulo. 2019. "Graft Vasculopathy of Vascularized Composite Allografts in Humans: A Literature Review and Retrospective Study." *Transplant International* 32 (8): tri.13421. https://doi.org/10.1111/tri.13421.

Niederhaus, S V, G E Leverson, D F Lorentzen, D J Robillard, H W Sollinger, J D Pirsch, J R Torrealba, and J S Odorico. 2013. "Acute Cellular and Antibody-Mediated Rejection of the Pancreas Allograft: Incidence, Risk Factors and Outcomes." *American Journal of Transplantation* 13 (11): 2945–55. https://doi.org/10.1111/ajt.12443.

Oda, Hiroki, Ryosuke Ikeguchi, Tomoki Aoyama, Souichi Ohta, Takashi Noguchi, Yukitoshi Kaizawa, Hirofumi Yurie, Hisataka Takeuchi, Koji Yamamoto, and Shuichi Matsuda. 2017. "MicroRNAs Are Potential Objective and Early Biomarkers for Acute Rejection of Transplanted Limbs in a Rat Model." *Microsurgery* 37 (8): 930–36. https://doi.org/10.1002/micr.30236.

Ok Oda, Hiroki, Ryosuke Ikeguchi, Hirofumi Yurie, Yukitoshi Kaizawa, Souichi Ohta, Koji Yamamoto, Tomoki Aoyama, and Shuichi Matsuda. 2016. "Plasma MicroRNAs Are Potential Biomarkers of Acute Rejection After Hindlimb Transplantation in Rats." *Transplantation Direct* 2 (11): e108. https://doi.org/10.1097/TXD.0000000000000620.

Oh, P L, I Martínez, Y Sun, J Walter, D A Peterson, and D F Mercer. 2012. "Characterization of the Ileal Microbiota in Rejecting and Nonrejecting Recipients of Small Bowel Transplants." *American Journal of Transplantation* 12 (3): 753–62. https://doi.org/10.1111/j.1600-6143.2011.03860.x.

Petruzzo, Palmina, Jean Kanitakis, Sylvie Testelin, Jean-Baptiste Pialat, Fanny Buron, Lionel Badet, Olivier Thaunat, Bernard Devauchelle, and Emmanuel Morelon. 2015. "Clinicopathological Findings of Chronic Rejection in a Face Grafted Patient." *Transplantation* 99 (12): 2644–50. https://doi.org/10.1097/TP.0000000000000765.

Petruzzo, Palmina, Claudia Sardu, Marco Lanzetta, and Jean Michel Dubernard. 2017. "Report (2017) of the International Registry on Hand and Composite Tissue Allotransplantation (IRHCTT)." *Current Transplantation Reports* 4 (4): 294–303. https://doi.org/10.1007/s40472-017-0168-3.

Petruzzo, Palmina, Sylvie Testelin, Jean Kanitakis, Lionel Badet, Benoit Lengelé, Jean-Pierre Girbon, Hélène Parmentier, et al. 2012. "First Human Face Transplantation." *Transplantation* 93 (2): 236–40. https://doi.org/10.1097/TP.0b013e31823d4af6.

Peyster, Eliot G, Chichung Wang, Felicia Ishola, Bethany Remeniuk, Clifford Hoyt, Michael D Feldman, and Kenneth B Margulies. 2020. "In Situ Immune Profiling of Heart Transplant Biopsies Improves Diagnostic Accuracy and Rejection Risk Stratification." *JACC: Basic to Translational Science* 5 (4): 328–40. https://doi.org/10.1016/j.jacbts.2020.01.015.

Pomahac, Bohdan, Julian Pribaz, Elof Eriksson, Ericka M Bueno, J Rodrigo Diaz-Siso, Frank J Rybicki, Donald J Annino, et al. 2011. "Three Patients with Full Facial Transplantation." *New England Journal of Medicine* 366: 715–37. https://doi.org/10.1056/NEJMoa1111432.

"Rationale for Additional Monitoring of the Hand." n.d. Accessed October 9, 2019. http://eknygos.lsmuni.lt/springer/673/Part 8/263-268.pdf.

Ren, Zhigang, Jianwen Jiang, Haifeng Lu, Xinhua Chen, Yong He, Hua Zhang, Haiyang Xie, Weilin Wang, Shusen Zheng, and Lin Zhou. 2014. "Intestinal Microbial Variation May Predict Early Acute Rejection after Liver Transplantation in Rats." *Transplantation* 98 (8): 844–52. https://doi.org/10.1097/TP.0000000000000334.

Robbins, Nicholas L, Matthew J Wordsworth, Bijaya K Parida, Bruce Kaplan, Vijay S Gorantla, Erik K Weitzel, and Warren C Breidenbach. 2019. "Is Skin the Most Allogenic Tissue in Vascularized Composite Allotransplantation and a Valid Monitor of the Deeper Tissues?" *Plastic and Reconstructive Surgery* 143 (4): 880e–6e. https://doi.org/10.1097/PRS.0000000000005436.

Rodrigo, E, M López-Hoyos, R Escallada, G Fernández-Fresnedo, J C Ruiz, C Piñera, J G Cotorruelo, J A Zubimendi, A L de Francisco, and M Arias. 2000. "Circulating Levels of Matrix Metalloproteinases MMP-3 and MMP-2 in Renal Transplant Recipients with Chronic Transplant Nephropathy." *Nephrology, Dialysis, Transplantation* 15 (12): 2041–45. https://doi.org/10.1093/ndt/15.12.2041.

Rowinska, Zuzanna, Simone Zander, Alma Zernecke, Michael Jacobs, Stephan Langer, Christian Weber, Marc W Merx, and Thomas A Koeppel. 2012. "Non- Invasive in Vivo Analysis of a Murine Aortic Graft Using High Resolution Ultrasound Microimaging." *European Journal of Radiology* 81 (2): 244–49. https://doi.org/10.1016/j.ejrad.2010.12.083.

Salvi, Samanta, Giorgia Gurioli, Ugo De Giorgi, Vincenza Conteduca, Gianluca Tedaldi, Daniele Calistri, and Valentina Casadio. 2016. "Cell-Free DNA as a Diagnostic Marker for Cancer: Current Insights." *OncoTargets and Therapy* 9 (October): 6549–59. https://doi.org/10.2147/OTT.S100901.

Sarhane, Karim A, Saami Khalifian, Zuhaib Ibrahim, Damon S Cooney, Theresa Hautz, Wei Ping Andrew Lee, Stefan Schneeberger, and Gerald Brandacher. 2014. "Diagnosing Skin Rejection in Vascularized Composite Allotransplantation: Advances and Challenges." *Clinical Transplantation* 28(3):277–85. https://doi.org/10.1111/ctr.12316.

Sarhane, Karim A, Sami H Tuffaha, Justin M Broyles, Amir E Ibrahim, Saami Khalifian, Pablo Baltodano, Gabriel F Santiago, Mohammed Alrakan, and Zuhaib Ibrahim. 2013. "A Critical Analysis of Rejection in Vascularized Composite Allotransplantation: Clinical, Cellular and Molecular Aspects, Current Challenges, and Novel Concepts." *Frontiers in Immunology* 4 (November): 406. https://doi.org/10.3389/fimmu.2013.00406.

Schneeberger, S, V S Gorantla, R P Van Riet, M Lanzetta, P Vereecken, C Van Holder, S Rorive, et al. 2008. "Atypical Acute Rejection after Hand Transplantation." *American Journal of Transplantation* 8 (3): 688–96. https://doi.org/10.1111/j.1600-6143.2007.02105.x.

Schneider, Michelle, Adela Rambi G Cardones, M Angelica Selim, and Linda C Cendales. 2016. "Vascularized Composite Allotransplantation: A Closer Look at the Banff Working Classification." *Transplant International* 29(6):663–71 https://doi.org/10.1111/tri.12750.

Schütz, Ekkehard, Anna Fischer, Julia Beck, Markus Harden, Martina Koch, Tilo Wuensch, Martin Stockmann, et al. 2017. "Graft-Derived Cell-Free DNA, a Noninvasive Early Rejection and Graft Damage Marker in Liver Transplantation: A Prospective, Observational, Multicenter Cohort Study." *PLoS Medicine* 14 (4): e1002286. https://doi.org/10.1371/journal.pmed.1002286.

Shores, Jaimie T, Gerald Brandacher, and W P Andrew Lee. 2015. "Hand and Upper Extremity Transplantation: An Update of Outcomes in the Worldwide Experience." *Plastic and Reconstructive Surgery* 135 (2): 351e–60e. https://doi.org/10.1097/PRS.0000000000000892.

Shores, Jaimie T, Veronika Malek, W P Andrew Lee, and Gerald Brandacher. 2017. "Outcomes after Hand and Upper Extremity Transplantation." *Journal of Materials Science: Materials in Medicine* 28 (5): 72. https://doi.org/10.1007/s10856-017-5880-0.

Siemionow, Maria. 2017. "The Decade of Face Transplant Outcomes." *Journal of Materials Science: Materials in Medicine* 28 (5): 64. https://doi.org/10.1007/s10856-017-5873-z.

Smith, C W 1993. "Endothelial Adhesion Molecules and Their Role in Inflammation." *Canadian Journal of Physiology and Pharmacology* 71:76–87. https://doi.org/10.1139/y93-012.

Soga, Shigeyoshi, Hale Ersoy, Dimitrios Mitsouras, Kurt Schultz, Amanda G Whitmore, Sara L Powers, Michael L Steigner, et al. 2010. "Surgical Planning for Composite Tissue Allotransplantation of the Face Using 320ydetector Row Computed Tomography." *Journal of Computer Assisted Tomography* 34 (5): 766–69. https://doi.org/10.1097/RCT.0b013e3181e9c133.

Spivey, Tara L, Lorenzo Uccellini, Maria L Ascierto, Gabriele Zoppoli, Valeria De Giorgi, Lucia G Delogu, Alyson M Engle, et al. 2011. "Gene Expression Profiling in Acute Allograft Rejection: Challenging the Immunologic Constant of Rejection Hypothesis." 174 (2011) *Journal of Translational Medicine*. https://doi.org/10.1186/1479-5876-9-174.

Tabibian, James H, and Saad S Kenderian. 2017. "The Microbiome and Immune Regulation After Transplantation." *Transplantation* 101 (1): 56–62. https://doi.org/10.1097/TP.0000000000001444.

Tasigiorgos, Sotirios, Branislav Kollar, Marvee Turk, Bridget Perry, Muayyad Alhefzi, Harriet Kiwanuka, Marie-Christine Nizzi, et al. 2019. "Five-Year Follow-up after Face Transplantation." *New England Journal of Medicine* 380 (26): 2579–81. https://doi.org/10.1056/NEJMc1810468.

Unadkat, J V, S Schneeberger, E H Horibe, C Goldbach, M G Solari, K M Washington, V S Gorantla, G M Cooper, A W Thomson, and W P Andrew Lee. 2010. "Composite Tissue Vasculopathy and Degeneration Following Multiple Episodes of Acute Rejection in Reconstructive Transplantation." *American Journal of Transplantation* 10 (2): 251–61. https://doi.org/10.1111/j.1600-6143.2009.02941.x.

Veríssimo Veronese, Francisco, Roberto Cerratti Manfro, Fernando Roberto Roman, Maria Isabel Edelweiss, David N Rush, Sylvia Dancea, Julio Goldberg, and Luiz Felipe Gonçalves. 2005. "Reproducibility of the Banff Classification in Subclinical Kidney Transplant Rejection." *Clinical Transplantation* 19 (4): 518–21. https://doi.org/10.1111/j.1399-0012.2005.00377.x.

Volokh, Maria, N Manturova, A Fisun, V Uyba, S Voskanyan, G Khubulava, N Kalakutskiy, and K Gubarev. 2019. "First Russian Experience of Composite Facial Tissue Allotransplantation." *Plastic and Reconstructive Surgery - Global Open* 7 (11): e2521. https://doi.org/10.1097/GOX.0000000000002521.

Weissenbacher, Annemarie, Theresa Hautz, Bernhard Zelger, Bettina G. Zelger, Verena Mayr, Gerald Brandacher, Johann Pratschke, and Stefan Schneeberger. 2014. "Antibody-Mediated Rejection in Hand Transplantation." *Transplant International* 27 (2): e13–17. https://doi.org/10.1111/tri.12233.

Weissenbacher A, Vrakas G, Chen M, et al. 2018. "De Novo Donor Specific HLA Antibodies after Combined Intestinal and Vascualrised Composite Allotransplantation." *Transplant International* 31 (4): 398–407. doi:10.1111/tri.13096

Whitehouse, Gavin, and Alberto Sanchez-Fueyo. 2014. "Postoperative Monitoring: Biomarkers and Alloimmune Responses and Their Relevance to Vascularized Composite Allotransplantation." *Current Transplantation Reports* 1 (3): 203–10. https://doi.org/10.1007/s40472-014-0022-9.

Win, Thet Su, Naoka Murakami, Thiago J Borges, Anil Chandraker, George Murphy, Christine Lian, Victor Barrera, et al. 2017. "Longitudinal Immunological Characterization of the First Presensitized Recipient of a Face Transplant." *JCI Insight* 2 (13). https://doi.org/10.1172/jci.insight.93894.

Wolfram, Dolores, Evi M Morandi, Nadine Eberhart, Theresa Hautz, Hubert Hackl, Bettina Zelger, Gregor Riede, et al. 2015. "Differentiation between Acute Skin Rejection in Allotransplantation and T-Cell Mediated Skin Inflammation Based on Gene Expression Analysis." *BioMed Research International* 2015: 259160. https://doi.org/10.1155/2015/259160.

Yang, Joshua Y C, Reuben D Sarwal, Tara K Sigdel, Izabella Damm, Ben Rosenbaum, Juliane M Liberto, Chitranon Chan-On, et al. 2020. "A Urine Score for Noninvasive Accurate Diagnosis and Prediction of Kidney Transplant Rejection." *Science Translational Medicine* 12 (535). https://doi.org/10.1126/scitranslmed.aba2501.

Zdichavsky, Marty, Jon W Jones, E Tuncay Ustuner, Xiaoping Ren, Jean Edelstein, Claudio Maldonado, Warren Breidenbach, Scott A Gruber, Mukunda Ray, and John H Barker. 1999. "Scoring of Skin Rejection in a Swine Composite Tissue Allograft Model." *Journal of Surgical Research* 85 (1): 1–8. https://doi.org/10.1006/jsre.1999.5673.

Section IV

Composite Tissue Graft
Manipulation and Engineering

8 Bioengineering Composite Tissue Constructs
Concepts and Challenges

*Kavit Amin, David Leonard,
Li Yenn Yong, Ralph Murphy,
Roxana Moscalu, Kirsten Liggat,
and Jason Wong*

CONTENTS

Introduction.. 149
    Competing Technologies for Composite Tissue Loss 150
The Substance 152
    Concept 152
    Strategy 154
    Challenge... 155
Nutrition... 156
    Concept 156
    Strategy 157
    Challenge... 158
The Scaffold.. 158
    Concept 158
    Strategy 159
    Challenge... 161
Conclusion 162
References... 163

INTRODUCTION

There is a growing need for replacement tissues after significant acute tissue loss following trauma, surgery or disease[1]. Reconstructive surgery aims to replace "like with like", highlighted by Millard as a key tenet of plastic surgery[2]. Increasingly, reconstructive microsurgery is used to perform surgeries to "fill in" defects that often involve loss of multiple tissue types. On one end of the spectrum is full thickness skin loss from injuries such as burns, where actually numerous components

DOI: 10.1201/9780429260179-12

of the integument are lost, including skin, fat, lymphatics, fascia, nerves and blood vessels. On the other side of the spectrum is loss of a whole limb, face or abdominal wall[3]. Replacing composite tissues is what defines the work of the reconstructive microsurgeon. At present, the state of the art is to "steal from Peter to give to Paul" by means of autologous replacement with free tissue transfer. The range of autologous composite tissues is finite, thus restricting the number of anatomical parts that can be sacrificed and donated for use[4]. Use of donated allogeneic vascularized composite tissues represents the ultimate sacrifice for replacing lost and damaged tissues, despite the immunological challenges, and this illustrates the need of sourcing like for like composite tissues. The potential risks of long-term immunosuppression and the paucity of donor tissue are clearly the main challenges that limit the availability of this technique. However, there are technologies that are competing with and complementary to transplantation in meeting this healthcare need. Replacing tissues with biological equivalents is a favorable approach, and thus tissue engineering and regenerative medicine strategies will be the focus of this chapter, with a specific emphasis on combined tissue types. Fundamental complexities of the cell biology, immunology and biointegration will be reviewed, alongside the translational challenges of introducing these technologies into the clinic.

COMPETING TECHNOLOGIES FOR COMPOSITE TISSUE LOSS

The current state of the art is with vascularized composite allotransplantation (VCA), where donor tissue composites are procured from an organ donor and transplanted to the recipient. Many different applications are now common, including hand, face[5] and abdominal wall[6] transplantation. More complex organs like penile and uterine[7] transplants have been described but are performed to serve specific functional needs in isolated cases. The main challenge for VCA remains the paucity of authorized donor tissue and the progressive combat with long-term immunosuppression and rejection[8].

Advanced prosthetics and bionics are not bound by the constraints of biology and have seen considerable developments over the years, with the development of lighter, stronger materials, haptic feedback and more energy-efficient mechanical components (Vujaklija and Farina 2018). In addition, the cost reductions and universal availability offered by 3D printing favors this technology for limb replacement[9,10]. The main challenge for bionics is the human tissue interface and how prosthetics can provide a more integrated replacement of the missing body composite[11]. Considerable work has been done to engineer better integration of the missing part by skeletal integration, and with the advancement and miniaturization of sensor technology, bionic parts can be activated by neuronal interfaces[12]. Tissue engineering has a potential role for adaptation to interfaces at the muscle, e.g., targeted muscle reinnervation[13], peripheral nerve, e.g., regenerative peripheral nerve interfaces[14,15], and brain, e.g., extracortical and intracortical electrodes[16].

Tissue regeneration is the plastic surgical panacea, from the promise of scarless healing to the complete recompositing of missing or damaged parts through to the recapitulation of the developmental process[17]. The signature process of this phenomena seen in primitive species is dedifferentiation of injured tissues leading to formation of a blastema and subsequent reformation of the missing parts. Although this is seen most frequently in amphibians like axolotl, some mammals like the MRL/MPJ mouse[18] or the African Spiny mouse[19] show regenerative properties. The challenge with regeneration is that the intrinsic processes are still not fully understood, and probably quite different across species. Studies point towards changes in inflammation[20], basic metabolic pathways[21], epigenetic phenomena[22] and reactive oxygen species signaling to trigger and maintain the regenerative phenotype[23]. Moreover, the ability to regenerate at a human scale is unlikely to be a potential solution given the process is rate limited by evolution. When scaled to human size, regeneration would take too long to be a practical clinical solution and would require dramatic shifts in biological pathways to permit it.

Tissue bioengineering probably provides a common platform for VCA, tissue regeneration and modern prosthetics to advance. The caveats of immunity and donor paucity can be met by manufactured, cell-specific tissues. The elements of scaling and reprogramming of tissue patterning could be met by rapid manufacturing of graded tunable materials and stem cells. Where problems exist with prosthetic attachments, better biointegration could be met by biomimicry and neuronal interfaces. Converging these paradigms across cell/matrix biology, biomaterial science, wound healing and microsurgery will be essential to bioengineer composite tissues (Figure 8.1).

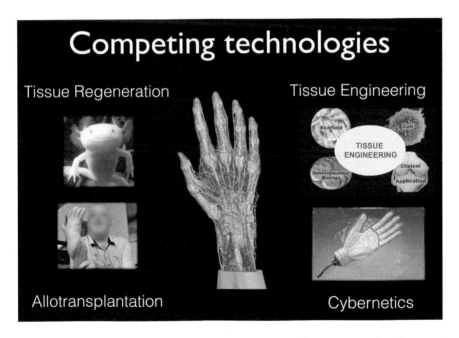

FIGURE 8.1 The "competing technologies" for tissue loss. Tissue regeneration, tissue engineering, vascularized composite allotransplantation and cybernetics each with differing steps towards clinical translation will ultimately provide the means to cater for any reconstructive challenge. Convergence of these technologies will hopefully see more impactful platforms being developed.

THE SUBSTANCE

CONCEPT

Increasingly, there is an appreciation that most tissues exist as a composite of different cellular and matrix contributions. As a consequence, composite tissue engineering is becoming more intricate and complex in order to resemble native tissues (Figure 8.2). An example of this is the move away from thin monocellular tissues like keratinocyte sheets[24] to bioengineered dermis and keratinocyte composites like Apligraf[25] (Table 8.1). Skin as a complex composite of more than just the epidermis requires an understanding of its structural nuances such as its mechanical, biological and functional properties[26]. Advanced features should see skin replacements facilitate thermoregulation, barrier function, immunoregulation, prevent water losses, provide UV protection and heal. One of the challenges is incorporating these functions with an adequate blood supply, lymphatic channels and with nervous system support[27].

Utility of simple engineered tissue composites in clinical practice is rare. At the time of writing (September 2021, www.clinicaltrials.gov), one research group is recruiting full-thickness burn patients in a phase IIb trials to evaluate a tissue-engineered dermo-epidermal autologous skin substitute (NCT03229564). Part of the reason is that engineered substitutes fall short of fulfilling the key functions of native skin and often do not have an inherent vascular supply, relying on the ingrowth of vessels from the host or angiogenesis[28]. In addition, most clinical cases do not

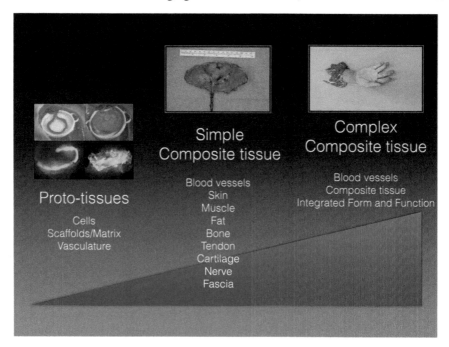

FIGURE 8.2 The developmental pathway to complex composite tissue replacements. Understanding the biological challenges of the basic assembly of proto-tissues will allow for the development of composite tissues that can be used to replace tissue loss. Ultimately, this will allow for more complex composite tissues to be fabricated.

TABLE 8.1
List of Current Commercially Available Skin Substitutes

Autologous Epidermis

EpiDex	Tissue engineered from autologous outer root sheath in chronic wounds and ulcers
EPIBASE	Cultured autologous keratinocytes from tissue biopsy
MySkin	Temporary silicone substrate to deliver autologous keratinocytes
Bioseed-S	Cultured autologous keratinocytes re-suspended in fibrin sealant
Epicel	Autologous epidermal keratinocytes on petroleum gauze
Vivoderm	Autologous keratinocytes on microperforated hyaluronic acid membrane
Autoderm	Cultured keratinocytes
Transderm	Cultured keratinocytes
Lyphoderm	Lyophilised neonatal keratinocytes
Cryoceal	Cryopreserved keratinocytes

Autologous Dermis

DenovoDerma	Neodermis-like regeneration graft
Hyalomatrix	Hyaluronic acid ester matrix
Hyalograft 3D	Fibroblasts seeded over esterified hyaluronic acid fibrous matrix

Allogenic * Xenogenic Dermis

Dermagraft	Ploygalactib mesh matrix seeded with human neonatal cryopreserved fibroblasts
Transcyte	Collagen nylon mesh seeded with allogenic neonatal human foreskin fibroblasts
Terudermis	Bovine lyophilised cross-linked collagen
Chitosan	Dermal matrix seeded with fibroblasts, nano-titanium oxide-chitosan artificial
Permacol	Porcine acellular dermis
Matroderm	Bovine non-cross-linked lyophilised dermis
EX Derm	Porcine aldehyde dermal collagen
Collatamp	Bovine collagen matrix

Synthetic Dermis

Chitosan membrane	PLGA chitosan nanofibrous membrane
Polyurethane	Biodegradeable microfibres

Autologous Composite

Permaderm	Autologous fibroblasts and keratinocytes with bovine collagen
Denovo Skin	Autologous full thickness composite
PolyActive	Cultured keratinocytes and fibroblasts

Allogenic * Xenogenic Composite

Apligraf OrCel	Collagen matrix seeded with neonatal foreskin fibroblasts/keratinocytes
Karoskin	Human cadaver skin with dermal and epidermal cells
Stratagraft	Full thickness skin substitute dermis/epidermis
AcuDress	Cultured keratinocytes
Oasis	Small intestine porcine matrix

have a paucity of donor autologous skin in the form of grafts, hence the demand for off-the-shelf solutions is limited, especially where cost restrictions preclude their use. Disruption to these barriers requires engineering platforms of scale, whereby a modular approach to tissue engineering allows fabrication of components that are missing. In this respect, assessment of the defect and composing like for like composites would utilize biofabrication and bioprinting to provide structure and spatial positioning of lost tissues. It is likely that neurovascular assembly and microsurgery will be the key enablers for clinical integration into the host environment.

STRATEGY

A number of strategies have been adopted to develop more complex tissue composites. Starting with skin, Miyazaki et al. engineered a prevascularized substitute with human fibroblasts, endothelial cells (ECs) and keratinocytes. At 7 days, vascular flow was evident compared with 14 days in a non-prevascularized substitute in nude mice[29]. This approach can form multilayer multicellular vascularized tissue. Vascular channels can be re-engineered into decellularized skin extracellular matrix with human adipose-derived stromal cells and human umbilical vein endothelial cells (HUVECs)[30]. It is also feasible to engineer artificial human lymphatics into composite skin constructs, providing immune channels for cell trafficking.

Building composites can use existing plastic surgical techniques including prefabrication and prelamination. Harnessing repair processes in vivo through in situ engineering is the obvious direction of reconstructive development. Flap prefabrication requires the transposition of a vascular pedicle into donor tissues whereas prelamination involves the addition of tissues to an established vascular bed[31]. Later, tissues are transferred, either "pedicled" or "free", to a secondary site requiring reconstruction. Fabrication of tissues is particularly useful at existing donor sites, where free flaps are frequently harvested and the vascular anatomy is well described. Clinical examples using this technique include recreating the ear[32] and nose[33]. This approach has been adapted for in situ tissue engineering of composites. All mesenchymal tissue types can be readily engineered. Fascia, muscle, bone, tendon and cartilage all have an engineered surrogate that mimics the native tissue well. Historically, they have been developed as homogenous tissues, but more recently, the synergistic effect of co-development gives rise to more functional tissue replacements.

Using connective tissue is a particularly useful way to build composites. For example, the material composition of fascia lends itself well for reconstruction, being highly vascular, composed predominantly of a structural collagen matrix and other hydrophilic glycosaminoglycans (GAGs)[34]. GAG-tissue extracellular matrix (ECM) hydrogels derived from fascia are particularly robust and biocompatible when used as fillers to preserve local architecture[35]. Engineering fascial templates has been attempted by combining laser patterned alginate-human collagen embedded with human mesenchymal stem cells (MSCs) for use in reconstructing abdominal wall defects[36]. A full thickness abdominal wall was also engineered using pre-seeded ECs with fibroblasts onto a porous biodegradable scaffold. The scaffold is perfused via the femoral vessels and transferred as an axial flap to reconstruct the abdominal wall[37]. The addition of native skeletal muscle potentiates vascularization of the muscle architecture and enhances abdominal wall function[38]. Further structural function can be achieved by engineering innervation into muscular constructs. Prefabrication of engineered muscle constructs with the sciatic and sural neurovascular bundle promotes neuromuscular junction development and increases force production and muscular tone[39].

Dynamic load and stress bearing composite tissues provide an even greater challenge to engineer. Not only do they have to be biologically active, but also have to resist high mechanical forces, in particular at tissue interfaces, like the entheses. In vitro fibroblast and myoblast cell line bioinks can be print fabricated into musculotendinous interfaces and achieve impressive biomechanical stability[40]. The bone tendon interface poses a different set of challenges, hence have been approached by combining fibrous elements derived by electrospinning and graded bone component through a combination of MSC seeding to gels and the addition of osteogenic growth factors into the constructs[41]. Matrix stiffness and tissue gradients permit the fabrication of these complex soft to hard tissue interfaces. In vivo, more robust tissue can be generated by exploiting the body's regenerative capabilities[42]. Periosteum has demonstrated significant value in generating hard tissues in vivo. Creating periosteal space by injecting 1% alginate and hyaluronic acid (HA) hydrogels at the fascial bone interface promotes large amounts of woven bone matrix formation. Interestingly, by inhibiting angiogenesis and creating a hypoxic environment, cartilage matrix is laid down instead[43], hence this approach can be used to engineer osteochondral tissue. Devitalized decellularized bone matrix can also be revitalized when wrapped with a vascularized pedicled periosteal flap[44] or when placing morcellized bone in small chambers beside the periosteum[45]. This demonstrates the potent osteogenic properties of this tissue. Omentum has also been used to induce osteogenesis when used to wrap hydroxyapatite blocks or autologous bone. Engineering long bones requires more vascularity than solely lamination can provide and, hence, can be achieved by combining devitalized cancellous bone filled with cartilage pellets, stromal vascular fraction, with the axial insertion of an arteriovenous bundle[46].

Surgical fabrication and in situ tissue engineering remains the most reliable method of generating specialized anatomy. Thus far, this has been reserved for laminated tubular structures. Multistep urethral reconstruction can be performed by combining prevascularized prelaminated buccal mucosa grafts on tissue-expanded groin flaps, which are far less prone to scarring and contraction.[47]. Prelamination of decellularized trachea with integra, and heterotopic implantation to the lateral thoracic artery flap at the first stage, followed by an autologous buccal mucosa graft at 21 days, can allow for restoration of the trachea[48]. The scope for complex tissue fabrication is limited only by the willingness, health and patience of the recipient, combined with the creativity and skill of the surgeon.

CHALLENGE

Adoption of biomaterials into the reconstructive toolset is slowly showing penetrance, with some clinical use. Acellular dermal matrices and biomaterial dermal substitutes, most widely used for breast reconstruction, can be prevascularized over vascular pedicles for free flap reconstruction[49], allowing for direct closure of the forearm donor site after harvest. Similarly, reconstructing a near total ear amputation with a prelaminated radial forearm flap with porous polyethylene implant allows the ear

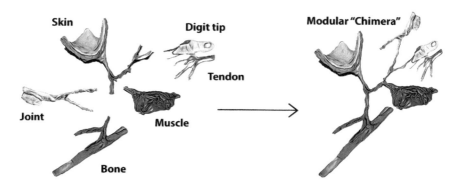

FIGURE 8.3 Modular "Chimeric" concept of composite tissue bioengineering. Different tissue types are fabricated in advance. Depending on the complex composite tissue requirements, "chimerising" the different tissues will allow bespoke composites to be composed and combined through microsurgery.

to be fabricated on the arm prior to transplantation[50]. The forearm, ankle, thigh and groin may be favored sites for heterotopic in situ engineering as vessels in these areas are relatively accessible for harvest.

Every surgical defect has unique tissue requirements that need careful planning prior to reconstruction. Having a modular tissue selection would facilitate preassembly in the laboratory setting. It is critical that preassembled tissues can be compatible not only with the recipient tissues, but also existing surgical approaches and techniques. Bespoke tissue composition requirements would be enabled by microsurgery, as seen in stacked[51] and chimeric flaps[52]. Complex defect requirements would necessitate preplanning and preassembly of different tissue types, but eventually the hope is full complex structures are developed in the laboratory (Figure 8.3). At present, tissue assembly is reliant on healing processes in vivo to vitalize engineered tissue. Future developments could see these inflammatory and healing processes provided by in vitro and ex vivo bioreactors. Early evidence for this being an effective approach can already be observed in co-cultures with activated macrophages that promote vascular sprouting in in vitro models of osteogenesis and bone healing[53].

NUTRITION

CONCEPT

With the exception of dense low metabolic tissues like cartilage and the lens of the eye, most engineered tissues without a nutrient blood supply necrose or fibrose. Nutrition is therefore a critical component of engineered tissues, especially in large composite tissues. The vascular tree, branching networks of blood vessels and the zonal units that each branch and perforator supplies, is a fundamental concept that reconstructive surgeons appreciate[54,55]. Each tissue type of the composite tissue should ideally have incorporated perforators by design to ensure its reliable perfusion. Perforators branch into a dense capillary network that are of a scale at the limit of current engineering. Fabricating vasculature channels, although feasible, needs to address the functional tubular hierarchies across a range of scales and sites, in addition to robust exchange of nutrients.

STRATEGY

Although experimentally creating tissues in small volume is feasibly maintained in culture conditions, there is an appreciation that if tissues are to be composed in clinically useful sizes, there needs evidence of early incorporation of a microvascular network. Without a vascular network, cells rely on a diffusion gradient, limiting the thickness of the construct to 200 μm[56]. The creation of native vasculature occurs through angiogenesis, where sprouting and remodeling occurs from existing vasculature, or vasculogenesis, where the formation of a primitive network arises de novo from circulating endothelial precursor cells[57,58]. Newly formed networks then undergo maturation by recruitment of mural cells and development of the surrounding supporting ECM and elastic laminae[59].

There is much to understand about the mechanisms governing angiogenesis and vasculogenesis in the adult, including the important cell contributions and recruitment dynamics after injury and repair[60]. Specific models have been developed to better understand their biological influence on tissue formation[61]. These effects can be augmented by pre-seeded ECs in scaffolds, creating the foundations of a capillary network which then undergoes inosculation with the host vasculature. As such, ECs have been widely used to prevascularize tissue constructs and form capillary networks in culture regardless of source of origin[62]. Coculture of ECs with vascular support cells such as pericytes or smooth muscle cells further help with maturation of the capillary network[63,64]. Together with MSCs, they have also been shown to be a paracrine source of angiogenic growth factors[65]. Pro-angiogenic growth factors such as vascular endothelial growth factor (VEGF), fibroblast growth factor 2 (FGF2), transforming growth factor-β1 (TGF-β1) and platelet-derived growth factor (PDGF-β) can be sequentially delivered exogenously in different combinations to enhance vascularization but is probably a less efficient approach[66]. Limits in generating autologous ECs needed to seed a scaffold have in part been allayed with the differentiation of human induced pluripotent stem cells (iPSCs) down the EC lineage, providing sufficient quantities for clinical translation but at some cost[67]. Whereas, isolation of all these cellular components is relatively straightforward from liposuction or lipectomy, which provides a plentiful resource for procurement[68].

Providing cells with the adequate structure and guidance to populate is essential for the correct distribution of vasculature in tissue. In development, the matrix grows at a rate dictated by vascular sprouting. This coordinated response relies on key patterning genes and gradients[69]. Bioengineering vascularized tissue constructs ex vivo requires the rapid and predictable creation of the microvascular network architecture. High-resolution printing of a three-dimensional capillary network can be achieved by inkjet printing and stereolithography. Kolesky et al. described a printing strategy where Pluronic F127-thrombin and a human MSC-laden gelatin-fibrinogen ink is dual extruded in a lattice pattern[70]. A gelatin, fibrinogen and human neonatal dermal fibroblasts, thrombin and transglutaminase matrix are then casted over the printed inks. Thrombin induces fibrinogen polymerization and transglutaminase crosslinks the gelatin and fibrin to provide adequate structural support. Cooling the construct to 4°C leaves behind microfluidic channels which are then perfused and endothelialized with HUVECs. Artificial tissue with a thickness of >1 cm can be printed with cell viability maintained for 6 weeks in vitro[70]. With methods established to produce channels, having stem cell plasticity in the native tissue allows for the development of a universal tissue platform. Generating tissue from iPSCs in a type 1 collagen and Matrigel solution, which incorporates sacrificial perfusion channels, can be used to form organ building blocks[71]. Many different tissue types could potentially be produced from these "plastic" units given the correct differentiation protocols.

Generating microcirculation by using in vivo strategies for angiogenesis often remains the most reliable approach. Early studies using a vascular pedicle consisting of an artery and a vein were seen to augment capillary sprouting when placed over or under nonvascularized tissue[72]. This evolved into numerous studies exploring the arterio-venous loop (AVL) chamber bioreactor for tissue generation[73]. When the AVL is inserted into a protected chamber space, spontaneous capillary sprouting occurs within the space, which generates new tissue whilst supporting vascularized tissue growth[74]. Various tissues have been successfully grown, including skeletal muscle, functional cardiac tissue, adipose tissue and bone[75–78].

CHALLENGE

The engineering of the vascular infrastructure into complex tissue can be likened to the plumbing of a house. In this respect, a nerve and lymphatic foundation should be considered as part of the intricate network that are key structural components to tissue homeostasis, sensory feedback and physiological control. There is an appreciation of the importance of neurovascular interactions, which are critical for regeneration[79], vascular tone[80] and tissue stability[81]. Studies have shown that nerve regeneration is better when they are vascularized[82,83], and tissue regeneration is deficient when nerve function is impaired[84].

Engineering the lymphatic system is seldom considered when developing tissue but may be crucial in maintaining long-term tissue homeostasis. Studies have shown that incorporating lymphatics into skin substitutes improve skin quality[85] and are essential in the management of tissue fluid balance, immune cell trafficking and tissue repair[86]. The next evolution in tissue engineering needs to consider these refinements in parallel to neurovascular development.

The long-term stability and safety of engineered vascular tissues are critical, and studies have shown that the vascular networks and tissues formed with the arteriovenous (AV) pedicle remained stable after a year in mouse models[87] and up to 6 months in humans[73]. However, clinical trials[88] with this approach indicate that the volume of tissue generated is variable. Reliable, consistent tissue generation that considers the finer intricacies of vascular anatomy is a significant challenge. Particular challenges include the development of functional basement membranes[89] and the reconstitution of the endothelial glycocalyx[90] as well as sympathetic regulation of vessel tone[91].

THE SCAFFOLD

CONCEPT

Tissues need to have defined boundaries, and in the mammalian species, this is provided by the endoskeleton, or fascial compartments[92]. Having been neglected from study for many years, there is now an appreciation of fascia, not only as a protective packing tissue but also as a key structure in compartmentalization, separating different tissues, and with a role in force transmission[93]. Fascia typically refers to two morphologies depending on whether it is superficial or deep fascia. Superficial fascia is a loose areolar tissue that has gel-like properties, whereas deep fascia is thick and fibrous and creates anatomical boundaries to tissue[94]. Each fulfill differing functional roles in structure and tissue dynamics. In addition, numerous critical cellular function roles have been realized, including its roles in wound healing[95] and regeneration[96].

Compartmentalization of fascia forms through natural cleavage planes and migration of fibroblasts at sites of mechanical force[97]. Fibrotic genes, such as TGF-β, are key regulators of its formation during development. Differentiated tissues also have a rudimentary "skin" rich in laminin, claudins, tight junctions and e-cadherin that forms a boundary layer between tissue types. When disrupted, this leads to the migration of cells and the formation of adhesions[98]. Whereas most differentiated cell populations will generate their own matrix, few will produce distinct fascial boundaries. This issue surrounding compartmentalization is therefore an important concept to consider when developing composite tissues.

STRATEGY

Preparation of bioartificial scaffolds by perfusion decellularization is a bioengineering approach which generates ECM scaffolds to serve as a structure for organ or tissue engineering. The donor organs may be allogeneic or xenogenic in origin, and perfusion aims to achieve comprehensive removal of antigenic, cellular material to generate a scaffold in which the complex architecture of the fibrous ECM is preserved, along with an intact three-dimensional map of the vascular network. There are a plethora of tissue-derived scaffolds that are already being utilized to support healing and regeneration of autologous tissues in the clinical setting, both commercial and through tissue biobanks, while the ultimate aim of research at the organ and composite tissue scale is to repopulate the scaffold with patient-compatible cells to restore organ function, or structural integrity, without the need of allogeneic transplantation and immunosuppression.

Decellularization removes the cellular and immunogenic components from tissue, while preserving the physical and biochemical properties of the ECM and the native ultra-structure. As yet, there is no consensus on a strict definition for decellularization, but it has been proposed that the final ECM scaffold should contain no more than 50 mg DNA per mg dry weight, that residual DNA fragments should not exceed 200 bp in length, and that the matrix should contain no visible nuclear components[99].

Donor antigenic motifs surviving decellularization would potentially predispose the engineered composite to immune mediated degradation following implantation, but this risk is not limited to intact cellular components, as residual cellular proteins and debris may function as damage-associated molecular patterns capable of triggering an innate inflammatory response through activation of toll-like receptors[100]. Thus, adequate removal of cellular components is necessary to ensure the avoidance of a deleterious inflammatory reaction to the scaffold following implantation.

However, any successful decellularization process must balance this against excess damage to the ECM, which would adversely impact recellularization, or result in functional impairment of the resulting construct[101].

A variety of decellularization techniques have been described, utilizing chemical, biological or physical processes. Each technique varies in the efficacy of cellular material removal achieved and the degree of disruption inflicted on the ECM[99]. In the context of vascularized tissue composites, the presence of a defined vasculature facilitates delivery of decellularizing agents, and removal of effluent and cellular debris, by perfusion. The combination of major vessels of adequate caliber for cannulation and a microvascular network widely distributed through the tissues allows for practical and efficient decellularization, particularly in tissues where high vascular density correlates with high cellular density[102]. Basic modular components around specific vascular territories would allow for individual functional units or compartments to be engineered.

Tissue-scale acellular scaffolds have already reached application to augment and support autologous tissue in reconstructive surgery[103]. A good example of this is decellularized human amniotic chorionic membranes, which not only contain a host of angiogenic growth factors (e.g., angiogenin, angiopoietin-2, EGF, bFGF, HBEGF, HGF, PDGF-BB, PlGF, and VEGF) but anti-inflammatory molecules and tissue inhibitors of metalloproteinases[104].

In relation to composite tissue, Ott and colleagues demonstrated the feasibility of producing a decellularized ECM scaffold of the rodent forelimb, utilizing flow-controlled detergent perfusion[105]. Following dissection and fasciotomy (to permit radial expansion and prevent flow restriction during perfusion), limbs were flushed with 5 mL phosphate buffered saline (PBS), prior to transfer to the organ chamber, where perfusion was performed at a constant 1 mL/min utilizing a sequential combination of 1% sodium dodecyl sulphate (SDS) (up to 50 hours), deionized water (1 hour) and 1% Triton-X100 (1 hour). Final debris washout was performed with a 124-hour perfusion of antibiotic-containing PBS. This protocol achieved successful decellularization of all tissues within the limb and preservation of mineral content and biochemistry of skeletal components.

Complete recellularization of any tissue with patient autologous cells is a highly complex task, requiring successful, functional integration of large numbers of cells, of diverse phenotypes, to achieve the required functions. Striking successes have been demonstrated, with evidence of both in vitro and rudimentary in vivo function in a number of solid organ systems[106,107]. Recellularization of rodent forelimbs has been achieved by a combination of techniques, including perfusion with HUVEC seeded culture media, and muscle compartment recellularized by direct injection of a combination of C_2C_{12} myoblasts, HUVECs and embryonic fibroblasts (Figure 8.4). Nuances such as perfusion stagnation for 60 minutes following HUVEC infusion to allow for vascular cell adhesion, and electrical stimulation of muscles to allow for greater muscle regeneration, at 6-ms 20V pulses at a frequency of 1 Hz enhanced cell-specific tissue uptake.

This strategy achieved a homogenous endothelial lining and development of histologically appropriate muscle, with demonstrable contractile activity and force generation approximately 80% of that of neonatal murine muscle, after only 14 days

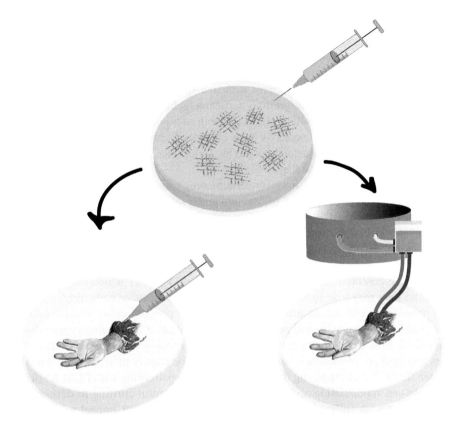

FIGURE 8.4 Schematic of revitalizing decellularized composite tissues with differentiated cell cultures. Cells are either directly delivered into tissue compartments or perfused into tissues using ex-vivo perfusion, expecting cells to home into their specific niches.

biomimetic culture. A chief challenge of composites is that each tissue will require their own unique differentiation protocols, adding complexity to their assembly. Transplantation into isogenic recipient rats confirmed patency of the vascular system (including recording of a pulsatile waveform from the radial artery) and provided in vivo demonstration of muscle contractility[108].

CHALLENGE

Decellularization and recellularization provides a promising strategy for fabricating composite tissues; however, at present the paucity of donor tissue limits its overall availability and universal application. Producing the structural intricacies of the ECM, especially the compartments and vasculature, provides the foundation and boundaries for these structural tissues. Although the fascial endoskeleton seems like a fairly simple tissue, there has been very little focus and research performed in this area[109]. The mechanical stiffness of each compartment heavily influences the development and cellular characteristics of each tissue[110] and part of the challenge will be tuning the mechanical attributes so that materials could be used to replicate its role.

Scale up of decellularization techniques has been the subject of significant research and development; indeed, detailed protocols have been published for perfusion decellularization of whole organs with size-specific modifications from murine to human scale[102]. The rodent forelimb perfusion technique outlined above has been successfully scaled for decellularization of both non-human primate and cadaveric human upper limbs[105,108]. There has been considerable recent progress with decellularization of complex tissue composites at clinical scale, including both limbs and fasciocutaneous and adipose flaps[111,112].

Major challenges remain, however, in achieving reliable, comprehensive recellularization, with the desired level of function and a safety profile suitable for clinical application. These challenges are both practical and regulatory, as any engineered cellular product with translational potential will have to demonstrate a robust safety profile. In practical terms, cell source remains a fundamental question; while patient-derived primary cell lines may be immunologically favorable, their limited proliferative potential substantially restricts the cell volumes which may be generated, and they may lose function in culture[113]. Embryonic stem cells, iPSCs, MSCs and progenitor cells are an attractive alternative to primary cells, given considerable proliferative capacity and potential for differentiation into multiple specialized lineages[114]. MSCs may be the most appropriate for reconstructive tissue as most tissues required are of mesenchymal origin and can be readily differentiated into the chosen tissue[115–117]. Combining the precision of tissue patterning with ECM scaffolds for structure, repopulation and reperfusion requires careful crafting to develop the desired tissues. A fully off-the-shelf solution with little donor impact will require combined fabrication approaches to fulfill multi-composite assembly.

Ex-vivo perfusion platforms can be steered towards facilitating biological processes by driving perfusion, reseeding, and removing byproducts of metabolism. By mimicking physiological circulation, it provides a bioreactor platform that allows tissues to be maintained and develop. This technology has been derived from clinical cardiopulmonary bypass circuits (heart bypass developed in the 1950s) and extracorporeal membrane oxygenation (lung bypass developed in the 1970s). The application of these circuits in clinical solid organ transplantation for prolonged preservation[118] and the "reconditioning" of marginal organs that were previously considered to be non-transplantable demonstrate their utility[119]. Though not currently used in clinical VCA practice, human cadaver limbs have been physiologically preserved for up to 24 hours[120]. The value these studies provide are the conditions, environment and critical mix of substrates that enable biological processes to thrive.

CONCLUSION

Tissue engineering still works on the premise of combining cells, scaffolds, and growth factors; however increasingly, biomimicry, hierarchy and tunability have been elements that focus the current generation of engineered tissue. Recapitulating anatomical, developmental and repair cues are the key next steps in generating clinically relevant tissues. In order to be relevant, most engineered tissues will need to be bespoke to the resultant defects, often involving different tissue types. Preparation of bioartificial scaffolds by perfusion decellularization offers the potential of engineering complex tissue constructs from patient-derived cells, while avoiding many of the challenges of a pure tissue engineering approach and preserving some of the structural function of the donor tissue. Producing the surgical technologies that are required to deliver this will inevitably need to be complemented with reconstructive microsurgery. Nonetheless, the aim towards an off-the-shelf solution for composite tissues remains a novel area of investigation, and further research is required to optimize all approaches for a range of solutions at human scale.

REFERENCES

1. Song, H. G., Rumma, R. T., Ozaki, C. K., Edelman, E. R. & Chen, C. S. Vascular Tissue Engineering: Progress, Challenges, and Clinical Promise. *Cell Stem Cell* **22**, 340–354, doi:10.1016/j.stem.2018.02.009 (2018).
2. Wolfe, S. A. D. Ralph Millard, Jr., M.D., 1919 to 2011. *Plast Reconstr Surg* **129**, 1214–1217, doi:10.1097/prs.0b013e31824a2e83 (2012).
3. Davidson, E. H. et al. Clinical Considerations for Vascularized Composite Allotransplantation of the Eye. *J Craniofac Surg* **27**, 1622–1628, doi:10.1097/SCS. 0000000000002985 (2016).
4. Wei, F. C. & Mardini, S. *Flaps and Reconstructive Surgery.* Second ed. (Elsevier, 2017).
5. Yanow, J., Pappagallo, M. & Pillai, L. Complex Regional Pain Syndrome (CRPS/RSD) and Neuropathic Pain: Role of Intravenous Bisphosphonates as Analgesics. *Sci World J* **8**, 229–236, doi:10.1100/tsw.2008.33 (2008).
6. Broyles, J. M. et al. Reconstruction of Large Abdominal Wall Defects Using Neurotized Vascular Composite Allografts. *Plast Reconstr Surg* **136**, 728–737, doi:10.1097/ PRS.0000000000001584 (2015).
7. Leonard, D. A., Kurtz, J. M. & Cetrulo, C. L., Jr. Vascularized Composite Allotransplantation: Towards Tolerance and the Importance of Skin-Specific Immunobiology. *Curr Opin Organ Transplant* **18**, 645–651, doi:10.1097/MOT. 0000000000000022 (2013).
8. Morelon, E., Petruzzo, P. & Kanitakis, J. Chronic Rejection in Vascularized Composite Allotransplantation. *Curr Opin Organ Transplant* **23**, 582–591, doi:10.1097/MOT. 0000000000000571 (2018).
9. Vujaklija, I. & Farina, D. 3D Printed Upper Limb Prosthetics. *Expert Rev Med Devices* **15**, 505–512, doi:10.1080/17434440.2018.1494568 (2018).
10. Hruby, L. A. et al. Bionic Upper Limb Reconstruction: A Valuable Alternative in Global Brachial Plexus Avulsion Injuries-A Case Series. *J Clin Med* **9**, 23, doi:10.3390/ jcm9010023 (2020).
11. Aman, M. et al. Bionic Hand as Artificial Organ: Current Status and Future Perspectives. *Artif Organs* **43**, 109–118, doi:10.1111/aor.13422 (2019).
12. Aman, M. et al. Bionic Reconstruction: Restoration of Extremity Function with Osseointegrated and Mind-Controlled Prostheses. *Wien Klin Wochenschr* **131**, 599–607, doi:10.1007/s00508-019-1518-1 (2019).
13. Kuiken, T. A. et al. Targeted Muscle Reinnervation for Real-Time Myoelectric Control of Multifunction Artificial Arms. *JAMA* **301**, 619–628, doi:10.1001/jama.2009.116 (2009).
14. Frost, C. M. et al. Regenerative Peripheral Nerve Interfaces for Real-Time, Proportional Control of a Neuroprosthetic Hand. *J Neuroeng Rehabil* **15**, 108, doi:10.1186/s12984-018-0452-1 (2018).

15. Rijnbeek, E. H., Eleveld, N. & Olthuis, W. Update on Peripheral Nerve Electrodes for Closed-Loop Neuroprosthetics. *Front Neurosci* **12**, 350, doi:10.3389/fnins.2018.00350 (2018).

16. Kwok, R. Neuroprosthetics: Once More, with Feeling. *Nature* **497**, 176–178, doi: 10.1038/497176a (2013).

17. Seifert, A. W. & Muneoka, K. The Blastema and Epimorphic Regeneration in Mammals. *Dev Biol* **433**, 190–199, doi:10.1016/j.ydbio.2017.08.007 (2018).

18. Clark, L. D., Clark, R. K. & Heber-Katz, E. A New Murine Model for Mammalian Wound Repair and Regeneration. *Clin Immunol Immunopathol* **88**, 35–45, doi:10.1006/ clin.1998.4519 (1998).

19. Seifert, A. W. et al. Skin Shedding and Tissue Regeneration in African Spiny Mice (Acomys). *Nature* **489**, 561–565, doi:10.1038/nature11499 (2012).

20. Panayidou, S. & Apidianakis, Y. Regenerative Inflammation: Lessons from Drosophila Intestinal Epithelium in Health and Disease. *Pathogens* **2**, 209–231, doi:10.3390/ pathogens2020209 (2013).

21. Iismaa, S. E. et al. Comparative Regenerative Mechanisms across Different Mammalian Tissues. *NPJ Regen Med* **3**, 6, doi:10.1038/s41536-018-0044-5 (2018).

22. Rouhana, L. & Tasaki, J. Epigenetics and Shared Molecular Processes in the Regeneration of Complex Structures. *Stem Cells Int* **2016**, 6947395, doi:10.1155/2016/6947395 (2016).

23. Love, N. R. et al. Amputation-Induced Reactive Oxygen Species are Required for Successful Xenopus Tadpole Tail Regeneration. *Nat Cell Biol* **15**, 222–228, doi:10.1038/ ncb2659 (2013).

24. Moustafa, M. et al. Randomized, Controlled, Single-Blind Study on Use of Autologous Keratinocytes on a Transfer Dressing to Treat Nonhealing Diabetic Ulcers. *Regen Med* **2**, 887–902, doi:10.2217/17460751.2.6.887 (2007).

25. Sabolinski, M. L., Alvarez, O., Auletta, M., Mulder, G. & Parenteau, N. L. Cultured Skin as a 'Smart Material' for Healing Wounds: Experience in Venous Ulcers. *Biomaterials* **17**, 311–320, doi:10.1016/0142-9612(96)85569-4 (1996).

26. Wong, R., Geyer, S., Weninger, W., Guimberteau, J. C. & Wong, J. K. The Dynamic Anatomy and Patterning of Skin. *Exp Dermatol* **25**, 92–98, doi:10.1111/exd.12832 (2016).

27. Lopez-Ojeda, W., Pandey, A., Alhajj, M. & Oakley, A. M. In *StatPearls*. In: StatPearls [Internet]. (Treasure Island, FL: StatPearls Publishing; 2021 Jan). Available from: https://www.ncbi.nlm.nih.gov/books/NBK441980/

28. Saberianpour, S. et al. Tissue Engineering Strategies for the Induction of Angiogenesis Using Biomaterials. *J Biol Eng* **12**, 36, doi:10.1186/s13036-018-0133-4 (2018).

29. Miyazaki, H. et al. A Novel Strategy to Engineer Pre-Vascularized 3-Dimensional Skin Substitutes to Achieve Efficient, Functional Engraftment. *Sci Rep* **9**, 7797, doi:10.1038/ s41598-019-44113-6 (2019).

30. Zhang, Q. et al. Decellularized Skin/Adipose Tissue Flap Matrix for Engineering Vascularized Composite Soft Tissue Flaps. *Acta Biomater* **35**, 166–184, doi:10.1016/j. actbio.2016.02.017 (2016).

31. Sinha, I., Guo, L. F. & Pribaz, J. J. *Flaps and Reconstructive Surgery* (Eds. F.C. Wei & S. Mardini), Ch. 5, 16–27 (Elsevier, 2017).

32. Zhou, G. et al. Free Prepared Composite Forearm Flap Transfer for Ear Reconstruction: Three Case Reports. *Microsurgery* **15**, 660–662, doi:10.1002/micr.1920150912 (1994).

33. Cavadas, P. C. & Torres, A. Total Nasal Reconstruction with Prefabricated and Prelaminated Free Flap. *Ann Plast Surg* **83**, e35–e38, doi:10.1097/SAP. 0000000000002077 (2019).

34. Guimberteau, J. C., Delage, J. P., McGrouther, D. A. & Wong, J. K. The Microvacuolar System: How Connective Tissue Sliding Works. *J Hand Surg Eur Vol* **35**, 614–622, doi:10.1177/1753193410374412 (2010).

35. Beachley, V. et al. Extracellular Matrix Particle-Glycosaminoglycan Composite Hydrogels for Regenerative Medicine Applications. *J Biomed Mater Res A* **106**, 147–159, doi:10.1002/jbm.a.36218 (2018).

36. Ayala, P. et al. Engineered Composite Fascia for Stem Cell Therapy in Tissue Repair Applications. *Acta Biomater* **26**, 1–12, doi:10.1016/j.actbio.2015.08.012 (2015).

37. Shandalov, Y. et al. An Engineered Muscle Flap for Reconstruction of Large Soft Tissue Defects. *Proc Natl Acad Sci U S A* **111**, 6010–6015, doi:10.1073/pnas.1402679111 (2014).

38. Juhas, M., Engelmayr, G. C., Jr., Fontanella, A. N., Palmer, G. M. & Bursac, N. Biomimetic Engineered Muscle with Capacity for Vascular Integration and Functional Maturation In Vivo. *Proc Natl Acad Sci U S A* **111**, 5508–5513, doi:10.1073/pnas.1402723111 (2014).

39. Williams, M. L., Kostrominova, T. Y., Arruda, E. M. & Larkin, L. M. Effect of Implantation on Engineered Skeletal Muscle Constructs. *J Tissue Eng Regen Med* **7**, 434–442, doi:10.1002/term.537 (2013).

40. Merceron, T. K. et al. A 3D Bioprinted Complex Structure for Engineering the Muscle-Tendon Unit. *Biofabrication* **7**, 035003, doi:10.1088/1758-5090/7/3/035003 (2015).

41. Baldino, L., Cardea, S., Maffulli, N. & Reverchon, E. Regeneration Techniques for Bone-to-Tendon and Muscle-to-Tendon Interfaces Reconstruction. *Br Med Bull* **117**, 25–37, doi:10.1093/bmb/ldv056 (2016).

42. Birkenfeld, F. et al. Scaffold Implantation in the Omentum Majus of Rabbits for New Bone Formation. *J Craniomaxillofac Surg* **47**, 1274–1279, doi:10.1016/j.jcms.2019.04.002 (2019).

43. Stevens, M. M. et al. In Vivo Engineering of Organs: The Bone Bioreactor. *Proc Natl Acad Sci U S A* **102**, 11450–11455, doi:10.1073/pnas.0504705102 (2005).

44. Huang, R. L. et al. Prefabrication of a Functional Bone Graft with a Pedicled Periosteal Flap as an In Vivo Bioreactor. *Sci Rep* **7**, 18038, doi:10.1038/s41598-017-17452-5 (2017).

45. Tatara, A. M. et al. Autologously Generated Tissue-Engineered Bone Flaps for Reconstruction of Large Mandibular Defects in an Ovine Model. *Tissue Eng Part A* **21**, 1520–1528, doi:10.1089/ten.TEA.2014.0426 (2015).

46. Epple, C. et al. Prefabrication of a Large Pedicled Bone Graft by Engineering the Germ for De Novo Vascularization and Osteoinduction. *Biomaterials* **192**, 118–127, doi:10.1016/j.biomaterials.2018.11.008 (2019).

47. Guo, H. L. et al. Tubularized Urethral Reconstruction Using a Prevascularized Capsular Tissue Prelaminated with Buccal Mucosa Graft in a Rabbit Model. *Asian J Androl* **21**, 381–386, doi:10.4103/aja.aja_43_19 (2019).

48. Den Hondt, M., Vanaudenaerde, B. M., Verbeken, E. K. & Vranckx, J. J. Epithelial Grafting of a Decellularized Whole-Tracheal Segment: An In Vivo Experimental Model. *Interact Cardiovasc Thorac Surg* **26**, 753–760, doi:10.1093/icvts/ivx442 (2018).

49. Medina, C. R., Patel, S. A., Ridge, J. A. & Topham, N. S. Improvement of the Radial Forearm Flap Donor Defect by Prelamination with Human Acellular Dermal Matrix. *Plast Reconstr Surg* **127**, 1993–1996, doi:10.1097/PRS.0b013e31820cf427 (2011).

50. Horta, R. et al. Reconstruction of a Near Total Ear Amputation with a Neurosensorial Radial Forearm Free Flap Prelaminated with Porous Polyethylene Implant and Delay Procedure. *Microsurgery* **38**, 203–208, doi:10.1002/micr.30249 (2018).

51. Ali, R. S., Garrido, A. & Ramakrishnan, V. Stacked Free Hemi-DIEP Flaps: A Method of Autologous Breast Reconstruction in a Patient with Midline Abdominal Scarring. *Br J Plast Surg* **55**, 351–353, doi:10.1054/bjps.2002.3834 (2002).

52. Hallock, G. G. Simultaneous Transposition of Anterior Thigh Muscle and Fascia Flaps: An Introduction to the Chimera Flap Principle. *Ann Plast Surg* **27**, 126–131, doi:10.1097/00000637-199108000-00006 (1991).

53. Dohle, E. et al. Macrophage-Mediated Angiogenic Activation of Outgrowth Endothelial Cells in Co-Culture with Primary Osteoblasts. *Eur Cell Mater* **27**, 149–164; discussion 164–165, doi:10.22203/ecm.v027a12 (2014).
54. Taylor, G. I. & Palmer, J. H. The Vascular Territories (Angiosomes) of the Body: Experimental Study and Clinical Applications. *Br J Plast Surg* **40**, 113–141, doi: 10.1016/0007-1226(87)90185-8 (1987).
55. Saint-Cyr, M., Wong, C., Schaverien, M., Mojallal, A. & Rohrich, R. J. The Perforasome Theory: Vascular Anatomy and Clinical Implications. *Plast Reconstr Surg* **124**, 1529–1544, doi:10.1097/PRS.0b013e3181b98a6c (2009).
56. Folkman, J. & Hochberg, M. Self-Regulation of Growth in Three Dimensions. *J Exp Med* **138**, 745–753, doi:10.1084/jem.138.4.745 (1973).
57. Carmeliet, P. Mechanisms of Angiogenesis and Arteriogenesis. *Nat Med* **6**, 389–395, doi:10.1038/74651 (2000).
58. Drake, C. J. Embryonic and Adult Vasculogenesis. *Birth Defects Res C Embryo Today* **69**, 73–82, doi:10.1002/bdrc.10003 (2003).
59. Roostalu, U. & Wong, J. K. Arterial Smooth Muscle Dynamics in Development and Repair. *Dev Biol* **435**, 109–121, doi:10.1016/j.ydbio.2018.01.018 (2018).
60. Roostalu, U. et al. Distinct Cellular Mechanisms Underlie Smooth Muscle Turnover in Vascular Development and Repair. *Circ Res* **122**, 267–281, doi:10.1161/CIRCRESAHA.117.312111 (2018).
61. Wong, R. et al. Angiogenesis and Tissue Formation Driven by an Arteriovenous Loop in the Mouse. *Sci Rep* **9**, 10478, doi:10.1038/s41598-019-46571-4 (2019).
62. Kim, S. & von Recum, H. Endothelial Stem Cells and Precursors for Tissue Engineering: Cell Source, Differentiation, Selection, and Application. *Tissue Eng Part B Rev* **14**, 133–147, doi:10.1089/teb.2007.0304 (2008).
63. Hegen, A. et al. Efficient In Vivo Vascularization of Tissue-Engineering Scaffolds. *J Tissue Eng Regen Med* **5**, e52–e62, doi:10.1002/term.336 (2011).
64. Sundberg, C., Kowanetz, M., Brown, L. F., Detmar, M. & Dvorak, H. F. Stable Expression of Angiopoietin-1 and Other Markers by Cultured Pericytes: Phenotypic Similarities to a Subpopulation of Cells in Maturing Vessels During Later Stages of Angiogenesis In Vivo. *Lab Invest* **82**, 387–401, doi:10.1038/labinvest.3780433 (2002).
65. Caporali, A. et al. Contribution of Pericyte Paracrine Regulation of the Endothelium to Angiogenesis. *Pharmacol Ther* **171**, 56–64, doi:10.1016/j.pharmthera.2016.10.001 (2017).
66. Lee, K., Silva, E. A. & Mooney, D. J. Growth Factor Delivery-Based Tissue Engineering: General Approaches and a Review of Recent Developments. *J R Soc Interface* **8**, 153–170, doi:10.1098/rsif.2010.0223 (2011).
67. Williams, I. M. & Wu, J. C. Generation of Endothelial Cells from Human Pluripotent Stem Cells. *Arterioscler Thromb Vasc Biol* **39**, 1317–1329, doi:10.1161/ATVBAHA.119.312265 (2019).
68. Papadopulos, N. A. et al. The Impact of Harvesting Systems and Donor Characteristics on Viability of Nucleated Cells in Adipose Tissue: A First Step Towards a Manufacturing Process. *J Craniofac Surg* **30**, 716–720, doi:10.1097/SCS.0000000000005310 (2019).
69. Shamloo, A., Xu, H. & Heilshorn, S. Mechanisms of Vascular Endothelial Growth Factor-Induced Pathfinding by Endothelial Sprouts in Biomaterials. *Tissue Eng Part A* **18**, 320–330, doi:10.1089/ten.TEA.2011.0323 (2012).
70. Kolesky, D. B., Homan, K. A., Skylar-Scott, M. A. & Lewis, J. A. Three-Dimensional Bioprinting of Thick Vascularized Tissues. *Proc Natl Acad Sci USA* **113**, 3179, doi:10.1073/pnas.1521342113 (2016).
71. Skylar-Scott, M. A. et al. Biomanufacturing of Organ-Specific Tissues with High Cellular Density and Embedded Vascular Channels. *Sci Adv* **5**, eaaw2459, doi:10.1126/sciadv.aaw2459 (2019).

72. Erol, O. O. & Sira, M. New Capillary Bed Formation with a Surgically Constructed Arteriovenous Fistula. *Plast Reconstr Surg* **66**, 109–115, doi:10.1097/00006534-198007000-00021 (1980).

73. Yap, K. K., Yeoh, G. C., Morrison, W. A. & Mitchell, G. M. The Vascularised Chamber as an In Vivo Bioreactor. *Trends Biotechnol* **36**, 1011–1024, doi:10.1016/j.tibtech.2018.05.009 (2018).

74. Lokmic, Z., Stillaert, F., Morrison, W. A., Thompson, E. W. & Mitchell, G. M. An Arteriovenous Loop in a Protected Space Generates a Permanent, Highly Vascular, Tissue-Engineered Construct. *FASEB J* **21**, 511–522, doi:10.1096/fj.06-6614com (2007).

75. Messina, A. et al. Generation of a Vascularized Organoid Using Skeletal Muscle as the Inductive Source. *FASEB J* **19**, 1570–1572, doi:10.1096/fj.04-3241fje (2005).

76. Dolderer, J. H. et al. Spontaneous Large Volume Adipose Tissue Generation from a Vascularized Pedicled Fat Flap Inside a Chamber Space. *Tissue Eng* **13**, 673–681, doi:10.1089/ten.2006.0212 (2007).

77. Buehrer, G. et al. Combination of BMP2 and MSCs Significantly Increases Bone Formation in the Rat Arterio-Venous Loop Model. *Tissue Eng Part A* **21**, 96–105, doi:10.1089/ten.TEA.2014.0028 (2015).

78. Tee, R. et al. Transplantation of Engineered Cardiac Muscle Flaps in Syngeneic Rats. *Tissue Eng Part A* **18**, 1992–1999, doi:10.1089/ten.TEA.2012.0151 (2012).

79. Partyka, P. P. et al. Harnessing Neurovascular Interaction to Guide Axon Growth. *Sci Rep* **9**, 2190, doi:10.1038/s41598-019-38558-y (2019).

80. Burnstock, G. & Ralevic, V. New Insights into the Local Regulation of Blood Flow by Perivascular Nerves and Endothelium. *Br J Plast Surg* **47**, 527–543, doi:10.1016/0007-1226(94)90136-8 (1994).

81. Mukouyama, Y. S., Shin, D., Britsch, S., Taniguchi, M. & Anderson, D. J. Sensory Nerves Determine the Pattern of Arterial Differentiation and Blood Vessel Branching in the Skin. *Cell* **109**, 693–705, doi:10.1016/s0092-8674(02)00757-2 (2002).

82. Muangsanit, P., Shipley, R. J. & Phillips, J. B. Vascularization Strategies for Peripheral Nerve Tissue Engineering. *Anat Rec (Hoboken)* **301**, 1657–1667, doi:10.1002/ar.23919 (2018).

83. Casal, D. et al. Reconstruction of a 10-mm-Long Median Nerve Gap in an Ischemic Environment Using Autologous Conduits with Different Patterns of Blood Supply: A Comparative Study in the Rat. *PLOS ONE* **13**, e0195692, doi:10.1371/journal.pone.0195692 (2018).

84. Buckley, G., Wong, J., Metcalfe, A. D. & Ferguson, M. W. Denervation Affects Regenerative Responses in MRL/MpJ and Repair in C57BL/6 Ear Wounds. *J Anat* **220**, 3–12, doi:10.1111/j.1469-7580.2011.01452.x (2012).

85. Frueh, F. S. et al. Prevascularization of Dermal Substitutes with Adipose Tissue-Derived Microvascular Fragments Enhances Early Skin Grafting. *Sci Rep* **8**, 10977, doi:10.1038/s41598-018-29252-6 (2018).

86. Null, M. & Agarwal, M. in *StatPearls*. In: StatPearls [Internet]. (Treasure Island, FL: StatPearls Publishing, 2021). Available from: https://www.ncbi.nlm.nih.gov/books/NBK513247/ (2019).

87. Findlay, M. W., Messina, A., Thompson, E. W. & Morrison, W. A. Long-Term Persistence of Tissue-Engineered Adipose Flaps in a Murine Model to 1 Year: An Update. *Plast Reconstr Surg* **124**, 1077–1084, doi:10.1097/PRS.0b013e3181b59ff6 (2009).

88. Morrison, W. A. et al. Creation of a Large Adipose Tissue Construct in Humans Using a Tissue-Engineering Chamber: A Step Forward in the Clinical Application of Soft Tissue Engineering. *EBioMedicine* **6**, 238–245, doi:10.1016/j.ebiom.2016.03.032 (2016).

89. Liliensiek, S. J., Nealey, P. & Murphy, C. J. Characterization of Endothelial Basement Membrane Nanotopography in Rhesus Macaque as a Guide for Vessel Tissue Engineering. *Tissue Eng Part A* **15**, 2643–2651, doi:10.1089/ten.TEA.2008.0284 (2009).

90. Dimitrievska, S. et al. Glycocalyx-Like Hydrogel Coatings for Small Diameter Vascular Grafts. *Advanced Functional Materials*, **30**(23), 1908963, doi:10.1002/adfm.201908963 (2020).

91. Sheng, Y. & Zhu, L. The Crosstalk Between Autonomic Nervous System and Blood Vessels. *Int J Physiol Pathophysiol Pharmacol* **10**, 17–28 (2018).

92. Varela, F. & Frenk, S. The Organ of Form: Towards a Theory of Biological Shape. *J Soc Biol Syst* **10**, 73–83, doi:10.1016/0140-1750(87)90035-2 (1987).

93. Wilke, J., Schleip, R., Yucesoy, C. A. & Banzer, W. Not Merely a Protective Packing Organ? A Review of Fascia and Its Force Transmission Capacity. *J Appl Physiol (1985)* **124**, 234–244, doi:10.1152/japplphysiol.00565.2017 (2018).

94. Stecco, C. et al. Histological Study of the Deep Fasciae of the Limbs. *J Bodyw Mov Ther* **12**, 225–230, doi:10.1016/j.jbmt.2008.04.041 (2008).

95. Correa-Gallegos, D. et al. Patch Repair of Deep Wounds by Mobilized Fascia. *Nature* **576**, 287–292, doi:10.1038/s41586-019-1794-y (2019).

96. Currie, J. D. et al. Live Imaging of Axolotl Digit Regeneration Reveals Spatiotemporal Choreography of Diverse Connective Tissue Progenitor Pools. *Dev Cell* **39**, 411–423, doi:10.1016/j.devcel.2016.10.013 (2016).

97. Aldeiri, B. et al. Transgelin-Expressing Myofibroblasts Orchestrate Ventral Midline Closure Through TGF-beta Signalling. *Development* **144**, 3336–3348, doi:10.1242/dev.152843 (2017).

98. Taylor, S. H. et al. Tendon is Covered by a Basement Membrane Epithelium that is Required for Cell Retention and the Prevention of Adhesion Formation. *PLOS ONE* **6**, e16337, doi:10.1371/journal.pone.0016337 (2011).

99. Crapo, P. M., Gilbert, T. W. & Badylak, S. F. An Overview of Tissue and Whole Organ Decellularization Processes. *Biomaterials* **32**, 3233–3243, doi:10.1016/j.biomaterials.2011.01.057 (2011).

100. Badylak, S. F. Decellularized Allogeneic and Xenogeneic Tissue as a Bioscaffold for Regenerative Medicine: Factors that Influence the Host Response. *Ann Biomed Eng* **42**, 1517–1527, doi:10.1007/s10439-013-0963-7 (2014).

101. Hillebrandt, K. H. et al. Strategies Based on Organ Decellularization and Recellularization. *Transpl Int* **32**, 571–585, doi:10.1111/tri.13462 (2019).

102. Guyette, J. P. et al. Perfusion Decellularization of Whole Organs. *Nat Protoc* **9**, 1451–1468, doi:10.1038/nprot.2014.097 (2014).

103. Maan, Z. N. et al. Cell Recruitment by Amnion Chorion Grafts Promotes Neovascularization. *J Surg Res* **193**, 953–962, doi:10.1016/j.jss.2014.08.045 (2015).

104. Koob, T. J. et al. Angiogenic Properties of Dehydrated Human Amnion/Chorion Allografts: Therapeutic Potential for Soft Tissue Repair and Regeneration. *Vasc Cell* **6**, 10, doi:10.1186/2045-824X-6-10 (2014).

105. Jank, B. J. et al. Engineered Composite Tissue as a Bioartificial Limb Graft. *Biomaterials* **61**, 246–256, doi:10.1016/j.biomaterials.2015.04.051 (2015).

106. Ott, H. C. et al. Perfusion-Decellularized Matrix: Using Nature's Platform to Engineer a Bioartificial Heart. *Nat Med* **14**, 213–221, doi:10.1038/nm1684 (2008).

107. Song, J. J. et al. Regeneration and Experimental Orthotopic Transplantation of a Bioengineered Kidney. *Nat Med* **19**, 646–651, doi:10.1038/nm.3154 (2013).

108. Gerli, M. F. M., Guyette, J. P., Evangelista-Leite, D., Ghoshhajra, B. B. & Ott, H. C. Perfusion Decellularization of a Human Limb: A Novel Platform for Composite Tissue Engineering and Reconstructive Surgery. *PLOS ONE* **13**, e0191497, doi:10.1371/journal.pone.0191497 (2018).

109. Benias, P. C. et al. Structure and Distribution of an Unrecognized Interstitium in Human Tissues. *Sci Rep* **8**, 4947, doi:10.1038/s41598-018-23062-6 (2018).
110. Engler, A. J., Sen, S., Sweeney, H. L. & Discher, D. E. Matrix Elasticity Directs Stem Cell Lineage Specification. *Cell* **126**, 677–689, doi:10.1016/j.cell.2006.06.044 (2006).
111. Giatsidis, G., Guyette, J. P., Ott, H. C. & Orgill, D. P. Development of a Large-Volume Human-Derived Adipose Acellular Allogenic Flap by Perfusion Decellularization. *Wound Repair Regen* **26**, 245–250, doi:10.1111/wrr.12631 (2018).
112. Jank, B. J. et al. Creation of a Bioengineered Skin Flap Scaffold with a Perfusable Vascular Pedicle. *Tissue Eng Part A* **23**, 696–707, doi:10.1089/ten.TEA.2016.0487 (2017).
113. Scarritt, M. E., Pashos, N. C. & Bunnell, B. A. A Review of Cellularization Strategies for Tissue Engineering of Whole Organs. *Front Bioeng Biotechnol* **3**, 43, doi:10.3389/fbioe.2015.00043 (2015).
114. Yu, J. et al. Induced Pluripotent Stem Cell Lines Derived from Human Somatic Cells. *Science* **318**, 1917–1920, doi:10.1126/science.1151526 (2007).
115. Jiang, W. C. et al. Cryo-Chemical Decellularization of the Whole Liver for Mesenchymal Stem Cells-Based Functional Hepatic Tissue Engineering. *Biomaterials* **35**, 3607–3617, doi:10.1016/j.biomaterials.2014.01.024 (2014).
116. Qian, H. et al. Bone Marrow Mesenchymal Stem Cells Ameliorate Rat Acute Renal Failure by Differentiation into Renal Tubular Epithelial-Like Cells. *Int J Mol Med* **22**, 325–332 (2008).
117. Toma, C., Pittenger, M. F., Cahill, K. S., Byrne, B. J. & Kessler, P. D. Human Mesenchymal Stem Cells Differentiate to a Cardiomyocyte Phenotype in the Adult Murine Heart. *Circulation* **105**, 93–98, doi:10.1161/hc0102.101442 (2002).
118. Guibert, E. E. et al. Organ Preservation: Current Concepts and New Strategies for the Next Decade. *Transfus Med Hemother* **38**, 125–142, doi:10.1159/000327033 (2011).
119. Whitson, B. A. & Black, S. M. Organ Assessment and Repair Centers: The Future of Transplantation is Near. *World J Transplant* **4**, 40–42, doi:10.5500/wjt.v4.i2.40 (2014).
120. Werner, N. L. et al. Ex Situ Perfusion of Human Limb Allografts for 24 Hours. *Transplantation* **101**, e68–e74, doi:10.1097/TP.0000000000001500 (2017).

9 Advances in Biomaterials for Reconstructive Transplantation

Ashish Dhayani and Praveen Kumar Vemula

CONTENTS

Introduction 172
   History of VCA 172
   Immunotherapy in VCA and its Limitations 173
   Need for Localized Therapy and Use of Topical Creams 174
   Biomaterials for Localized Drug Delivery in VCA 174
   Future of Biomaterials and Immunotherapy in Reconstructive
   Transplantation 176
Systemic and Topical Drug Delivery in VCA 177
   Topical Delivery of Immunosuppressants to Prevent Skin Allograft
   Rejection 177
Implantable Materials for Prolonged Drug Delivery and Targeted
Immune Therapies 178
   Nanoparticle-Based Delivery of MPA Upregulated PD-L1 on
   Dendritic Cells and Prolongs Murine Skin Allograft Survival 178
   Sustained Delivery Using Implantable Biomaterials for Corneal
   Allografts 179
On-Demand Drug Delivery Using Biomaterials 180
   Enzyme-Responsive, Injectable Hydrogels for Drug Delivery
   in Limb Allografts 181
   An Ultrasound-Responsive Ionically Crosslinked Hydrogel for
   Targeted Immunotherapy 183
   Macrophage-Targeted Therapy to Induce Hematopoietic Chimerism
   and Long-Term Donor Tolerance 183
Biomaterials for Multi-Drug Therapies to Target Various
Immunomodulatory Pathways 184
   In Situ Forming, Rapamycin-Loaded Implants for Low-Dose
   Immunosuppression in Hindlimb Rodent Allograft 184
   Multi-Stimuli Responsive Hydrogels for Ocular Delivery 185
   Treg-Inducing Microparticles Promote Tolerance and Indefinite
   Graft Survival without Systemic Immunosuppression 185
   Sustained Delivery of CCL22 for Local Recruitment of Tregs
   to Induce Donor-Specific Tolerance in VCA 186

DOI: 10.1201/9780429260179-13

Scope for Future 188
    The Choice of Biomaterial(s) 188
    Early Diagnosis and Better Treatment Options to Prevent
    Rejection Episodes 188
    New Biomaterials for Combination Therapy 188
    Developing Patient Compliant Approaches 189
Conclusion 189
Acknowledgments 190
References 190

INTRODUCTION

HISTORY OF VCA

Reconstructive transplantation, also known as vascularized composite allotransplantation (VCA) or composite tissue transplantation (CTA) is the transplantation of multiple types of tissues as a functional unit such as a hand, face or uterus. Ever since reconstructive surgery had been practiced, an Italian plastic surgeon, Gaspare Tagliacozzi (1547–1599) is recognized as the pioneer of the field of plastic surgery (portrait, Figure 9.1)[1]. Tagliacozzi popularized the field of plastic surgery,

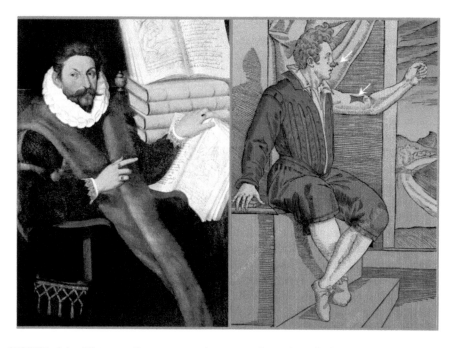

FIGURE 9.1 History of reconstructive transplantation. Left: Portrait of Gaspare Tagliacozzi. Right: One of Gaspare Tagliacozzi's methods for replacing a missing nose. Here we see the healed patient with a new nose and a missing section of skin on his upper arm (white arrows). This skin has been used to form his new nose.

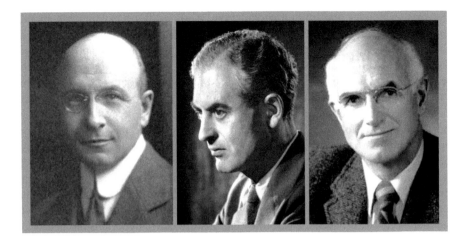

FIGURE 9.2   Pioneers in the field. Pioneering efforts from doctors and researchers in the field of transplantation surgery and immunology that paved the way for the future of VCA and also earned them Nobel Prizes in their respective fields. From left to right: Dr. Alexis Carrel, Dr. Peter Medawar and Dr. Joseph Murray.

and particularly rhinoplasty, in the 16th century. His book on plastic surgery is called *De Curtorum Chirurgia Per Institionem* (1597) (see illustration, Figure 9.1).

In the field of transplantation, contributions from three pioneers (Figure 9.2) have enormously impacted. Alexis Carrel in 1900s carried out the first successful orthotropic hindlimb transplants in dogs. For his pioneering efforts, he received a Nobel Prize in 1912[2]. Peter Medawar studied and demonstrated that the specific characteristics of rejection process such as latency, memory and specificity were a consequence of an active immune response mounted on the donor graft by the recipient. These studies laid the foundation of the study of modern immunology and the basis of immunological tolerance and earned Peter Medawar a Nobel Prize in 1960[3]. Another surgeon, Joseph Murray, performed the first successful kidney transplantation study in identical twins[4]. For his pioneering efforts in organ transplantation, Joseph Murray was awarded a Nobel Prize in Physiology and Medicine in 1990. However, the first successful limb allograft transplantation was performed in Lyon, France, in 1998. Since then, several such tissues have been allografted, ranging from pharynx, abdominal wall, uterus, penis, tongue, ear and scalp, bone and joint, upper and lower extremities[5].

IMMUNOTHERAPY IN VCA AND ITS LIMITATIONS

VCA is not a life-saving surgery as opposed to solid organ transplantation (SOT). Hence, the clinicians' major dilemma is if they can justify the lifelong daily use of immunosuppressants and their co-morbidities with the aesthetic and functional outcomes seen in the patients. In other words, what is the cost-benefit ratio? The holy grail in VCA is to develop an immunomodulation protocol to induce indefinite donor-specific tolerance, without the need for long-term systemic immunosuppression.

The first principles for immunomodulation in allograft transplants are mostly derived from that of SOT. Thus, various strong immunosuppressive drugs such as tacrolimus (FK506), cyclosporine A (CsA), sirolimus (rapamycin), anti-thymocyte globulin (ATG) and various monoclonal antibodies (mAbs) were used before the transplantation is performed and administered for several months thereafter[6]. This is to ensure that the graft is not rejected within the first-year post-surgery since the chances of graft rejection are extremely high during this time period (~85–90%)[7]. This high dose is followed by maintenance therapy, where the doses of stronger immunosuppressive drugs are tapered along with administration of milder drugs such as rapamycin and mycophenolate mofetil (MMF). Depending on the severity, the immunotherapy is modified thereafter but has to be carried out daily and lifelong. This poses a high risk for a VCA patient where side effects of the immunotherapy such as abnormal hair growth, nephrotoxicity, hepatotoxicity, electrolyte and metabolic disturbances, gastrointestinal disturbances, hypertension, neurotoxicity, various malignancies, increased risk of opportunistic infections and multi-organ failure further lead to increased risk of graft loss[8,9]. This plethora of side effects present us an opportunity to design newer and innovative ways of performing immunotherapy that are different from conventional approaches and increase patient compliance.

NEED FOR LOCALIZED THERAPY AND USE OF TOPICAL CREAMS

The advantage of VCA over SOT is that the VCA graft offers a unique opportunity for visual monitoring of the graft. Thus, the signs of rejection can be spotted early on, and doctors can intervene accordingly. Thus, topical creams of tacrolimus (0.1% w/w, Protopic)[10,11], pimecrolimus (Elidel)[12] and clobetasol propionate[13] have already been approved by US Food and Drug Administration (FDA) for use as adjunctive to routine systemic immunosuppression for various diseases. Moreover, since the skin is considered to be the most immunogenic component of VCA, there is a need to develop topical creams for various drugs such as CsA, rapamycin and MMF. However, not all of them are equally effective. Localized delivery of immunosuppressive drugs can selectively inhibit several immune responses such as T cell priming, activation of antigen-presenting cells, production of antibodies from B cells and antigen presentation at secondary lymphoid organs. Thus, it enables a reduction in drug dosage and controlling the immune reaction[14,15].

BIOMATERIALS FOR LOCALIZED DRUG DELIVERY IN VCA

Localized immunosuppression with biomaterials has several advantages compared to conventional systemic drug delivery, especially in VCA (Figure 9.3)[16].

Most oral capsules/systemically delivered drugs are rapidly cleared by the first-pass metabolism and excreted out, making them less bioavailable. Typically, in the oral route, drugs are degraded in gastric fluids by low pH, various enzymes and bacteria present in the gastrointestinal tract. Hence, a small portion of the drugs actually reaches the targeted organ, thus requiring frequent dosing, strict patient compliance and close monitoring of drug levels. This can be overcome by site-specific drug

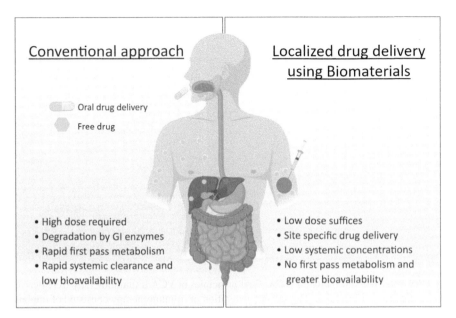

FIGURE 9.3   Conventional versus localized drug delivery using biomaterials. Schematic showing how local delivery of drugs can help overcome the limitations of systemic drug delivery.

delivery using biomaterials, where the drug is released and acts locally, with a tiny portion reaching the systemic circulation[14–17]. The drug can be maintained for a long time without the need for frequent dosing, thus improving patient compliance while mitigating the side effects.

The first-generation of immunotherapy comprises systemic immunotherapy and local adjunctive therapy with the use of topical creams, emulsions and eye drops (Figure 9.4). These would serve well in only skin grafts or corneal transplants but were not always effective since they did not reach the deeper tissues and hence needed conventional systemic therapy.

The second-generation immunotherapy comprises local immunotherapy with implantable biomaterials for long-term delivery of immunosuppressants in various allografts, including cornea, with prolonged survival of grafts in various animal models. These systems indeed reduced the toxic effects of systemic immunosuppressants. Some of the biomaterials have since shown efficacy in clinical studies and are discussed later in the chapter[18,19]. The biggest limitation of these drug delivery systems (DDSs) was continuous delivery and no control over the release kinetics of the drugs along with the invasive procedure, which posed a significant problem.

The third generation of biomaterials designed to sense and titrate the right amount of drug depending on the physiological need or the severity of the disease addresses the problems mentioned above. This approach provided control over the unwanted release of the drug when it is not needed and reduced side effects. This approach has been demonstrated successfully in preclinical studies.

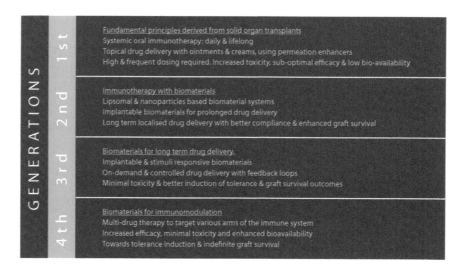

GENERATIONS

1st
Fundamental principles derived from solid organ transplants
Systemic oral immunotherapy: daily & lifelong
Topical drug delivery with ointments & creams, using permeation enhancers
High & frequent dosing required. Increased toxicity, sub-optimal efficacy & low bio-availability

2nd
Immunotherapy with biomaterials
Lipsomal & nanoparticles based biomaterial systems
Implantable biomaterials for prolonged drug delivery
Long term localised drug delivery with better compliance & enhanced graft survival

3rd
Biomaterials for long term drug delivery.
Implantable & stimuli responsive biomaterials
On-demand & controlled drug delivery with feedback loops
Minimal toxicity & better induction of tolerance & graft survival outcomes

4th
Biomaterials for immunomodulation
Multi-drug therapy to target various arms of the immune system
Increased efficacy, minimal toxicity and enhanced bioavailability
Towards tolerance induction & indefinite graft survival

FIGURE 9.4 Biomaterials for VCA. First principles of VCA immunotherapy were derived from solid organ transplants. The second generation of immunotherapy consisted of implantable biomaterials for long-term drug delivery. The third generation had stimuli-responsive materials developed for on-demand drug delivery. The fourth generation focuses on multi-drug therapy along with delivery of bio-therapeutics.

The fourth generation of biomaterials are designed based on an understanding of the immunobiology of the disease to deliver biomolecules as therapeutics in extremely minute quantities yet achieve the right efficacy when administered with conventional immunotherapy. Moreover, various drug combinations and multiple stimuli-triggered drug release have been developed along with short induction protocols similar to clinical therapies and can be easily adapted if successful.

FUTURE OF BIOMATERIALS AND IMMUNOTHERAPY IN RECONSTRUCTIVE TRANSPLANTATION

The need for site-specific drug delivery in VCA was realized very early in the time since the SOT field faced the same problem. However, clinicians and researchers had to address several problems pertaining to VCA, such as the choice of the biomaterial, immunomodulation therapy, encapsulation of right drug(s) combo, fine-tuned release kinetics, biodegradability, biocompatibility, site of administration and patient compliance, among others. Hence, even though several preclinical studies have shown the efficacy of the drug and the importance of biomaterial for drug delivery, we still have a long way to go before anything reaches to the clinics. As we gather more knowledge from the immunobiology of the disease, it would be interesting to apply them in the context of the better design of drug delivery vehicles. Also, biological molecules as therapeutics need to be carefully studied since they have multiple interacting partners. Thus, multiple approaches culminating into a single standard of care might benefit the patients and help change the risk-benefit ratio in favor of patients.

SYSTEMIC AND TOPICAL DRUG DELIVERY IN VCA

Since the first principles governing immunotherapy were adopted from SOT, systemic delivery of drugs was practiced. The approval of new immunosuppressive agents in the 1990s, such as tacrolimus, cyclosporine microemulsion, rapamycin and MMF led to rapid advances in VCA immunobiology and immunopharmacology. It increased the choice of drugs that can be used for maintenance immunosuppression. The immunomodulation post-transplantation began with induction therapy using anti-lymphocyte serum (ALS) or ATG to deplete the patient's lymphocytes, followed by maintenance immunosuppression using tacrolimus, rapamycin, MMF, CsA and corticosteroids such as prednisolone[6,20]. VCA involves multiple tissue types with different tissues having different antigenicity. Skin and muscle are typically the most immunogenic, and they are more accessible to immunotherapy. Hence, a lot of topical formulations were developed and approved. However, not everything worked as effectively as it should, and most topical creams are used only as adjunctive therapies. Moreover, most immunosuppressive agents had a plethora of side effects, but the huge choice of drugs meant that many could be tried depending on the patients' reaction to a particular drug. Limitations of individual drugs led clinicians to try combinations of drugs, and several synergistic partners were discovered to improve rejection prophylaxis[21–23]. This allowed a reduction in dosage with broadening of the therapeutic window.

TOPICAL DELIVERY OF IMMUNOSUPPRESSANTS TO PREVENT SKIN ALLOGRAFT REJECTION

In one of the first studies of local immunotherapy, Billingham et al. reported that the topical use of cortisone acetate administered at a lower than systemic dose protected the skin grafts in rabbits[24]. However, it was not until several decades of research and discovery of new immunosuppressants that something became clinically successful. One of the first successful clinical studies showing the safety and efficacy of local immunotherapy was demonstrated using aerosolized Cyclosporin A (CsA) in acute[25] and chronic[26] lung transplants. Bertelmann and colleagues showed that topical MMF could not prevent rejection of rodent corneal allografts in an experimental keratoplasty model[27]. Very recently, a study by Feturi et al. described a topical formulation of mycophenolic acid (MPA) with optimal skin permeation characteristics[28]. The release of MPA was studied *in vitro* and *in vivo* such that no systemic side effects were observed. However, the formulation needs to be studied in an animal model of skin allograft to study its feasibility in preventing skin rejection.

Another study by Solari et al. showed the efficacy of topical tacrolimus in preventing acute skin rejection[11]. In a Wistar-Furth to Lewis orthotropic rat hindlimb transplantation model, they showed that only topical tacrolimus was insufficient to prevent rejection. All animals rejected their grafts by day 9. In another group, ALS induction (two doses) along with 21-day systemic CsA could sustain the graft on an average up to 40 days. The group with the combination of induction protocol and systemic immunosuppression along with topical tacrolimus showed rejection of two grafts on post-operative day (POD) 35 and 56, respectively, with the rest four animals reaching 100-day graft survival, rejection free. Upon histological examination of the two rejected grafts, it was found that the rejecting animals showed a severe immune reaction to the hypodermis and muscle tissue, sparing the epidermis. Also, the systemic levels of tacrolimus were low or undetectable with skin levels being 100-fold higher than the underlying muscle tissue. The induction protocol was the one typically followed during conventional immunotherapy, which included T cell depletion (ALS induction therapy) along with systemic immunosuppression (using CsA). This showed the feasibility of using topical tacrolimus as an adjunct therapy to prevent acute rejection of the skin component of composite tissue allograft, reducing the morbidity associated with systemic immunosuppression.

IMPLANTABLE MATERIALS FOR PROLONGED DRUG DELIVERY AND TARGETED IMMUNE THERAPIES

By recognizing the importance of site-specific drug delivery, various groups have designed biomaterials to release drugs long-term for maintenance therapies. Attempts were also made to tackle the local immune system at the graft to control the overall immune reaction better and, at the same time, keep the global immune response intact to fight off various other pathogens. Several examples of corneal transplants, skin grafts and hindlimb VCAs have been described and studied in detail. Some of these have even reached clinical trials and are discussed below.

NANOPARTICLE-BASED DELIVERY OF MPA UPREGULATED PD-L1 ON DENDRITIC CELLS AND PROLONGS MURINE SKIN ALLOGRAFT SURVIVAL

Nanoparticles (NPs) are an excellent choice of drug delivery vehicle for VCA since they are highly tunable, can be used for targeting specific locations, can preferentially accumulate at sites of inflammation due to increased permeability of blood vessels, can be cleared by the reticuloendothelial system and transported to secondary lymphoid organs where immune cell maturation occurs. Delivery of an immunosuppressive agent at such sites can have significant benefits since it can alter immune cell maturation, hence control the immune reaction before it starts. Moreover, the effect is more localized, leading to local immunosuppression, sparing the global immune response. Poly lactic-co-glycolic acid (PLGA) is an FDA-approved safe and biocompatible polymer used in various biomedical applications. The study by Shirali et al. demonstrated the fabrication of MPA-encapsulated PLGA NPs[29]. Conventional systemic MPA maintenance immunosuppression is associated with adverse gastrointestinal toxicity, anemia and splenic cytopenia. Localized or targeted MPA delivery can prevent the systemic effects due to reduced drug dosages along with the selective effect on immune cells, thus leading to better outcomes. The study showed a significant allograft survival, where NPs loaded with MPA were administered intermittently (NP-MPA, 5 doses of 5 mg NP-MPA, ~250 µg MPA total dose), compared to intermittent injections of i.p. administered MPA (5 doses of 5 mg MPA giving total dose of 25 mg MPA). Even though the amount of MPA in NPs was 100-fold lower than conventional treatment (daily administered MPA group from day 1–14, 5 mg MPA/day, total dose of 70 mg MPA), significantly higher allograft survival was observed in NP-MPA treated group. Moreover, endocytosis of NP-MPA by dendritic cells led to upregulation of PD-L1, which reduced the priming of alloreactive T cells, further leading to improved graft survival outcomes. Combining NP-MPA with co-stimulatory blockade using CTLA-4Ig and anti-CD154 further improved skin allograft survival, indicating that the use of multiple therapeutics might help to achieve better graft outcomes.

SUSTAINED DELIVERY USING IMPLANTABLE BIOMATERIALS FOR CORNEAL ALLOGRAFTS

Systemic delivery of drugs in the cornea is difficult because of its avascular nature. It is also an immune-privileged site because of the blood-ocular barrier. Hence, a high dose of systemic drug administration is required, leading to side effects. Local delivery using implantable materials will help overcome these barriers and long-term sustained release leading to improved patient compliance.

A study by Shi et al. using tacrolimus containing PGLC implants in a rabbit model of high-risk penetrating keratoplasty showed survival for >180 days without rejection in corneal allografts (Figure 9.5)[30]. The implant contained 0.5 mg of tacrolimus mixed with PGLC and made into a cylinder, 1.5 mm long and 1 mm in diameter. The implant could sustain drug levels of ~10–20 ng/mL in aqueous humor up to the study period, explaining the prevention of graft rejection. Systemic blood levels were <0.3 ng/mL, which prevented the toxic side effects of tacrolimus caused by conventional delivery. Moreover, there was a complete absence of neovascularization, which is the most prevalent cause of corneal allograft rejection, and the sustained drug levels were maintained up to 24 weeks.

Follow up study by the same group reported the use of rapamycin-loaded PGLC polymer-based intraocular DDS in a rabbit model of high-risk penetrating keratoplasty[31]. A 0.5 mg rapamycin-loaded PGLC implantable DDS was successful in

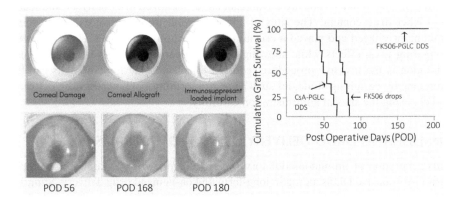

FIGURE 9.5 **Implantable biomaterials for corneal allografts.** The top left shows a schematic for implantable materials for corneal transplantation. Kaplan-Meier survival plots showing FK-loaded poly glycolide-co-lactide-co-caprolactone (PGLC) implants led to no rejection of corneal allografts up to 180 days. The bottom left shows representative images from the FK-PGLC implant group at various PODs.

preventing corneal allograft rejection in New Zealand rabbits with a median survival time (MST) of >90 days compared to four times daily administered rapamycin eye drops that showed graft survival of only 36 days. Pro-inflammatory markers such as interleukin-2R (IL-2R), monocyte chemoattractant protein-1 (MCP-1), tumor necrosis factor α (TNF-α) and vascular endothelial growth factor (VEGF) were detectable in all groups but were not detected in the rapamycin-PGLC group. Moreover, a high concentration of rapamycin in the aqueous humor is crucial for preventing rejection. This was shown by maintaining steady levels in the implant group (7–12 ng/mL). On the contrary, rapamycin was undetectable in the eye drop group and the two animals from the implant group that were rejecting.

An earlier study from the same group using CsA-PGLC implants showed graft survival of 90 days compared to using eye drops containing the same drug[32]. A long-term clinical study was undertaken in patients with corneal blindness, from 2003 to 2011, to test the feasibility of corneal allograft survival using CsA-loaded PGLC implants[18]. CsA was chosen based on its superior pharmacological profile. A total of 92 patients underwent corneal transplantation wherein each implant containing 1 mg CsA was placed in the anterior chamber of the eye. The implant was found to degrade between the 5- and 13-month range (average 7.6±4.3 months) depending on individual rather than disease condition. Thus, 6-month survival was considered successful, considering the biodegradability of implants. Out of the 92 eyes that underwent surgery, 88% (81 eyes) were considered successful, while 7.6% (seven eyes) showed partial success and 4.3% (four eyes) were a failure. Overall mean graft survival time was 36.1±17.7 months (12.3 to the 61.6-month range). The corneal endothelial cell density is considered as a read-out of the toxicity of the implant. The initial and 6-month post keratoplasty endothelial cell numbers had not changed significantly, indicating the non-toxic nature of the implants. The anterior chamber as the site for implantation was the perfect choice as it could help maintain the therapeutic drug amount for an extended period locally without any toxic effects.

Implantable biomaterials are advantageous for localized drug delivery and loading higher drug content. The sites of administration in the above examples were immune-privileged and played a crucial role in sustaining the drug release without generating toxic effects while showing efficient clearance. However, their biggest limitation is the invasive procedure required for placing the implant. This can be overcome by designing strategies such as *in situ* forming implants for drug delivery and choosing the sites of administration carefully.

ON-DEMAND DRUG DELIVERY USING BIOMATERIALS

This generation of immunomodulatory therapy comprised of examples of the first stimuli-responsive DDSs aiding in long-term and on-demand drug delivery. Stimuli-responsive systems (SRS) typically identify a physiological marker that is used as a cue for drug delivery (Figure 9.6). Various types of physiological markers have been identified and used as triggers for drug delivery. Some of these markers include enzymes that are over/under-expressed during individual disease conditions[33,34], pH changes occurring during certain disease states (tumors, wound healing, gastric delivery)[35,36], redox[37], hyperthermia, adenosine triphosphate[38] and other

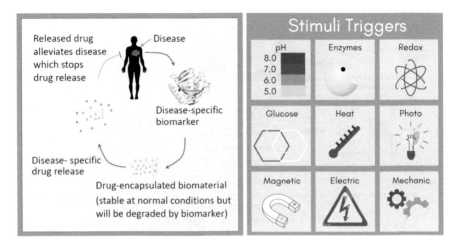

FIGURE 9.6   Stimuli-responsive drug delivery. Left: Schematic showing disease marker-specific drug release from the biomaterial. Right: Various types of stimuli triggers can be identified to design on-demand drug delivery vehicles. Some of these are shown here.

metabolites[39,40]. Various external stimuli can also be used to trigger drug delivery *in vivo*. Such stimuli would include ultrasound-mediated drug delivery[41], light-triggered drug release[42], electric[43] and magnetic field[44] triggered drug release systems.

ENZYME-RESPONSIVE, INJECTABLE HYDROGELS FOR DRUG DELIVERY IN LIMB ALLOGRAFTS

Hydrogels comprise of small amphiphilic molecules that can self-assemble due to weak intermolecular forces such as H-bonding, electrostatic interactions, π-π interactions, hydrophobicity and van der Waals forces to form 3D matrices. In turn, these matrices can trap one or more drug molecules, and release them in response to physiological cues. Gajanayake et al. reported one such enzyme-responsive hydrogel-based system that was prepared from an amphiphile, triglycerolmonostearate (TGMS) (Figure 9.7)[45]. TGMS was chosen from several FDA-approved *generally recognized as safe agents* for two major reasons: (a) It has the ability to self-assemble into hydrogels and encapsulate immunosuppressants, and (b) it has an ester group that can be cleaved by the action of esterases and matrix metalloproteinases, overexpressed during the rejection episodes of an allograft. Thus, the overexpressed enzymes during rejection episodes will mediate the degradation of the hydrogel, thus releasing the drug that can control the rejection episode. Eventually, it leads to lowering the enzyme concentration, providing a feedback loop to reduce the drug release. The *in vitro* release kinetics clearly showed that the purified enzymes could trigger the release of the tacrolimus from TGMS hydrogels. Activated macrophage culture media, used as a proxy for inflammation, triggered the release of tacrolimus from TGMS hydrogels in a dose-dependent manner. On the contrary, conditioned media from non-activated macrophages could not degrade gel to release the drug. In a later study published by Dzhonova et al., it was conclusively shown that tacrolimus

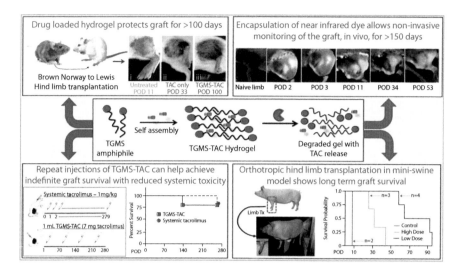

FIGURE 9.7   On demand, inflammatory enzyme-triggered drug release using TGMS-Tacrolimus (TAC) hydrogels. Development of the TGMS-TAC hydrogel system and results of graft survival in various animal models.

release could be mediated by inflammatory enzymes, *in vivo*[46]. Moreover, loading of a near-infrared dye (NIRD) in tacrolimus-containing hydrogels enabled non-invasive monitoring of TGMS drug depot, *in vivo*. It was observed that a single dose of this hydrogel containing 7 mg tacrolimus injected locally could enhance graft survival to >100 days, whereas the control group given free tacrolimus showed a MST of only 33 days. Moreover, the group with no treatment or only vehicle injection rejected the grafts within 11 days.

In another series of experiments performed by Dzhonova et al., it was shown that long-term side effects of tacrolimus systemic therapy could be mitigated by using TGMS-TAC-based localized drug delivery. Repeat injections of TGMS-TAC hydrogels once every 70 days could enhance the graft survival up to 280 days[47]. In another group of rats, a systemic daily dose of 1 mg/kg tacrolimus was required for the same effect, essentially showing the hydrogel-based therapy to be more patient compliant. The hydrogel group showed lower systemic drug levels and four times lower total drug amount compared to the systemic group. Blood urea nitrogen and creatinine levels were significantly lower in the hydrogel group, indicating no renal toxicity compared to the systemic group. The systemic drug group also showed lymphoma in one animal and bacterial infection in another animal, common side effects of systemic immunosuppression. On the other hand, the hydrogel group showed an absence of malignancies or opportunistic infections and a stable graft.

As an extension of the above studies, TGMS-TAC hydrogels were tested in a study by Fries et al. in a mini-swine orthotopic forelimb allograft model[48]. The idea of the study was to determine a tolerable dose to prolong graft survival in a large animal model. A high dose (91 mg tacrolimus) and a low dose (49 mg tacrolimus) groups were chosen for the study, respectively. Surprisingly, the low dose group showed graft survival ranging from 56 to 93 days, whereas the high dose group showed an allograft survival of 24–42 days. Untreated animals showed Banff Grade IV acute rejection by POD 6. This validates that the TGMS-TAC system could be developed as a potential therapeutic for future clinical studies with a few caveats in mind. Long-term studies with low dose immunosuppression, say every 30–40 days, should be carried out in large animal studies to check for drug toxicity, efficacy and graft tolerance. Moreover, adjunctive therapy, such as topical tacrolimus or rapamycin, can be used to prevent acute rejection. The study did not use any adjunctive therapies to prevent the confounding effects of these to TGMS-TAC therapy. Also, the dosing of individual immunosuppressants needs to be optimized according to the animal model used. Lastly, to reach closer to a clinical setting, multi-drug immunosuppression needs to be carried out, which might require further optimization.

AN ULTRASOUND-RESPONSIVE IONICALLY CROSSLINKED HYDROGEL FOR TARGETED IMMUNOTHERAPY

Ionically crosslinked alginate system has been well studied and adapted for various biomedical applications. Mooney's group had reported an ultrasound responsive alginate system to deliver mitoxantrone for enhanced chemotherapy in breast cancer[49]. The same system was later used in collaboration with Gorantla's group for mono and dual drug therapy in Brown Norway (BN) to Lewis hindlimb VCA[50]. A study by Feturi et al. showed that alginate-based hydrogels can be used for encapsulation of either tacrolimus (10 mg/1 mL gel), rapamycin (10 mg/mL) or tacrolimus + rapamycin (10 mg/mL each) and followed their release *in vivo* using LC-MS/MS. The system could provide continuous drug delivery without stimulation and in an on-demand manner depending on the ultrasound pulse. The rapamycin group showed an MST of 21 days, whereas both the other groups showed an increased graft survival of >100 days. Interestingly, dual drug encapsulation could not enhance graft survival compared to tacrolimus monotherapy. Systemic toxicity was monitored by percent body weight change and creatinine clearance tests. There was only ≤15% body weight change in the first 2 weeks post-transplantation, which was stabilized and increased thereafter. Additionally, there was no significant difference in the rate of creatinine clearance, which showed a lack of systemic toxicity.

These examples suggest that by using SRS, we could address the need of timely drug delivery with minimal side effects of drugs. These systems may increase patient compliance due to less frequent administration. TGMS-based system showed reliance in a rodent as well as porcine models of allograft transplantation. There is an urgent need for further preclinical trials for dose optimization in both the ultrasound-responsive and enzyme-responsive systems so that they can be further translated to clinics.

MACROPHAGE-TARGETED THERAPY TO INDUCE HEMATOPOIETIC CHIMERISM AND LONG-TERM DONOR TOLERANCE

Li et al. showed that selective targeting and depletion of macrophages using clodronate-loaded liposomes could induce hematopoietic chimerism and donor-specific allograft tolerance in a murine model of skin allograft[51]. After the bone marrow transplantation, transplantation of skin allografts on day 90 and day 180 showed no rejection of donor skin, without any systemic immunosuppression therapy, which suggests the induction of tolerance to donor skin. Moreover, third-party allografts were quickly rejected, suggesting the tolerance was specific only to the donor skin from which bone marrow transplant (BMT) had been carried out. The study showed that small molecule targeted therapy could be used to prevent rejection of the most immunogenic component of the allograft, the skin. However, clodronate is a toxic compound and led to ~30% mortality. Another agent with lesser mortality or use of milder dose or a different slow-releasing platform can be used to study this further. Moreover, the study should be repeated in a rodent hindlimb model to confirm its applicability in VCA.

BIOMATERIALS FOR MULTI-DRUG THERAPIES TO TARGET VARIOUS IMMUNOMODULATORY PATHWAYS

The current generation of immunotherapy desires the need to design and test multi-drug therapies using various biomaterials. Multiple drugs act on different immune cells for enhanced immunomodulatory effects and long-term graft survival. This can be achieved using prodrug-based biomaterials or materials that can encapsulate and deliver bio-therapeutics to tackle various arms of the immune system. Some of the examples presented here have already shown promise in the preclinical stage and are ready to be taken forward in larger animal models.

Tolerance induction using regulatory T cells (Tregs) has received a major attention in the past decade for most disorders with the immune system in hyperdrive. Webster et al. described an *in vivo* Treg expansion protocol using IL-2-mAb complexes[52]. An injection daily for 3 days induced a 10-fold increase in Tregs, which were found in the liver, gut, spleen and lymph nodes. Pretreatment with IL-2-mAb complexes rendered the mice resistant to induction of experimental autoimmune encephalo-myelitis. Pretreatment also allowed long-term acceptance of islet allografts with-out immunosuppression. Xu and colleagues have used the same strategy to prevent graft rejection in a murine model of orthotropic hindlimb transplant[53]. Using the complexes pre and post-treatment significantly increased the graft survival time, with pretreatment showing significantly prolonged time compared to even the post-transplant group. The complexes also led to the reduction of CD4 and CD8 effector T cells (Teffs) and IFN-γ.

IN SITU FORMING, RAPAMYCIN-LOADED IMPLANTS FOR LOW-DOSE IMMUNOSUPPRESSION IN HINDLIMB RODENT ALLOGRAFT

Sutter et al. demonstrated the development of an *in situ* forming PLGA implant-able system loaded with rapamycin[54]. *In situ* forming implants give us the flexibility to load multiple therapeutic molecules without any harsh treatment and the ease of injectability and rapid clearance. The therapy could prevent graft rejection for >100 days (5 mg rapamycin), which was comparable to systemic rapamycin ther-apy administered daily (0.5 mg/kg), leading to a much higher amount of overall dose. Moreover, even though systemic therapy prevented graft rejection for a similar period, most animals developed graft versus host disease (60%). The implant group also showed durable tolerance induction as well as myeloid and lymphoid chimerism by POD 21. There was an induction of Tregs in peripheral blood and VCA skin. The depot was cleared much rapidly from the system without any signs of foreign body reaction, typically seen in hydrogels and other biomaterials. However, the *in situ* forming implants could have been loaded with biotherapeutics such as proteins, which could play a role in regulating Tregs and thus improve graft survival. Multiple drug loading can be optimized, as well.

MULTI-STIMULI RESPONSIVE HYDROGELS FOR OCULAR DELIVERY

Most neuroprotective medications for optic neuropathies are administered as eye drops. However, the bioavailability of drugs is significantly lowered in corneal penetration, which is <5%. Thus, there is an unmet clinical need for the development of trans-corneal drug delivery vehicles. Kabiri et al. reported the development of a stimuli-responsive, *in situ* forming hydrogel for the delivery of cannabigerolic acid (CBGA) to treat glaucoma[55]. The hydrogel was a composite of hyaluronic acid and methylcellulose, both of which are FDA approved. The hydrogel was loaded with polylactic acid and polyethyleneoxide NPs, which were loaded with CBGA. The formulation was optimized to have a switch between temperature-dependent rheopexy (thickening) and thixotropy (shear thinning). The thickening was important for rapid gelation upon contact with the ocular surface and shear thinning behavior was to release the drug with mechanical movement such as the blinking movement of the eye. The study achieved >300% trans-corneal penetration of CBGA compared to control eye drops, showing the efficacy of the treatment. However, its efficacy remains to be established in experimental disease models and follow up in large animal models.

Treg-INDUCING MICROPARTICLES PROMOTE TOLERANCE AND INDEFINITE GRAFT SURVIVAL WITHOUT SYSTEMIC IMMUNOSUPPRESSION

Jhunjhunwala et al. reported a triple therapy formulation for the induction of Tregs *in vivo* from naïve CD4+ cells and reduced inflammation in various experimental disease models[7]. Indeed, Tregs are potent immunomodulators in the body. However, they are a tiny percent (only 2–3%) of total lymphocytes. Hence, the clinical use of Tregs would require their culture and expansion *ex vivo* followed by reinfusion in the patient. This would pose certain challenges such as a need for good manufacturing practices facilities, the natural propensity of Tregs to transdifferentiate into proinflammatory effectors and their relative instability. Natural induction of Tregs is mediated by tolerogenic dendritic cells and certain malignant tumors from CD4+ T cells, as a means to evade the immune system, by using certain Treg-trophic factors such as TGF-ß1 and IL-2. Moreover, rapamycin is a commonly used immunosuppressive drug known to suppress TH1 and TH17 Teff differentiation and regulate Treg suppression maintenance.

Fisher et al. reported a PLGA microparticle (MP) based system encapsulating TGF-ß1, IL-2 and rapamycin (TRI-MP) for induction of Tregs to promote long-term

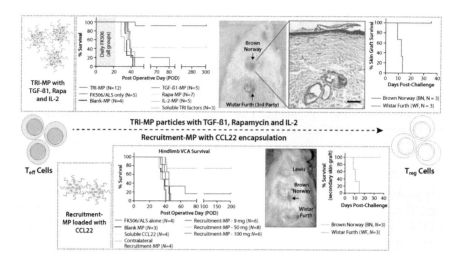

FIGURE 9.8   Induction of Tregs from Teff cells for maintaining immune homeostasis.
The top panel shows the development of the TRI-MP system for graft survival up to 300 days
and donor-specific tolerance induction as shown by acceptance of secondary grafts. Bottom
panels show a similar design of MPs loaded with CCL22, termed as Recruitment MPs with a
graft survival of >200 days. The study showed similar donor-specific tolerance induction as
shown by acceptance of secondary skin grafts and rejection of third-party skin grafts.

allograft tolerance in a BN to Lewis, complete major histocompatibility complex
mismatched hindlimb model (Figure 9.8)[56]. Their immunotherapy consisted of
induction protocol using tacrolimus from 0–21 days along with treatment with rabbit anti-rat ALS (antilymphocyte serum) on day (-4) and day 1. Their experimental
group consisted of the induction protocol along with an injection of TRI-MP on
days 0 and 21. Compared to the controls with only induction protocol, where the
grafts were rejected within 2–3 weeks, the TRI-MP treatment group showed indefinite graft survival (11/12 animals) for >300 days. Moreover, it also imparted donor-
specific tolerance in immunocompetent rats, which was confirmed by acceptance of
secondary skin grafts from donor strains. In contrast, skin grafts from third party
donor strains were rejected. This was one of the first examples of multidrug therapy
for immunomodulation in VCA. The TRI-MP treatment reduced the expression of
inflammatory markers and increased the expression of Treg-associated cytokines
in the allograft tissue. The treatment also leads to a reduction in TH1 populations in
the allografts with an expansion in the number of Tregs, thus showing benefit at
multiple levels. Efficacy and dose optimization for large animals is further required
to translate this approach to the clinic.

Sustained Delivery of CCL22 for Local Recruitment of Tregs to Induce Donor-Specific Tolerance in VCA

The deficiency of Tregs is known to cause destructive inflammation and many autoimmune conditions due to a loss of immune homeostasis. Several reports suggest that

small changes in the number of Tregs are sufficient to dramatically alter favorable local immune response. CCL22 is a chemokine, typically used by various tumors to control the immune response by controlling the number of Tregs. Inspired by the ability of these tumor cells to recruit Tregs using CCL22, Jhunjhunwala et al. developed a PLGA-based system loaded with CCL22 for continuous release and recruitment of Tregs *in vitro* and *in vivo* to restore immune homeostasis[57].

The same formulation was later adapted by Fisher et al. for recruiting Tregs locally in a BN to Lewis model, completely mismatched hindlimb allograft transplants (Figure 9.8, bottom panel)[58]. As per their previous study, they followed the same induction protocol using ALS (day -4 and day 1) and maintenance immunosuppression using tacrolimus from 0 to 21 days. The treatment group further included PLGA MPs loaded with CCL22, Recruitment MPs, which could show sustained CCL22 release of up to 40 days. A 50 mg dose of Recruitment MPs on day 0 and day 21 could prolong graft survival for >200 days (75% animals) compared to baseline immunosuppression, which rejected the grafts between 2–3 weeks post 21-day systemic immunotherapy. The long-term surviving allografts showed enriched Tregs in allograft skin and draining lymph nodes along with enhanced Treg function without affecting the proliferation of conventional T cells, thus maintaining homeostasis. The levels of pro-inflammatory cytokines such as TNF-α, INF-γ, IL-17A, Perforin-1 and serglycin was found to be significantly less than that of skin biopsies from actively rejecting grafts. Furthermore, Recruitment MPs confer donor antigen-specific tolerance in long-term surviving grafts. This was confirmed by challenging long-term BN allografts with non-vascularized, full-thickness skin grafts from Brown Norway (BN) animals (allogeneic) and Wistar Furth (WF) animals (third party, allogeneic) donors. Recruitment MP-treated animals accepted BN allografts as observed by hair growth and wound healing, whereas the third-party WF allografts were rejected as shown by necrosis of the tissue.

Like TRI-MP therapy, dose optimization in larger animal models of VCA should be well studied, and these models are required to translate this strategy for human VCAs. Tuning the right doses is a challenge. Too high a concentration of CCL22 might saturate/lead to internalization of the receptors, inhibiting Treg chemotaxis. On the other hand, too low a concentration might not be capable of affecting and sustaining the migration of Tregs.

Utmost care needs to be taken to evaluate biological molecules as therapeutics since they have multiple interacting partners in their microenvironment. For example, CCL22 can recruit natural killer cells, plasmacytoid dendritic cells, and also enhance the overexpression of CTLA4 on Tregs, which can further lead to immunosuppression. Excessive immunosuppression is also a challenge and is associated with secondary bacterial and viral infections, which might lead to graft loss. Treg induction using TRI-MP can become a limitation if the Tregs transdifferentiate into Teffs, thus losing all advantages of optimal immunosuppression. Therefore, one needs to be cognizant of small changes in doses and how they might affect overall function along with remedies to tackle the problem if and when it happens to salvage the situation without leading to graft loss. We also need to understand that under normal circumstances, there is a balanced immune response. Shifting the balance towards prolonged immunosuppression could mean other abnormalities such as malignancies in long-term usage. This, however, needs to be addressed by long-duration studies along with conventional therapies if required.

SCOPE FOR FUTURE

The unique scenario in the field provides a huge opportunity to develop advanced approaches to tackle issues in VCA.

THE CHOICE OF BIOMATERIAL(S)

Selecting the correct type of biomaterial undeniably plays the most important role in determining the survival of the allograft. Most biomaterials used for drug delivery may lead to unwanted immune activation, especially when present *in vivo* for a long period of time. The right selection of material ensures correct drug release kinetics and adequate clearance without leading to foreign body response. Hence, it could lead to a better scope for clinical translation[59,60].

EARLY DIAGNOSIS AND BETTER TREATMENT OPTIONS TO PREVENT REJECTION EPISODES

Recently, implantable fluorescent hydrogel fibers generated from polyethylene glycol (PEG) and polyacrylamide (PAM) were designed for continuous glucose monitoring for up to 140 days, *in vivo*[61]. Encapsulation of NIRD in TGMS hydrogels was used for non-invasive monitoring of tacrolimus drug depot, *in vivo*[46]. These advanced systems could be used to detect rejection episodes, which will enable better control of immunotherapy and monitoring patients. Conventional monitoring of graft rejection requires a painful and invasive allograft tissue biopsy. Detection of new biomarkers, as well as the use of sentinel flaps, can be employed for monitoring rejection episodes[62]. Kueckelhaus et al. reported a method of non-invasive monitoring of chronic rejection by measuring the facial artery to radial artery intimal thickness ratio using ultrasound bio-microscopy[63].

NEW BIOMATERIALS FOR COMBINATION THERAPY

Although we have developed several materials for on-demand delivery of multi-drugs, which have shown success in preclinical studies, we are yet to optimize these for humans. Encapsulation of multiple drugs is a challenging process. It depends on a variety of factors such as type of material, type of drug(s), amounts of respective drugs and eliminating burst/non-specific release, among others. Therefore, the use of multiple vehicles or approaches that can effectively accommodate multiple drugs with ease, such as prodrug-based approaches[64] and in situ gelation approaches, can be used, where multiple drug depots can be injected at multiple locations[54,65]. In certain cases, the prodrug as well as *in situ* gelation approach can be combined, as shown by Wang et al. for enhanced chemotherapy[66]. They described a prodrug-based supramolecular hydrogelator as a reservoir for long-term, responsive release of both camptothecin and anti-PD-1 antibody, leading to immune stimulation and

PD-1 blockade, showing 100% survival in mice models of GL-261 brain cancer and CT 26 colon cancer models.

DEVELOPING PATIENT COMPLIANT APPROACHES

The biggest hurdle faced by pharma and healthcare is patient non-compliance. Most therapies fail because patients cannot adhere to their medicine routines as they need to take for years. As researchers, we can develop therapies which can be easily followed and efficiently tracked so that the patients do not get bogged down by complicated routines.

Recently, a gastric resident system was described for multi-drug, multi-gram dosing of tuberculosis drugs, which could sustain drug release for at least a month in a porcine model[67]. This would be a highly patient compliant approach even in VCA if we could reduce the dosing frequency from once daily to once monthly. Stimuli-responsive microneedle-based patches have been developed for insulin delivery. They can be easily adapted for rapid drug release and topical drug application in VCA patients[37]. Refillable drug depots have been described in multiple studies by Brudno et al., which can be used to refill drugs with minimal invasion, *in vivo*[68,69]. A similar approach was shown by Wang et al. for refilling immunosuppressive drugs tacrolimus, rapamycin and MPA[70]. However, their efficacy in the VCA model remains to be validated.

Although a series of critical examples have been discussed here, there is a need to extend this list. Various parameters need to be considered to achieve the overall outcome of allograft survival. For example, those aspects include i) tolerance induction using Tregs and mesenchymal stem cells, ii) refined graft preservation procedures, iii) immunosuppression minimization protocols, iv) minimally invasive microsurgical techniques, v) refined rejection criteria and better guidelines to assess the outcomes of graft survival, vi) improved selection criteria, vii) engineering immune tolerant biomaterials, viii) augmenting adaptive and innate immune responses and ix) better human leukocyte antigen (HLA) and cytomegalovirus (CMV) matching[71-74]. The best approach should be developed considering the combination of these factors.

CONCLUSION

Even though the history of VCA is short, multiple studies have shown that the dilemma between graft survival and the co-morbidities of adverse side effects can be avoided by using relevant site-specific DDSs. Even though a small number of VCA surgeries have been performed so far, there is a greater unmet need for more VCA surgeries if the immunosuppression protocols can be optimized to increase patient compliance. Currently used immunosuppressive agents are indispensable in conventional immunosuppression protocols, and immunomodulation protocols are complex. Simplified and individually optimized immunomodulation is possible using biomaterial-based strategies and will play a crucial role in upcoming immunomodulatory therapies. Moreover, there is a scope to adopt these therapeutic regimes for solid organ transplant patients as well if they are successful for VCA patients.

ACKNOWLEDGMENTS

Ashish Dhayani thanks University Grant Commission for Senior Research Fellowship. We thank Devayani Khare for editorial suggestions. Praveen Kumar Vemula thanks in Stem for core funds. The authors have no other relevant affiliations or financial involvement with any organization or entity with a financial interest in or financial conflict with the subject matter or materials discussed in the manuscript apart from those disclosed.

REFERENCES

1. Gander, B. et al. Composite tissue allotransplantation of the hand and face: A new frontier in transplant and reconstructive surgery. *Transpl. Int.* **19**, 868–880 (2006).
2. Toledo-pereyra, L. H. Classics of modern surgery: The unknown man of Alexis Carrel-father of transplantation. *J. Investig. Surg.* **16**, 243–246 (2003).
3. Medawar, P. B. Immunological tolerance. *Nature.* **189**, 14–17 (1961).
4. Murray, J. E., Merrill, J. P. & Harrison, J. H. Renal homotransplantation in identical twins. *J. Am. Soc. Nephrol.* **12**, 201–204 (2001).
5. Taddeo, A., Tsai, C., Vögelin, E. & Rieben, R. Novel targeted drug delivery systems to minimize systemic immunosuppression in vascularized composite allotransplantation. *Curr. Opin. Organ Transplant.* **23**, 1–9 (2018).
6. Gorantla, V. S. et al. Immunosuppressive agents in transplantation: Mechanisms of action and current anti-rejection strategies. *Microsurgery.* **20**, 420–429 (2000).
7. Yang, J. H. & Eun, S. C. Therapeutic application of T regulatory cells in composite tissue allotransplantation. *J. Transl. Med.* **15**, 85–90 (2017).
8. Gruber, S. A. The case for local immunosuppression. *Transplantation.* **54**, 1–11 (1992).
9. Covvey, J. R. & Mancl, E. E. Pharmaceutical care in transplantation: Current challenges and future opportunities. *Nanomedicine.* **14**, 2651–2658 (2019).
10. Lebwohl, M. et al. Tacrolimus ointment is effective for facial and intertriginous psoriasis. *J. Am. Acad. Dermatol.* **51**, 723–730 (2004).
11. Solari, M. G. et al. Daily topical tacrolimus therapy prevents skin rejection in a rodent hind limb allograft model. *Plast. Reconstr. Surg.* **123**, 17–25 (2009).
12. Ang-tiu, C. U., Meghrajani, C. F. & Maano, C. C. Pimecrolimus 1% cream for the treatment of seborrheic dermatitis : A systematic review of randomized controlled trials. *Expert Rev. Clin. Pharmacol.* **5**, 91–97 (2012).
13. Gharb, B. B. et al. Effectiveness of topical immunosuppressants in prevention and treatment of rejection in face allotransplantation. *Transplantation* (2013). doi:10.1097/TP.0b013e31828bca61
14. Schnider, J. T. et al. Site-specific immunosuppression in vascularized composite allotransplantation: prospects and potential. *Clinical and Developmental Immunology* (2013). doi:10.1155/2013/495212
15. Ormerod, A. D., Shah, S. A. A., Copeland, P., Omar, G. & Winfield, A. Treatment of psoriasis with topical sirolimus: Preclinical development and a randomized, double-blind trial. *Br. J. Dermatol.* **152**, 758–764 (2005).
16. Dhayani, A., Kalita, S., Mahato, M., Srinath, P. & Praveen, K. Biomaterials for topical and transdermal drug delivery in reconstructive transplantation. *Nanomedicine.* **20**, 2713–2733 (2019).
17. Al-Lawati, H., Aliabadi, H. M., Makhmalzadeh, B. S. & Lavasanifar, A. Nanomedicine for immunosuppressive therapy: achievements in pre-clinical and clinical research. *Expert Opinion on Drug Delivery* (2018). doi:10.1080/17425247.2018.1420053

18. Shi, W. et al. A novel cyclosporine a drug-delivery system for prevention of human corneal rejection after high-risk keratoplasty: A clinical study. *Ophthalmology.* **120**, 695–702 (2013).

19. Islam, M. M. et al. Biomaterials-enabled cornea regeneration in patients at high risk for rejection of donor tissue transplantation. *NPJ Regen. Med.* **3**, 2 (2018).

20. Kueckelhaus, M. et al. Vascularized composite allotransplantation: current standards and novel approaches to prevent acute rejection and chronic allograft deterioration. *Transplant International* (2016). doi:10.1111/tri.12652

21. Li, Z. et al. CD8+ T-Cell depletion and rapamycin synergize with combined coreceptor/stimulation blockade to induce robust limb allograft tolerance in mice. *American Journal of Transplantation* (2008). doi:10.1111/j.1600-6143.2008.02419.x

22. Zhao, X.-F., Alexander, J. W., Schroeder, T., Babcock, G. F. The synergistic effect of low-dose cyclosporine and flucinolone acetonide on the survival of rat allogeneic skin grafts. *Transplantation.* **46**, 490–492 (1988).

23. Alemdar, A. Y., Sadi, D., McAlister, V. C. & Mendez, I. Liposomal formulations of tacrolimus and rapamycin increase graft survival and fiber outgrowth of dopaminergic grafts. *Cell Transplant.* **13**, 263–271 (2004).

24. Billingham, R. E., Krohn, P. L. & Medawar, P. B. Effect of locally applied cortisone acetate on survival of skin homografts in rabbits. *Br. Med. J.* **2**, 4739 (1951).

25. Keenan, R. J. et al. Treatment of refractory acute allograft rejection with aerosolized Cyclosporine in lung transplant recipients. *J. Throracic Cardiovasc. Surg.* **113**, 335–341 (1997).

26. Iacono, A. T. et al. Aerosolized cyclosporine in lung recipients with refractory chronic rejection. *Am. J. Respir. Crit. Care Med.* **153**, 1451–1455 (1996).

27. Bertelmann, E., de Ruijter, M., Gong, N., Knapp, S. & Pleyer, U. Survival of corneal allografts following topical treatment with the immunomodulator mycophenolate mofetil. *Ophthalmologica.* **224**, 38–41 (2009).

28. Feturi, F. G. et al. Mycophenolic acid for topical immunosuppression in vascularized composite allotransplantation: Optimizing formulation and preliminary evaluation of bioavailability and pharmacokinetics. *Front. Surg.* **5**, 1–11 (2018).

29. Shirali, A. C. et al. Nanoparticle delivery of mycophenolic acid upregulates PD-L1 on dendritic cells to prolong murine allograft survival. *Am. J. Transplant.* **11**, 2582–2592 (2011).

30. Shi, W., Liu, T., Xie, L. & Wang, S. FK506 in a biodegradable glycolide-co-clatide-co-caprolactone polymer for prolongation of corneal allograft survival. *Curr. Eye Res.* **30**, 969–976 (2005).

31. Shi, W., Gao, H., Xie, L. & Wang, S. Sustained intraocular rapamycin delivery effectively prevents high-risk corneal allograft rejection and neovascularization in rabbits. *Investig. Ophthalmol. Vis. Sci.* **47**, 3339–3344 (2006).

32. Wang, S. G., Xie, L. X., Bei, J. Z., Shi, W. Y. & Cai, Q. An implantable immuno-suppressive cyclosporine drug delivery system. *Key Eng. Mater.* **288–289**, 125–128 (2005).

33. Gu, Z. et al. Injectable nano-network for glucose-mediated insulin delivery. *ACS Nano.* **7**, 4194–4201 (2013).

34. Zhang, S. et al. An inflammation-targeting hydrogel for local drug delivery in inflammatory bowel disease. *Sci Transl Med.* **7**, 300ra128 (2015).

35. Guo, H., Tan, S., Gao, J. & Wang, L. Sequential release of drugs form a dual-delivery system based on pH-responsive nanofibrous mats towards wound care. *Journal of Materials Chemistry B* (2020). doi:10.1039/c9tb02522g

36. Zhang, S. et al. A pH-responsive supramolecular polymer gel as an enteric elastomer for use in gastric devices. *Nat. Mater.* **14**, 1065–1073 (2015).

37. Yu J., Zhang, Y., Ye, Y., DiSanto, R., Sun W., Ranson D., Ligler, F. S., Buse, J. B., Zhen., G. Microneedle-array patches loaded with hypoxia-sensitive vesicles provide fast glucose-responsive insulin delivery. *Proc. Natl. Acad. Sci.* **112**, 8260–8265 (2015).

38. Mo, R., Jiang, T., Disanto, R., Tai, W. & Gu, Z. ATP-triggered anticancer drug delivery. *Nat. Commun.* **5**, 1–10 (2014).

39. Gu, Z. et al. Glucose-responsive microgels integrated with enzyme nanocapsules for closed-loop insulin delivery. *ACS Nano* (2013). doi:10.1021/nn401617u

40. Hu, X. et al. H2O2-responsive vesicles integrated with transcutaneous patches for glucose-mediated insulin delivery. *ACS Nano* (2017). doi:10.1021/acsnano.6b06892

41. Di, J. et al. Ultrasound-triggered regulation of blood glucose levels using injectable nano-network. *Adv. Healthc. Mater.* **3**, 811–816 (2014).

42. Luo, D. et al. Doxorubicin encapsulated in stealth liposomes conferred with light-triggered drug release. *Biomaterials* **75**, 193–202 (2016).

43. Kolosnjaj-Tabi, J., Gibot, L., Fourquaux, I., Golzio, M. & Rols, M. P. Electric field-responsive nanoparticles and electric fields: Physical, chemical, biological mechanisms and therapeutic prospects. *Adv. Drug Deliv. Rev.* **138**, 56–67 (2019).

44. Liu, J. F., Jang, B., Issadore, D. & Tsourkas, A. Use of magnetic fields and nanoparticles to trigger drug release and improve tumor targeting. *Wiley Interdiscip. Rev. Nanomed. Nanobiotechnol.* **11**, 1–18 (2019).

45. Gajanayake, T. et al. A single localized dose of enzyme-responsive hydrogel improves long-term survival of a vascularized composite allograft. *Sci. Transl. Med.* **6**, 249ra110 (2014).

46. Dzhonova, D. et al. Local release of tacrolimus from hydrogel- based drug delivery system is controlled by inflammatory enzymes in vivo and can be monitored non-invasively using in vivo imaging. *PLOS ONE.* **13**, 1–16 (2018).

47. Dzhonova, D. V. et al. Local injections of tacrolimus-loaded hydrogel reduce systemic immunosuppression-related toxicity in vascularized composite allotransplantation. *Transplantation* **102**, 1684–1694 (2018).

48. Anton Fries, C. et al. Graft-implanted, enzyme responsive, tacrolimus-eluting hydrogel enables long-term survival of orthotopic porcine limb vascularized composite allografts: A proof of concept study. *PLOS ONE.* **14**, 1–15 (2019).

49. Huebsch, N. et al. Ultrasound-triggered disruption and self-healing of reversibly cross-linked hydrogels for drug delivery and enhanced chemotherapy. *Proc. Natl. Acad. Sci. U. S. A.* **111**, 9762–9767 (2014).

50. Feturi, F. G. et al. Ultrasound-mediated on-demand release from ionically cross-linked hydrogel: New approach for targeted Immunotherapy in Vascularized Composite Allotransplantation. *PRS Glob. Open.* 18–19 (2017).

51. Li, Z., Xu, X., Feng, X. & Murphy, P. M. The Macrophage-depleting Agent Clodronate Promotes Durable Hematopoietic Chimerism and Donor-specific Skin Allograft Tolerance in Mice. *Sci. Rep.* **6**, 1–10 (2016).

52. Webster, K. E. et al. In vivo expansion of T reg cells with IL-2-MAB complexes: Induction of resistance to EAE and long-term acceptance of islet allografts without immunosuppression. *J. Exp. Med.* **206**, 751–760 (2009).

53. Xu, H. et al. Utility of IL-2 complexes in promoting the survival of murine orthotopic forelimb vascularized composite allografts. *Transplantation.* **102**, 70–78 (2018).

54. Sutter, D. et al. Delivery of rapamycin using in situ forming implants promotes immunoregulation and vascularized composite allograft survival. *Sci. Rep.* **9**, 1–16 (2019).

55. Kabiri, M. et al. A stimulus-responsive, in-situ forming, nanoparticle-laden hydrogel for ocular drug delivery. *Drug Deliv. Transl. Res.* **8**, 484–495 (2018).

56. Fisher, J. D. et al. Treg-inducing microparticles promote donor-specific tolerance in experimental vascularized composite allotransplantation. *PNAS.* 1–6 (2019). doi:10.1073/pnas.1910701116

57. Jhunjhunwala, S. et al. Bioinspired controlled release of CCL22 recruits regulatory T cells in vivo. *Adv. Mater.* **24**, 4735–4738 (2012).

58. Fisher, J. D. et al. In situ recruitment of regulatory T cells promotes donor-specific tolerance in vascularized composite allotransplantation. *Sci. Adv.* **6**, 1–11 (2020).

59. Li, C. et al. Design of biodegradable, implantable devices towards clinical translation. *Nat. Rev. Mater.* **5**, 61–81 (2020).

60. Juillerat-Jeanneret, L., Aubert, J. D., Mikulic, J. & Golshayan, D. Fibrogenic disorders in human diseases: from inflammation to organ dysfunction. *Journal of Medicinal Chemistry* (2018). doi:10.1021/acs.jmedchem.8b00294

61. Heo, Y. J., Shibata, H., Okitsu, T., Kawanishi, T. & Takeuchi, S. Fluorescent hydrogel fibers for long-term in vivo glucose monitoring. *PNAS.* **108**, 13399–13403 (2011).

62. Kueckelhaus, M. et al. Vascularized composite allotransplantation: Current standards and novel approaches to prevent acute rejection and chronic allograft deterioration. *Transpl. Int.* **29**, 655–662 (2016).

63. Kueckelhaus, M. et al. Noninvasive monitoring of immune rejection in face transplant recipients. *Plast. Reconstr. Surg.* **136**, 1082–1089 (2015).

64. Vemula, P. K. et al. On-demand drug delivery from self-assembled nanofibrous gels: A new approach for treatment of proteolytic disease. *J. Biomed. Mater. Res. A.* **97 A**, 103–110 (2011).

65. Jain, A., Dhiman, S., Dhayani, A., Vemula, P. K. & George, S. J. Chemical fuel-driven living and transient supramolecular polymerization. *Nat. Commun.* **10**, 1–9 (2019).

66. Wang, F. et al. Supramolecular prodrug hydrogelator as an immune booster for checkpoint blocker-based immunotherapy. *Sci. Adv.* **6**, 1–13 (2020).

67. Verma, M. et al. A gastric resident drug delivery system for prolonged gram-level dosing of tuberculosis treatment. *Sci. Transl. Med.* **11**, eaau6267 (2019).

68. Brudno, Y. et al. Refilling drug delivery depots through the blood. *Proc. Natl. Acad. Sci. U. S. A.* **111**, 12722–12727 (2014).

69. Brudno, Y. et al. Replenishable drug depot to combat post-resection cancer recurrence. *Biomaterials.* **178**, 373–382 (2018).

70. Wang, H. et al. Clickable, acid labile immunosuppressive prodrugs for in vivo targeting. *Biomater. Sci.* **8**, 266–277 (2020).

71. Iske, J. et al. Composite tissue allotransplantation: Opportunities and challenges. *Cell. Mol. Immunol.* **16**, 343–349 (2019).

72. Tostanoski, L. H. & Jewell, C. M. Engineering self-assembled materials to study and direct immune function. *Advanced Drug Delivery Reviews* (2017). doi:10.1016/j.addr.2017.03.005

73. Gammon, J. M. & Jewell, C. M. Engineering immune tolerance with biomaterials. *Adv. Healthc. Mater.* **1801419**, 1–19 (2019).

74. Weissenbacher, A. et al. Meeting report of the 13th Congress of the International Society of Vascularized Composite Allotransplantation. *Transplantation.* **102**, 1250–1252 (2018).

10 Gene Editing Strategies for Immunomodulation
Translation from Cells to Vascularized Tissues

Fatih Zor, Esra Goktas, and Vijay Gorantla

CONTENTS

Introduction 195
Standard Methods for Gene Delivery to Tissues 196
    Viral Vectors 196
    Non-Viral Gene Transfection 197
    Genomic Editing 197
CRISPR Technology for Gene Editing 197
Target Tissues for Gene Therapy 198
Gene Editing of Vascularized Tissues 198
Gene Editing for Immunomodulation 200
Future Perspectives 201
References 201

INTRODUCTION

Both solid organ transplantation (SOT) and vascularized composite allotransplantation (VCA) recipients require lifelong immunosuppression to avoid graft rejection. Such immunosuppression increases vulnerability to metabolic, infectious and neoplastic complications. Most ongoing research in transplantation surgery is focused on attempts to optimize immunosuppressive regimens by cell-mediated immunomodulation or depletional strategies to tolerize recipients to mismatched donor antigens. Unlike other solid organs, VCA involves visible grafts (such as hand/face), requiring age, gender, size, shape and color matching of donors and recipients. Such phenotypic matching potentially restricts the pool of available donors for VCA. Thus, additional human leucocyte antigen (HLA) matching is not currently considered mandatory in VCA. However, data from the United Network for Organ Sharing (UNOS) show that long-term graft survival of deceased donor renal transplants with zero HLA-A, -B, and -DR mismatch was nearly 20% better than fully mismatched grafts with a proportional reduction in survival with increasing degrees of mismatch[1]. Emerging evidence in VCA confirms that HLA mismatch increases the risk of acute rejection (AR) or chronic rejection (CR), hampering graft survival[2].

DOI: 10.1201/9780429260179-14

The primary targets of the immune response to allogeneic tissues are the major histocompatibility complex (MHC) molecules, which are present on all donor cells. Indeed, the term MHC highlights the fact that MHC molecules were discovered in the context of tissue transplantation between incompatible individuals. Recipient T cells recognize alloantigens via two distinct, but not mutually exclusive, pathways: direct and indirect. Direct recognition occurs when recipient T cells recognize intact donor MHC molecules complexed with peptide on donor stimulator cells. In contrast, indirect recognition occurs when the recipient antigen presenting cells (APCs) process the donor MHC molecules prior to presentation to recipient T cells in a self-restricted manner. This recognition of allograft MHC antigen is the primary event that ultimately leads to graft rejection[3].

The skin is the most antigenic component of VCA with its complement of Langerhans cells, dermal dendritic cells and keratinocytes[4]. The MHC Class I and II molecules on these cells are key for direct and indirect allorecognition for VCA. Transcription and translation of MHC Class I and Class II genes is controlled by several regulatory genes. Editing, silencing or suppression of these genes on donor cells results in reduced or absent presentation of MHC Class I and MHC Class II molecules at the cell surface. There are several studies indicating that blocking of MHC molecules mitigates AR[5,6].

The emerging fields of genomics and proteomics offer unparalleled opportunities for systemic, objective, quantitative, biology-oriented analysis and manipulation of molecular mechanisms involved in a wide variety of diseases. The "clustered regularly interspaced short palindromic repeats (CRISPR) associated nuclease 9" (CRISPR/Cas9) system has been recently adapted from a mechanism of prokaryotic adaptive immunity to targeted genome editing of sequence-specific DNA in mammalian cells[7]. When compared with other gene editing technologies, CRISPR/Cas9 system is easy to customize and has a higher editing efficiency[8]. In this chapter, we want to overview the current techniques of gene editing and their application in vascularized composite tissues, especially in the field of transplantation.

STANDARD METHODS FOR GENE DELIVERY TO TISSUES

Genome editing can be achieved ex vivo or in vivo by delivering the editing system to target cells, which cause addition, ablation or correction of the target cell genome. On the other hand, there are two primarily different gene delivery systems: viral and non-viral systems. Both methods and systems have their own advantages and drawbacks[9,10].

VIRAL VECTORS

Whether used ex vivo or in vivo, viral vectors are frequently used for gene delivery because of their natural ability to infect certain target cells and transfer their genetic material. There are several viral vectors used for gene delivery[11–13]. However, retroviruses (lentiviruses), adenoviruses (AdV) and adeno-associated viruses (AAV) are among the most popular viral vectors for gene editing, and almost all clinical trials and treatment protocols that have been approved by regulatory agencies are based on viral vectors[14–17]. Although each viral vector has specific advantages and disadvantages such as target tissue specificity and effectivity, viral vectors in general have some drawbacks. These are mostly related to triggering immunogenic responses, transgene mis-insertion risks, difficulty of packaging large nucleic acids and problems with large-scale production[18].

Non-Viral Gene Transfection

Because of the potential risks of viral vectors, non-viral methods of gene editing strategies have been developed. These techniques are simpler and offer lower infection risk in expense of less specific and more variable gene expression in target tissues. Non-viral gene delivery is a broad term, including various heterogenous techniques such as liposomes, nucleic acid containing nanoparticles, polymers and naked nucleic acid[14,19]. The major disadvantage of these techniques is the low efficacy. Thus, methods to increase the efficacy of these techniques, such as micro-seeding, "gene guns," ultrasounds, microbubbles, or electroporation, have been developed.

Genomic Editing

Genomic editing is an alternative way of modifying the mammalian genome using targeted endonucleases and provides the possibility of directly targeting and modifying genomic sequences in almost all eukaryotic cells.

These techniques include zinc finger nucleases (ZFNs), transcription activator-like effector nuclease (TALEN) and CRISPR. Both ZFN and TALEN require engineering of a protein component for each gene locus, which causes double-strand breaks (DSBs) in target DNA. This break point, however, is not specific enough and may have off-target effects in ZFN while TALEN is highly specific. CRISPR/Cas9 system basically uses RNA-guided DNA cleavage module and induces DSBs in target DNA. These DSBs can be repaired either by homology-directed repair (HDR) and nonhomologous end-joining (NHEJ), enabling targeted integration or gene disruptions, respectively[7,20].

CRISPR TECHNOLOGY FOR GENE EDITING

The CRISPR/Cas9 system has been recently adapted from a mechanism of prokaryotic adaptive immunity to targeted genome editing of sequence-specific DNA in mammalian cells[7]. The simplicity, versatility, high specificity and efficiency of the technique made it one of the most robust platforms in basic biomedical research and therapeutic applications.

This technique consists of Cas9 nuclease and a guide RNA (gRNA) that is a fusion of a crispr RNA (crRNA) and a constant trans-activating crispr RNA (tracrRNA). Generally, gRNA can be easily replaced by a synthetic chimeric single guide RNA (sgRNA). The Cas9 nuclease can be directed by an sgRNA to any targeted genomic locus based on base pairing. Binding of Cas9 to the DNA is mediated by a partially complementary tracrRNA and cleavage is directed. Targeted integration or gene disruption occurs during the NHEJ or HDR pathways[7,20,21]. This CRISPR/Cas9 system can be delivered using viral or non-viral vectors[22].

Although widely accepted as a simple, specific and effective technique, CRISPR/Cas9-based genome editing also has some challenges and limitations. First of all, the off-target effects of Cas9 nuclease needs to be reduced before translation to clinical application. Moreover, setting and reaching the target site with efficiency and accuracy of both cleavage and repair could be challenging. The control of the DSB repair, either by NHEJ or HDR, is another challenge of the CRISPR/Cas9-based genome editing[23].

TARGET TISSUES FOR GENE THERAPY

The target tissue for the gene delivery or editing is extremely important because the decision of performing ex vivo or in vivo delivery or using viral or non-viral delivery techniques depends on the target tissue for the gene delivery. Technically, gene editing can be performed in any tissue. Most of the studies are focusing on gene editing of a certain cell types of a particular tissue.

Tissues with a large surface area with minimal thickness such as skin are favorable for genetic manipulation because of accessibility[10,12]. Moreover, if the main target of the cells in that particular tissue have high self-renewing capacity (such as fibroblasts and keratinocytes in skin), then the gene editing will be more efficient and easier[12,24].

Deep tissues with low self-renewing capacity (such as bone tissue, including osteoblasts, or cartilage tissue, including chondrocytes) need special techniques for gene delivery such as tissue-engineered scaffolds or transplanting genetically modified stem cells/chondrocytes in target tissues[25,26]. Gene transfer of neurotrophic factors, mostly in combination with cell therapies and scaffolds, has also been investigated as a method to promote nerve repair and stimulate the regenerative capacity of peripheral nerves[19,27].

Gene editing of composite tissues, including more than one tissue types, is also a challenge, as every gene editing strategy is more effective in certain tissue type. For example, gene editing using naked DNA or plasmids is more successful in skeletal muscle tissue due to its capacity to endocytosis[19]. Certain vectors, on the other hand, have more affinity to certain types of tissues. AAV-2, for example, has tropism allowing the efficient transduction of skin[28,29]. These challenges may play a role in why genetic modification of vascularized tissues or composite tissues is not a popular method. However, there are increasing numbers of studies focusing on gene therapy of vascularized tissues, as the vascular pedicle of these tissues may provide an access to all cells and potentially enables genetic modification of the whole tissue[30–33].

GENE EDITING OF VASCULARIZED TISSUES

Gene therapy may offer novel strategies for treatment of diseased organs such as kidney, liver and heart or modification of composite tissues which are used during reconstructive procedures[34,35]. Moreover, it can provide an opportunity to modify the immune response and prolong the survival of solid organ and vascularized composite allotransplants[34,36].

Microvascular free tissue transfer (also called free flaps or vascularized grafts) includes transfer of bulk tissue or organ based on a single arterial and venous pedicle to a distant recipient site and providing blood circulation by microvascular vessel anastomosis. The technique provides the basis for extensive reconstruction, SOT and VCAs[35,37]. The isolation of the arterial and venous pedicle provides a therapeutic opportunity for delivering target molecules (such as gene editing material) to the whole tissue, either by in situ or ex vivo perfusion[30].

During free tissue transfer and organ transplantation, the total ischemia (cold and warm) time is limited by the metabolism of the transferred tissue, and technically, the skeletal tissue is one of the most ischemia vulnerable tissue in the human body[38,39]. Generally speaking, we have at least 60–120 minutes of ischemia time, where gene editing strategies may be applied to the procured tissue[30,39,40].

Using vascular pedicle for delivering genetic material was described more than two decades ago. Yang et al. successfully delivered CTLA4Ig gene to heart via intra-arterial infusion using recombinant AdV as a vector[36]. A similar approach was used for liver by Olthoff et al., where AdV-mediated transduction of liver was successfully achieved by portal vein injection of the viral vector[41].

Other routes of genetic material delivery to vascularized organs are also possible. For example, transfection of kidney has been achieved by retrograde administration of the vector into the ureter or directly into the renal interstitial parenchyma[42]. The available route of the gene delivery depends on the organ or tissue. Although artery seems to be the main route, ureter for kidney, portal vein for liver and transdermal application for skin flaps are additional routes[31,34,41,42].

The success of gene therapy is also dependent on the use of an efficient gene transfer system to allow the expression of the therapeutic gene in a specific organ or composite tissue. However, the most important disadvantage of genetic editing of organs or vascularized tissues was the fairly poor transduction rates into various cells or structures of the particular organ or composite tissue regardless of the route of the delivery of the vector. Thus, novel gene editing technologies are getting investigated for the successful outcomes[34].

Novel gene editing techniques such as TALEN and CRISPR/Cas9 have the potential to overcome this problem as it is possible to generate a tissue specific vector and increase the transduction rate of in vivo model systems[43]. For example, CRISPR/Cas9-mediated genome editing has been successfully used in a mouse model of Duchenne muscular dystrophy where the mutated exon 23 from the dystrophin gene was removed[44]. Actually, there are also preclinical studies focusing on therapeutic applications of CRISPR/Cas9 in model organisms such as hemoglobinopathies (β-thalassemia and sickle cell disease), inherited eye disease (Leber congenital amaurosis), genetic liver disease (hereditary tyrosinemia, α1-antitrypsin deficiency), congenital genetic lung diseases (cystic fibrosis) and genetic deafness[45].

Several of these preclinical studies have been translated to clinical trials. CRISPR, TALEN and ZFN trials (https://clinicaltrials.gov) are ongoing for treatment of diseases like β-thalassemia, sickle cell disease, Leber congenital amaurosis, hemophilia, HIV, mucopolysaccharidosis and various forms of cancer[43,45].

GENE EDITING FOR IMMUNOMODULATION

Although the main popular area of gene editing is genetic diseases and cancers, there are also studies focusing on modification of immune response using gene editing strategies for treatment of transplant rejection, primary immune deficiencies and autoimmune diseases[46]. T cells function at the center of the adaptive immunity, and one way to modify the immune response is to genetically modify the T cell subpopulation[47]. Studies showed that infusion of donor-derived regulatory T cells (Tregs) or antigen-specific Tregs are effective in controlling the preventing organ or tissue graft rejection or autoimmune inflammation[48,49]. Other T cells can also be genetically modified to exert immunomodulatory effects. Genetically modified living T cells with chimeric antigen receptors can be used for treatment of certain malignancies. T cells can also be redirected to target tumors by transferring with a T cell receptor[50,51].

One of the main application field of gene editing is transplantation research. It is well known that the primary targets of the immune response to allogeneic tissues are the MHC molecules, which are present on all donor cells. Recipient T cells recognize MHC antigens, and this recognition of allograft MHC antigen is the primary event that ultimately leads to graft rejection[3]. It is shown that the degree of the MHC mismatch between the donor and the recipient has great impact on long-term graft survival of deceased donor renal transplants[1]. Recent studies in VCA also confirms that MHC mismatch increases the risk of AR or CR, hampering graft survival[2]. Most ongoing research in VCA is focused on attempts to optimize immunosuppressive regimens by cell-mediated immunomodulation or depletional strategies to tolerize recipients to mismatched donor antigens[52]. Gene editing in transplantation field primarily focuses on modification of the antigenicity of the allograft or the immune response against alloantigens[53,54].

The first techniques of genetic engineering of the allograft was performed by transfection of cells with antisense oligodeoxynucleotides, which prevent translation of certain proteins by specifically binding to mRNA. Other mechanisms such as splicing inhibition and translational arrest have also been tried[55–58]. Later, several viral vectors were used to deliver CTLA4Ig gene to the allograft, including heart, kidney and VCA during the ischemia period[36,59–61].

Later efforts focused on modifying or silencing the MHC genes using CRISPR/Cas9. Das et al. used CRISPR/Cas9 technology to create murine cell lines, lacking MHC Class I or MHC Class II surface expression by targeting β2 microglobulin and IAb molecule, respectively. They successfully generated MHC knockout murine cells, shown by flow cytometry[62]. Merola et al. showed that CRISPR/Cas9-mediated dual ablation of β2-microglobulin and Class II transactivator in human endothelial colony-forming cells provided silencing of both Class I and II MHC genes and preserved the endothelial cell functions related to blood flow and circulatory roles. However, these MHC Class I and II ablated cells were not able to bind to donor specific antigens and activate allogeneic CD4+ T cells. Moreover, these cells were resistant to killing by CD8+ alloreactive cytotoxic T lymphocytes in vitro and in vivo[63].

Chang et al. studied ex vivo genomic editing of allografts using small interfering RNA (siRNA) targeted against MHC-I (siMHC-I). Following procurement, the endothelial cells of the allograft were transfected with siMHC-I, and the success of the transfection was shown by quantitative polymerase chain reaction and flow cytometry. By using a rat model of VCA, they showed that siMHC-I-guided MHC knockdown resulted in significant (at least 50%) reduction of MHC Class I expression in all tissue compartments. Additionally, siMHC-I-guided MHC knockdown caused prolonged rejection-free survival of rat VCA[64].

Another technique for gene silencing is RNA interference (RNAi) where double-stranded RNA (dsRNA) molecules are used to silence the gene carrying the same code. In organ transplantation, the target genes are generally related to ischemia-reperfusion injury or graft rejection. There are several preclinical studies reporting encouraging results of using siRNA in liver, kidney, lung and heart transplantation[65–68]. The success of RNAi therapeutics in preclinical studies yielded clinical trials. First attempts have been made to decrease delayed graft failure after kidney transplantation by silencing the p53 gene using RNAi therapy. Although the results are promising, there are many unknowns such as small RNA dosage, treatment conditions and duration. RNAi as a therapeutic agent is still in its infancy but will definitely have an impact in the field of organ transplantation in the near future[69,70].

Another major development in the field of transplantation-related gene editing is reported by Kelton et al[71]. They performed a proof-of-concept study demonstrating reprogramming of MHC in APCs, using CRISPR/Cas-9 cassette exchange. This technique provided replacement of MHC genes instead of silencing them.

Gene editing technologies have also been used in xenotransplantation. Estrada et al. have used CRISPR-based approach to knock down three porcine surface antigens to prevent hyper AR with promising results[72]. Silencing of porcine MHC Class I antigens has also been shown to increase survival of pig kidneys in non-human primate transplant recipients from days to months[73,74]. However, despite these encouraging results, there is a long way to achieve sufficient tolerance to xenotransplanted kidneys or other organs in humans to compete with the gold standard of human allograft.

FUTURE PERSPECTIVES

Genetic engineering of the vascularized tissues is still a developing field with a potentially considerable clinical impact. The ultimate goal of transplantation is providing donor-specific tolerance to allograft, and gene editing strategies propose such an effect by modulating the allograft to evade it from immune surveillance and protecting it from either AR or CR without systemic immunosuppression. However, there are many unknowns such as vector efficiency, vector toxicity, control of gene expression and biosecurity. Our current understanding shows that advances in novel or more specific or sensitive methods of genomic editing may open a new era for organ transplantation.

REFERENCES

1. Danovitch, G. M. & Cecka, J. M. Allocation of deceased donor kidneys: past, present, and future. *American Journal of Kidney Diseases* **42**, 882–890, doi:10.1016/j.ajkd.2003.07.017 (2003).
2. Bonastre, J., Landin, L., Diez, J., Casado-Sanchez, C. & Casado-Perez, C. Factors influencing acute rejection of human hand allografts. *Annals of Plastic Surgery* **68**, 624–629, doi:10.1097/sap.0b013e318255a411 (2012).

3. Game, D. S. & Lechler, R. I. Pathways of allorecognition: implications for transplantation tolerance. *Transplant Immunology* **10**, 101–108, doi:10.1016/s0966-3274(02)00055-2 (2002).

4. Fukunaga, A., Khaskhely, N. M., Sreevidya, C. S., Byrne, S. N. & Ullrich, S. E. Dermal dendritic cells, and not Langerhans cells, play an essential role in inducing an immune response. *Journal of Immunology* **180**, 3057–3064, doi:10.4049/jimmunol.180.5.3057 (2008).

5. Abrahimi, P. et al. Blocking MHC class II on human endothelium mitigates acute rejection. *JCI Insight* **1**, e85293, doi:10.1172/jci.insight.85293 (2016).

6. Torikai, H. et al. Toward eliminating HLA class I expression to generate universal cells from allogeneic donors. *Blood* **122**, 1341–1349, doi:10.1182/blood-2013-03-478255 (2013).

7. Heintze, J., Luft, C. & Ketteler, R. A CRISPR CASe for high-throughput silencing. *Frontiers in Genetics* **4**, 193–193, doi:10.3389/fgene.2013.00193 (2013).

8. Ran, F. A. et al. Genome engineering using the CRISPR-Cas9 system. *Nature Protocols* **8**, 2281–2308, doi:10.1038/nprot.2013.143 (2013).

9. Giatsidis, G., Venezia, E. D. & Bassetto, F. The role of gene therapy in regenerative surgery. *Plastic and Reconstructive Surgery* **131**, 1425–1435, doi:10.1097/prs.0b013e31828bd153 (2013).

10. Tepper, O. M. & Mehrara, B. J. Gene therapy in plastic surgery. *Plastic and Reconstructive Surgery* **109**, 716–734, doi:10.1097/00006534-200202000-00047 (2002).

11. Athanasopoulos, T., Munye, M. M. & Yáñez-Muñoz, R. J. Nonintegrating gene therapy vectors. *Hematology/Oncology Clinics of North America* **31**, 753–770, doi:10.1016/j.hoc.2017.06.007 (2017).

12. Balaji, S. et al. Adenoviral-mediated gene transfer of insulin-like growth factor 1 enhances wound healing and induces angiogenesis. *The Journal of Surgical Research* **190**, 367–377, doi:10.1016/j.jss.2014.02.051 (2014).

13. Dunbar, C. E. et al. Gene therapy comes of age. *Science* **359**, eaan4672, doi:10.1126/science.aan4672 (2018).

14. Foldvari, M. et al. Non-viral gene therapy: gains and challenges of non-invasive administration methods. *Journal of Controlled Release* **240**, 165–190, doi:10.1016/j.jconrel.2015.12.012 (2016).

15. Trono, D. Lentiviral vectors: turning a deadly foe into a therapeutic agent. *Gene Therapy* **7**, 20–23, doi:10.1038/sj.gt.3301105 (2000).

16. Wang, D., Tai, P. W. L. & Gao, G. Adeno-associated virus vector as a platform for gene therapy delivery. *Nature Reviews Drug Discovery* **18**, 358–378, doi:10.1038/s41573-019-0012-9 (2019).

17. Zabner, J. et al. Adenovirus-mediated gene transfer transiently corrects the chloride transport defect in nasal epithelia of patients with cystic fibrosis. *Cell* **75**, 207–216, doi:10.1016/0092-8674(93)80063-k (1993).

18. Thomas, C. E., Ehrhardt, A. & Kay, M. A. Progress and problems with the use of viral vectors for gene therapy. *Nature Reviews Genetics* **4**, 346–358, doi:10.1038/nrg1066 (2003).

19. Zor, F. et al. Effect of VEGF gene therapy and hyaluronic acid film sheath on peripheral nerve regeneration. *Microsurgery* **34**, 209–216, doi:10.1002/micr.22196 (2013).

20. Li, H. et al. Applications of genome editing technology in the targeted therapy of human diseases: mechanisms, advances and prospects. *Signal Transduction and Targeted Therapy* **5**, 1–1, doi:10.1038/s41392-019-0089-y (2020).

21. Jinek, M. et al. A programmable dual-RNA-guided DNA endonuclease in adaptive bacterial immunity. *Science* **337**, 816–821, doi:10.1126/science.1225829 (2012).

22. Li, L., Hu, S. & Chen, X. Non-viral delivery systems for CRISPR/Cas9-based genome editing: challenges and opportunities. *Biomaterials* **171**, 207–218, doi:10.1016/j.biomaterials.2018.04.031 (2018).

23. Eid, A. & Mahfouz, M. M. Genome editing: the road of CRISPR/Cas9 from bench to clinic. *Experimental & Molecular Medicine* **48**, e265–e265, doi:10.1038/emm.2016.111 (2016).

24. Mofazzal Jahromi, M. A. et al. Nanomedicine and advanced technologies for burns: preventing infection and facilitating wound healing. *Advanced Drug Delivery Reviews* **123**, 33–64, doi:10.1016/j.addr.2017.08.001 (2018).

25. Bougioukli, S. et al. Gene therapy for bone repair using human cells: superior osteogenic potential of bone morphogenetic protein 2-transduced mesenchymal stem cells derived from adipose tissue compared to bone marrow. *Human Gene Therapy* **29**, 507–519, doi:10.1089/hum.2017.097 (2018).

26. Grol, M. W. & Lee, B. H. Gene therapy for repair and regeneration of bone and cartilage. *Current Opinion in Pharmacology* **40**, 59–66, doi:10.1016/j.coph.2018.03.005 (2018).

27. Busuttil, F., Rahim, A. A. & Phillips, J. B. Combining gene and stem cell therapy for peripheral nerve tissue engineering. *Stem Cells and Development* **26**, 231–238, doi:10.1089/scd.2016.0188 (2017).

28. Büning, H., Braun-Falco, M. & Hallek, M. Progress in the use of adeno-associated viral vectors for gene therapy. *Cells Tissues Organs* **177**, 139–150, doi:10.1159/000079988 (2004).

29. Keswani, S. G. et al. Pseudotyped adeno-associated viral vector tropism and transduction efficiencies in murine wound healing. *Wound Repair and Regeneration* **20**, 592–600, doi:10.1111/j.1524-475X.2012.00810.x (2012).

30. Agrawal, V. K. et al. Microvascular free tissue transfer for gene delivery: in vivo evaluation of different routes of plasmid and adenoviral delivery. *Gene Therapy* **16**, 78–92, doi:10.1038/gt.2008.140 (2008).

31. Dempsey, M. P. et al. Using genetically modified microvascular free flaps to deliver local cancer immunotherapy with minimal systemic toxicity. *Plastic and Reconstructive Surgery* **121**, 1541–1553, doi:10.1097/prs.0b013e31816ff6aa (2008).

32. Michaels, J. et al. Biologic brachytherapy: ex vivo transduction of microvascular beds for efficient, targeted gene therapy. *Plastic and Reconstructive Surgery* **118**, 54–65, doi: 10.1097/01.prs.0000220466.27521.22(2006).

33. Michaels, J. T. et al. Ex vivo transduction of microvascular free flaps for localized peptide delivery. *Annals of Plastic Surgery* **52**, 581–584, doi:10.1097/01.sap.0000122652.81844.37 (2004).

34. Isaka, Y. Gene therapy targeting kidney diseases: routes and vehicles. *Clinical and Experimental Nephrology* **10**, 229–235, doi:10.1007/s10157-006-0442-7 (2006).

35. Seth, R., Khan, A. A., Pencavel, T., Harrington, K. J. & Harris, P. A. Targeted gene delivery by free-tissue transfer in oncoplastic reconstruction. *The Lancet Oncology* **13**, e392–e402, doi:10.1016/s1470-2045(12)70235-8 (2012).

36. Yang, Z., Rostami, S., Koeberlein, B., Barker, C. F. & Naji, A. Cardiac allograft tolerance induced by intraarterial infusion of recombinant adenoviral CTLA4Ig1. *Transplantation* **67**, 1517–1523, doi:10.1097/00007890-199906270-00004 (1999).

37. Siemionow, M. Z. & Zor, F. in *Plastic and Reconstructive Surgery* 3–10 (Springer London, 2014).

38. Blaisdell, F. The pathophysiology of skeletal muscle ischemia and the reperfusion syndrome: a review. *Cardiovascular Surgery* **10**, 620–630, doi:10.1016/s0967-2109(02)00070-4 (2002).

39. Zor, F., Meric, C. & Siemionow, M. Effects of hPTPβ inhibitor on microcirculation of rat cremaster muscle flap following ischemia-reperfusion injury. *Microsurgery* **37**, 624–631, doi:10.1002/micr.30131 (2016).

40. Amin, K. R., Wong, J. K. F. & Fildes, J. E. Strategies to reduce ischemia reperfusion injury in vascularized composite allotransplantation of the limb. *The Journal of Hand Surgery* **42**, 1019–1024, doi:10.1016/j.jhsa.2017.09.013 (2017).

41. Olthoff, K. M. et al. Adenovirus-mediated gene transfer into cold-preserved liver allografts: survival pattern and unresponsiveness following transduction with CTLA4Ig. *Nature Medicine* **4**, 194–200, doi:10.1038/nm0298-194 (1998).
42. Akbulut, T. & Park, F. Gene therapy to the kidney using viral vectors. *Paidiatrike* **71**, 177–185 (2008).
43. WareJoncas, Z. et al. Precision gene editing technology and applications in nephrology. *Nature Reviews Nephrology* **14**, 663–677, doi:10.1038/s41581-018-0047-x (2018).
44. Nelson, C. E. et al. In vivo genome editing improves muscle function in a mouse model of Duchenne muscular dystrophy. *Science* **351**, 403–407, doi:10.1126/science.aad5143 (2016).
45. Wu, S.-S., Li, Q.-C., Yin, C.-Q., Xue, W. & Song, C.-Q. Advances in CRISPR/Cas-based gene therapy in human genetic diseases. *Theranostics* **10**, 4374–4382, doi:10.7150/thno.43360 (2020).
46. Xiong, X., Chen, M., Lim, W. A., Zhao, D. & Qi, L. S. CRISPR/Cas9 for human genome engineering and disease research. *Annual Review of Genomics and Human Genetics* **17**, 131–154, doi:10.1146/annurev-genom-083115-022258 (2016).
47. Chae, W.-J. & Bothwell, A. L. M. Therapeutic potential of gene-modified regulatory T cells: from bench to bedside. *Frontiers in Immunology* **9**, 303, doi:10.3389/fimmu.2018.00303 (2018).
48. Joffre, O. et al. Prevention of acute and chronic allograft rejection with CD4+ CD25+Foxp3+ regulatory T lymphocytes. *Nature Medicine* **14**, 88–92, doi:10.1038/nm1688 (2008).
49. Liu, X. et al. Cell-penetrable mouse forkhead box protein 3 alleviates experimental arthritis in mice by up-regulating regulatory T cells. *Clinical and Experimental Immunology* **181**, 87–99, doi:10.1111/cei.12630 (2015).
50. Morgan, R. A. et al. Cancer regression in patients after transfer of genetically engineered lymphocytes. *Science* **314**, 126–129, doi:10.1126/science.1129003 (2006).
51. Porter, D. L., Levine, B. L., Kalos, M., Bagg, A. & June, C. H. Chimeric antigen receptor-modified T cells in chronic lymphoid leukemia. *The New England Journal of Medicine* **365**, 725–733, doi:10.1056/NEJMoa1103849 (2011).
52. Montgomery, R. A., Tatapudi, V. S., Leffell, M. S. & Zachary, A. A. HLA in transplantation. *Nature Reviews Nephrology* **14**, 558–570, doi:10.1038/s41581-018-0039-x (2018).
53. Itano, H. et al. Lipid-mediated ex vivo gene transfer of viral interleukin 10 in rat lung allotransplantation. *The Journal of Thoracic and Cardiovascular Surgery* **122**, 29–38, doi:10.1067/mtc.2001.114636 (2001).
54. Sato, M. & Keshavjee, S. Gene therapy in lung transplantation. *Current Gene Therapy* **6**, 439–458, doi:10.2174/156652306777934810 (2006).
55. Mathieu, P. et al. Genetic engineering in allotransplantation of vascularized organs. *Current Gene Therapy* **2**, 9–21, doi:10.2174/1566523023348147 (2002).
56. Myers, K. J. & Dean, N. M. Sensible use of antisense: how to use oligonucleotides as research tools. *Trends in Pharmacological Sciences* **21**, 19–23, doi:10.1016/s0165-6147(99)01420-0 (2000).
57. Walder, R. Y. & Walder, J. A. Role of RNase H in hybrid-arrested translation by antisense oligonucleotides. *Proceedings of the National Academy of Sciences of the United States of America* **85**, 5011–5015, doi:10.1073/pnas.85.14.5011 (1988).
58. Wood, K. J. Gene therapy and allotransplantation. *Current Opinion in Immunology* **9**, 662–668, doi:10.1016/s0952-7915(97)80046-5 (1997).
59. Akamaru, Y. et al. Ex vivo and systemic transfer of adenovirus-mediated CTLA4Ig gene combined with a short course of FK506 therapy prolongs islet graft survival. *Transplant Immunology* **11**, 91–100, doi:10.1016/s0966-3274(02)00153-3 (2003).

60. Xiao, B. et al. Ex vivo transfer of adenovirus-mediated CTLA4Ig gene combined with a short course of rapamycin therapy prolongs free flap allograft survival. *Plastic and Reconstructive Surgery* **127**, 1820–1829, doi:10.1097/prs.0b013e31820cf264 (2011).

61. Tomasoni, S. et al. CTLA4Ig gene transfer prolongs survival and induces donor-specific tolerance in a rat renal allograft. *Journal of the American Society of Nephrology* **11**, 747–752 (2000).

62. Das, K. et al. Generation of murine tumor cell lines deficient in MHC molecule surface expression using the CRISPR/Cas9 system. *PLOS ONE* **12**, e0174077, doi:10.1371/journal.pone.0174077 (2017).

63. Merola, J. et al. Progenitor-derived human endothelial cells evade alloimmunity by CRISPR/Cas9-mediated complete ablation of MHC expression. *JCI Insight* **4**, e129739, doi:10.1172/jci.insight.129739 (2019).

64. Chang, J. B. et al. Ex vivo major histocompatibility complex I knockdown prolongs rejection-free allograft survival. *Plastic and Reconstructive Surgery – Global Open* **6**, e1825, doi:10.1097/GOX.0000000000001825 (2018).

65. Gillooly, A. R., Perry, J. & Martins, P. N. First report of siRNA uptake (for RNA interference) during ex vivo hypothermic and normothermic liver machine perfusion. *Transplantation* **103**, e56–e57, doi:10.1097/tp.0000000000002515 (2019).

66. Ichim, T. E. et al. RNA interference: a potent tool for gene-specific therapeutics. *American Journal of Transplantation* **4**, 1227–1236, doi:10.1111/j.1600-6143.2004.00530.x (2004).

67. Wang, H. et al. Prevention of allograft rejection in heart transplantation through concurrent gene silencing of TLR and kinase signaling pathways. *Scientific Reports* **6**, 33869, doi:10.1038/srep33869 (2016).

68. Yang, C. et al. Serum-stabilized naked caspase-3 siRNA protects autotransplant kidneys in a porcine model. *Molecular Therapy* **22**, 1817–1828, doi:10.1038/mt.2014.111 (2014).

69. Brüggenwirth, I. M. A. & Martins, P. N. RNA interference therapeutics in organ transplantation: the dawn of a new era. *American Journal of Transplantation* **20**, 931–941, doi:10.1111/ajt.15689 (2020).

70. *I5NP for Prophylaxis of Delayed Graft Function in Kidney Transplantation*, https://clinicaltrials.gov/ct2/show/NCT00802347

71. Kelton, W. et al. Reprogramming MHC specificity by CRISPR-Cas9-assisted cassette exchange. *Scientific Reports* **7**, 45775, doi:10.1038/srep45775 (2017).

72. Estrada, J. L. et al. Evaluation of human and non-human primate antibody binding to pig cells lacking GGTA1/CMAH/beta4GalNT2 genes. *Xenotransplantation* **22**, 194–202, doi:10.1111/xen.12161 (2015).

73. Higginbotham, L. et al. Pre-transplant antibody screening and anti-CD154 costimulation blockade promote long-term xenograft survival in a pig-to-primate kidney transplant model. *Xenotransplantation* **22**, 221–230, doi:10.1111/xen.12166 (2015).

74. Iwase, H. et al. Pig kidney graft survival in a baboon for 136 days: longest life-supporting organ graft survival to date. *Xenotransplantation* **22**, 302–309, doi:10.1111/xen.12174 (2015).

Index

A

Acute rejection (AR)
  antigenicity, 122
  challenges, 137
  clinical and histopathological assessment, 123–124
  donor-derived cell-free DNA, 128–129
  gene expression profiling, 126–128
  imaging, 130–131
  immune phenotyping, 137
  microbiome, 136–137
  miRNAs profiling, 129
  phenotypes, *see* Cell phenotypes
  proteomics, 129–130
  serum, tissue biomarkers and surrogates, 122–123
  SSFs, 131–136
  tissue loss, 122
Adenosine triphosphate (ATP), 61
Adjunctive rapamycin therapy, 28
Adoptive transfer, 35–36
Allograft growth, 82
ALS, *see* Anti-lymphocyte serum (ALS)
Amniotic band syndrome, 84
Amphiphile, 181
Amputation, 80–81
AMR, *see* Antibody-mediated rejection (AMR)
Angiogenesis, 152, 155, 157, 158
Antibody-mediated rejection (AMR), 123
Antigen-presenting cells (APCs), 11, 196
Antigen-specific immune suppression, 29
Antigen-specific (Ag-specific) Tregs, 10–11
Anti-lymphocyte serum (ALS), 177
Antioxidants, 64
Anti-thymocyte globulin (ATG), 8
APCs, *see* Antigen-presenting cells (APCs)
Apoptosis, 61
Arteriosclerosis, 28
Arterio-venous loop (AVL), 158
ATG, *see* Anti-thymocyte globulin (ATG)
ATP, *see* Adenosine triphosphate (ATP)
Autoimmune diseases, 37
AVL, *see* Arterio-venous loop (AVL)
Axonal regeneration, 102, 103

B

Banff grading scale, 50, 52, *53*, 54
Belatacept, 85
Bioengineering composite tissue constructs
  competing technologies, 150–151, *151*
  composite tissues, 150
  long-term immunosuppression, 150
  nutrition, 156–158
  replacement tissues, 149
  scaffold, 158–162
  substance, 152–156
Biomarkers, 50, 52, 54, 107, 122–138
Biomaterials
  choice of, 188
  combination therapy, 188–189
  immunotherapy, 176
  localized drug delivery
    conventional *vs.*, 175
    first-generation immunotherapy, 175
    fourth generation, 176
    oral capsules/systemically delivered drugs, 174
    second-generation immunotherapy, 175
    third generation, 175
  multi-drug therapies, 184–188
  on-demand drug delivery, 180–184
Bionics, 150
Bioreactor system, 16
Blood-brain barrier, 111, 112
BMT, *see* Bone marrow transplant (BMT)
Bone marrow transplant (BMT), 6, 184

C

Cannabigerolic acid (CBGA), 185
Capillary destruction, 51
CAR, *see* Chimeric antigen receptor (CAR)
Carbon nanotubes (CNTs), 110
CAR-modified T cells (CAR-T cells), 11
CBGA, *see* Cannabigerolic acid (CBGA)
CCI, *see* Chronic constriction injury (CCI)
Cell infusion, 15, 16
Cell phenotypes
  peripheral blood, 124–125
  tissue, 125–126
Cell seeding, 15, 16
Children's Hospital of Philadelphia, 91
Chimeric antigen receptor (CAR)
  allogeneic targets, 12
  allograft rejection, 13
  autoimmunity and transplant tolerance, 12
  cancer immunotherapy, 12
  CD8+ Tregs, 12
  clinical trials, 13
  immunodeficient mouse model, 12

inflammatory cytokines, 13
mAbCAR, 13
2nd generation, *11*
TCR, 29
Chronic constriction injury (CCI), 107–108, *108,*
109, 113
Chronic rejection (CR)
definition, 48–49
GV, 122
human transplantation, 47
IH, 47
invasive surrogate techniques, 49–50
non-invasive surrogate techniques, 50–52
non-specific clinicopathological findings, **48**
CIT, *see* Cold ischemia time (CIT)
Clustered regularly interspaced short palindromic
repeats/associated nuclease 9
(CRISPR/Cas9), 196–198
Coagulative myonecrosis, 63
Cold ischemia time (CIT), 63
Competing technologies, 150–151, *151*
Composite tissue transplantation (CTA), 172
Computed tomography–angiography (CT-A), 51
Corneal allografts, *179*, 179–180
Cortical plasticity, 84–85
Cortical reorganization, 84
Costimulation blockade (CoB), 7
CR, *see* Chronic rejection (CR)
Creeping substitution, 132
CsA, *see* Cyclosporin A (CsA)
CTA, *see* Composite tissue transplantation
(CTA)
CT-A, *see* Computed tomography-angiography
(CT-A)
Cyclosporin A (CsA), 35, 177
Cytokine release syndrome, 13, 80

D

Danger/damage-associated molecular patterns
(DAMPs), 62
DASH, *see* Disabilities of Arm Shoulder and
Hand (DASH)
DBM, *see* Donor bone marrow (DBM)
DCregs, *see* Regulatory dendritic cells
(DCregs)
DDSs, *see* Drug delivery systems (DDSs)
Decellularization/recellularization (DE/RE)
aim, 14
approaches, 15–16
methods, 14–15
scaffolds, 16–17
swine fasciocutaneous flap, *15*
vascularized composite allograft, 17–19, *18*
Deep wide biopsy (DWB), 50, 54
Delayed BMT protocol, 7
Dendritic cells (DCs), 32, 178–179

Disabilities of Arm Shoulder and Hand (DASH),
83
Dog leukocyte antigen (DLA), 6
Donor antigen specific Tregs, 29
Donor bone marrow (DBM), 6
Donor bone marrow cellular therapy, 85
Donor-derived cell-free DNA, 128–129
Donor specific antibodies (DSAs), 8, 48, 49, 50,
52, 54, *55*, 85, 136
Dorsal root ganglia (DRG), 111, 113
Double-strand breaks (DSBs), 197
Double stranded RNA (dsRNA), 201
Drug delivery
implantable materials
corneal allografts, *179*, 179–180
dendritic cells and murine skin allograft
survival, 178–179
on-demand, *see* On-demand drug delivery
systemic and topical
antigenicity, 177
immunosuppressants, skin allograft
rejection, 177–178
immunosuppressive agents, 177
Drug delivery systems (DDSs), 175
DSAs, *see* Donor specific antibodies
(DSAs)
Duchenne muscular dystrophy, 199
DWB, *see* Deep wide biopsy (DWB)

E

Embryonic stem cells (ESCs), 16, 104
End-stage renal disease (ESRD), 5
ESCs, *see* Embryonic stem cells (ESCs)
E-selectin, 128
ESRD, *see* End-stage renal disease (ESRD)
Ex-situ perfusion system, 68, *69*
Extracellular matrix (ECM), 14
Ex vivo expansion, 31, 35–36
Ex-vivo perfusion platforms, 162

F

Fibroblast growth factor 2 (FGF2), 157
FK506 therapy, 83
Flow magnetic resonance imaging, 50–51
Food and Drug Administration (FDA), 12, 174
Forkhead box protein 3 (FOXP3), 30, 31, 127
Free flaps, 199
Functional reinnervation, 83–84

G

Gastric resident system, 189
Gene editing strategies
CRISPR technology, 197–198
genomic editing, 197

genomics and proteomics, 196
immunomodulation, 200–201
immunosuppression, 195
MHC, 196
non-viral gene transfection, 197
target tissues, 198
transplantation surgery, 195
vascularized tissues, 198–199
viral vectors, 196–197
Gene expression profiling
  adhesion molecules, 128
  face transplant *vs.* solid organ transplant
      rejection, *127*
  rejection-related genes, 126–128
Genomic editing, 197
GITR, *see* Glucocorticoid-induced tumour
      necrosis factor receptor (GITR)
Glucocorticoid-induced tumour necrosis factor
      receptor (GITR), 127–128
GMP, *see* Good Manufacturing Practice (GMP)
GNPs, *see* Gold nanoparticles (GNPs)
Gold nanoparticles (GNPs), 105
Good Manufacturing Practice (GMP), 31
Graft vasculopathy (GV), 8, 86, 122
Graft-versus-host disease (GVHD), 8, 29
GV, *see* Graft vasculopathy (GV)
GVHD, *see* Graft-versus-host disease
      (GVHD)

H

Hair follicles, 104
Hand Transplant Score System, 86
Haploidentical swine model, 6
HCT, *see* Hematopoietic cell transplantation
      (HCT)
HDR, *see* Homology-directed repair (HDR)
Hematopoietic cell transplantation (HCT)
  clinical tolerance studies, 8
  co-stimulatory blockade and local
      immunosuppression technologies, 8–9
  delayed tolerance induction, 7–8
  mesenchymal stem cells and regulatory
      dendritic cells, 9
  preclinical work, 5–7
Hematopoietic chimerism, 183–184
Hematoxylin and eosin (H&E), 54
Histidine-tryptophan-ketoglutarate (HTK), 68
HLA, *see* Human leucocyte antigen (HLA)
HLA-A2, *see* Human leukocyte antigen-A2
      (HLA-A2)
Homology-directed repair (HDR), 197
HTK, *see* Histidine-tryptophan-ketoglutarate
      (HTK)
Human adipose-derived stromal cells, 154
Human leucocyte antigen (HLA), 195
Human leukocyte antigen-A2 (HLA-A2), 12

Human umbilical vein endothelial cells
      (HUVECs), 154, 157, 160
Hydrogels
  enzyme-responsive injectable, 181–183
  multi-stimuli responsive, 185
  ultrasound-responsive ionically crosslinked,
      183

I

Iatrogenic injuries, 101
IH, *see* Intimal hyperplasia (IH)
IL-2 interaction, 29–30
IL-2R, *see* Interleukin-2R (IL-2R)
Imaging immune cells, 106–107
Immune dysregulation, polyendocrinopathy,
      enteropathy, X-linked (IPEX)
      syndrome, 30
Immune modulating strategies, 6
Immune phenotyping, 137
Immune system, *62*
Immunogenicity, 5, 17
Immunomodulation, 28, 29, 30–32, 34, 36, 105,
      106–109, 113, 173–174, 176, 177, 186,
      189, 195, 200–201
Immunomodulatory pathways
  CCL22, 186–188
  hindlimb rodent allograft, 184–185
  ocular delivery, 185
  orthotropic hindlimb transplant, 184
  prodrug-based biomaterials, 184
  tolerance and indefinite graft survival,
      185–186
  tolerance induction, 184
Immunosuppression, 5–9, 10, 14, 18, 28, 29,
      31, 33, 34, 68, 76, 79, 80, 83, 85–86,
      89, 90, 91, 92, 122, 123, 150, 159,
      173–174, 177–178, 182, 183, 184–188,
      195
Immunosuppressive drugs, 32, 35
Immunotherapy, 173–176
Induced pluripotent stem cells (iPSCs), 17, 104,
      157
In situ forming implants, 184–185
Interleukin-2R (IL-2R), 180
International Society of VCA (ISVCA), 48, 54,
      55
Intimal hyperplasia (IH), 47, 50–52, 54, 56
Invasive surrogate techniques
  Banff grading scale, 50, 52, *53*, 54
  biomarkers, 50
  claims and controversies, 52–54
  DWB, 50, 54
  for-cause skin biopsy, 49, 50
  histopathologic and immunohistochemical
      findings, 49
  protocol biopsies, 49, **49**

iPSCs, *see* Induced pluripotent stem cells (iPSCs)
Ischemia-reperfusion injury, 36, 81, 132, 201
Ischemic flexion contracture, 63
Ischemic reperfusion syndrome, 79
ISVCA, *see* International Society of VCA (ISVCA)

K

Kidney transplant, 31

L

Laser Doppler flowmeter, 130
Long-term donor tolerance, 183–184
L-selectin, 128
Lymphatic system, 158

M

mAbs, *see* Monoclonal antibodies (mAbs)
Machine perfusion (MP), 64, 65
Macrophages, 102
Macrophage-targeted nanosystems, 107–110
Macrophage-targeted therapy, 183–184
Magnetic resonance imaging (MRI), 50–51, 76, 84–85, 107, 108, 112, 131
Magnetoencephalography, 79, 84
Major histocompatibility complex (MHC), 5, 6, 8, 9, 11, 13, 17, 69, 196, 200–201
Mammalian target of rapamycin (mTOR), 35
MCP-1, *see* Monocyte chemoattractant protein-1 (MCP-1)
Melatonin-stimulated MSC-derived exosomes (MT-Exo), 109
Mesenchymal stem cells (MSCs), 9, 104
Metal NPs, 111–112
Methylprednisolone, 35
MHC, *see* Major histocompatibility complex (MHC)
Microarrays, 126
Microbiome, 136–137
Microcirculatory dysfunction, 68
MicroRNAs (miRNAs), 129
Microvascular free tissue transfer, 199
MMF, *see* Mycophenolate mofetil (MMF)
Modular chimeric concept, *156*
Monoclonal antibodies (mAbs), 174
Monocyte chemoattractant protein-1 (MCP-1), 180
MP, *see* Machine perfusion (MP)
MPA, *see* Mycophenolic acid (MPA)
MSCs, *see* Mesenchymal stem cells (MSCs)
mTOR, *see* Mammalian target of rapamycin (mTOR)

Multistep urethral reconstruction, 155
Multi-walled carbon nanotubes (MWCNT), 110
MWCNT, *see* Multi-walled carbon nanotubes (MWCNT)
Myasthenia gravis, 30
Mycophenolate mofetil (MMF), 7, 174
Mycophenolic acid (MPA), 177

N

NAC, *see* Nipple-areolar complex (NAC)
Nailfold capillaroscopy, 86
Nanohorns, 110
Nanomedicine, 107–108, *109*, 113
Nanoparticles (NPs), 105–107, **106**, 110–111, 112, 113, 178–179
NanoString technology, 127
Nanosystems, 112–113
    macrophage-targeted, 107–110
Near-infrared fluorescence (NIRF), 107
Necrosis, 61
Nephrotoxicity, 90
Nerve transection/injury, 102–103
Neural stem cells, 104
Neuro immune interactions, 102
Neuroimmunomodulation, 106, 108, 113
Neuroinflammation, 102
Neurons
    carbon nanotubes, nanohorns and nanoparticles, 110–111
    metal NPs, 111–112
    QDs, 111
Neuropathic pain, 101, 113
Neuroregeneration
    cell therapy, 104–105
    cellular targets, 102–104
    definition, 101–102
    immunomodulation and imaging immune cells, 106–107
    macrophage-targeted nanosystems, 107–110
    nanoparticles, 105–107, **106**, 110–111, 112, 113
    nanosystems, 107–110, 112–113
    neurons, 110–112
Neurotrophic agents, 102
NHEJ, *see* Nonhomologous end-joining (NHEJ)
NHP, *see* Non-human primate (NHP)
Ninth Banff Conference on Allograft Pathology, 123
Nipple-areolar complex (NAC), 19
NMR, *see* Nuclear magnetic resonance (NMR)
Nonhomologous end-joining (NHEJ), 197
Non-human primate (NHP), 5–9, 28, 162, 201
Non-invasive surrogate techniques
    biomarkers, 52, 54
    capillary destruction, 51
    claims and controversies, 55–56

CT-A, 51
*flow*MRI, 50–51, 56
ultrasound biomicroscopy, 50, 56
vascular-functional diagnosis, 51
vessel elasticity and compliance, 52
Non-viral gene transfection, 197
Nuclear magnetic resonance (NMR), 107, *108*
Nutrition
  challenge, 158
  concept, 156
  strategy, 157–158

O

Ocular delivery, 185
Olfactory cells, 104
On-demand drug delivery
  enzyme-responsive, injectable hydrogels,
    181–183
  hematopoietic chimerism and long-term
    donor tolerance, 183–184
  inflammatory enzyme-triggered drug release,
    182
  physiological markers, 180
  SRS, 180, *181*
  ultrasound-responsive ionically crosslinked
    hydrogel, 183
Organ donors, 90
Orthopedics, 17
Orthotopic swine forelimb transplantation model,
  65

P

Pain hypersensitivity, 108, 113
PAT, *see* Photoacoustic tomography (PAT)
Patient compliant approaches, 189
Patient Generated Index, 89
Patient rehabilitation, 82–83
Pattern recognition receptors (PRRs), 62
PBMCs, *see* Peripheral blood mononuclear cells
  (PBMCs)
PBS, *see* Phosphate buffered saline (PBS)
PDGF-β, *see* Platelet-derived growth factor
  (PDGF-β)
Pediatric upper extremity
  ethical considerations
    consent, 91
    weighing risks and patient benefits,
      90–91
  indications, 91–92
  introduction, 76
  psychosocial issues, 86–90
  quadrimembral amputations, 76, *79*
  VCA recipients, *see* Pediatric VCA r
    ecipients
  worldwide experience, 76–80, **77–78**

Pediatric VCA recipients
  allograft growth, 82
  allograft size, selection and transport, 81
  cortical plasticity, 84–85
  etiology of amputation, 80–81
  failed trial of prostheses, 81
  functional reinnervation, 83–84
  immunosuppression, 85–86
  outcomes assessment tools, 86
  patient rehabilitation, 82–83
PEG, *see* Polyethylene glycol (PEG)
Perfluorocarbon nanoemulsions (PFCNEs), 107,
  108
Periosteum, 155
Peripheral blood mononuclear cells (PBMCs), 28
Peripheral nerve injuries (PNIs), 101, 103
PET, *see* Positron emission tomography (PET)
Phosphate buffered saline (PBS), 160
Photoacoustic tomography (PAT), 112
Placental embolus, 84
Platelet-derived growth factor (PDGF-β), 157
PLGA, *see* Poly(lactic-co-glycolic)acid (PLGA)
Pluripotent stem cells (PSCs), 16
PNIs, *see* Peripheral nerve injuries (PNIs)
Poly(lactic-co-glycolic)acid (PLGA), 32
Polyacrylamide (PAM), 188
Polyethylene glycol (PEG), 84, 188
Poly lactic-co-glycolic acid (PLGA), 178
Positron emission tomography (PET), 112, 131
Pro-inflammatory M1 macrophages, 106
Protocol biopsies, 49, **49**
PRRs, *see* Pattern recognition receptors (PRRs)
PSCs, *see* Pluripotent stem cells (PSCs)
P-selectin, 128
Psychosocial issues
  family and caregiver factors
    community and societal factors, 90
    family-centered care, 89–90
  individual child factors
    expectations and functionality, 89
    self-image, 89
    treatment adherence, 89
  perspectives, 86, **87–88**
Pulse wave velocity (PWV), 52

Q

Quantum dots (QDs), 111

R

Range of motion (ROM), 83
Rapamycin, 32, 174, 180
Rapamycin-loaded implants, 184–185
Reactive oxygen species (ROS), 62
Reconstructive transplantation, *see* Vascularized
  composite allotransplantation (VCA)

Regulatory dendritic cells (DCregs), 9
Regulatory T cells (Tregs)
 antigen specificity, 29
 classification and subtypes, 28
 contact-dependent and contact-independent
  mechanisms, 10
 ex vivo expansion, adoptive transfer and
  clinical trials, 35–36
 IL-2 interaction, 29–30
 immune homeostasis, *186*
 immunosuppressive drugs, 35
 lymphocytes, 9
 mechanisms, 28
 peripheral blood and allograft, 10
 recruiting microparticle systems, 32–34
 treatment, 10
 VCA, 30–32
Reperfusion injury
 introduction and mechanism, 61–62
 prevention and treatment
  adverse effects, 64
  antioxidants, 64
  blood gas analysis, 68
  brain-dead, heart-beating patients, *67*
  ex-situ perfusion, 65, 68, *69*
  ex-vivo/extracorporeal perfusion, 65
  limb chamber, *66*
  MP, 64, 65
  organ preservation solutions, 64
  swine forelimb transplantation, 65
 vascularized composite tissue allografts,
  62–63
Reticuloendothelial system, 178
Rheumatoid arthritis, 37
RNA interference (RNAi), 201
RNA-seq technologies, 126
Rodent forelimb perfusion technique, 162
ROM, *see* Range of motion (ROM)
ROS, *see* Reactive oxygen species (ROS)

S

Scaffold
 challenge, 161–162
 concept, 158–159
 revitalizing decellularized composite tissues,
  161
 strategy, 159–161
scFv, *see* Single-chain variable fragment (scFv)
Schwann cells (SCs), 102–103
Sciatic nerve myelination, 63
SDS, *see* Sodium dodecyl sulphate (SDS)
Sentinel skin flaps (SSFs), 123, 131–136, **133–135**
Silver nanoparticles (SNPs), 105, 106, 112
Single-chain variable fragment (scFv), 11
Single photon emission computed tomography
  (SPECT), 112

Single-wall carbon nanotubes (SWCNT), 110
Single-walled carbon-nanohorns (SNH), 110
Skin allograft rejection, 177–178
SNH, *see* Single-walled carbon-nanohorns
  (SNH)
SNPs, *see* Silver nanoparticles (SNPs)
Sodium dodecyl sulphate (SDS), 160
Solid organ transplantation (SOT), 4–5, 17, 18,
  28, 37, 50, 62, 173, 195
SPECT, *see* Single photon emission computed
  tomography (SPECT)
SPR, *see* Surface plasmon resonance (SPR)
SRS, *see* Stimuli responsive systems (SRS)
SSF, *see* Sentinel skin flap (SSF)
Stimuli responsive systems (SRS), 180, *181*
Substance
 challenge, 155–156
 concept, 152–154
 developmental pathway, *152*
 skin substitutes, **153**
 strategies, 154–155
Surface plasmon resonance (SPR), 111–112
SWCNT, *see* Single-wall carbon nanotubes
  (SWCNT)
Swine forelimb perfusion system, *64*
Systemic lupus erythematosus, 37

T

Tacrolimus (TAC), 7
Tacrolimus monotherapy, 85
Tacrolimus systemic therapy, 182
TBI, *see* Total body irradiation (TBI)
T cell-mediated rejection (TCMR), 124–125
T cell receptor (TCR), 29
T cells
 Ag-specific Tregs, 10–11
 CAR, 11–13
 Tregs, 9–10
T effector (Teff), 28
TGF-β1, *see* Transforming growth factor-β1
  (TGF-β1)
TGMS, *see* Triglycerolmonostrearate (TGMS)
TGMS-TAC hydrogel system, *182*
Thrombocytes, 62
Tissue bioengineering, 151
Tissue regeneration, 150
Tissue-scale acellular scaffolds, 160
TLRs, *see* Toll-like receptors (TLRs)
TNF-α, *see* Tumor necrosis factor α (TNF-α)
Toll-like receptors (TLRs), 62
Total body irradiation (TBI), 7
Tourniquet ischemia model, 63
Transaction/crushing injuries, 102
Transcription activator-like effector nuclease
  (TALEN), 197
Transcutaneous techniques, 56

Transforming growth factor-β1 (TGF-β1), 157
Transfusion-related acute lung injury, 79
Traumatic neuroma formation, 102
Treg-inducing microparticle systems, 34
Tregs, *see* Regulatory T cells (Tregs)
Triglycerolmonostrearate (TGMS), 181
TRI microparticles (TRI-MP), 34
Tumorigenicity, 105
Tumor necrosis factor α (TNF-α), 180

U

Ultrasound biomicroscopy (UBM), 50, 56, 131
United Network for Organ Sharing (UNOS),
        195

V

Vascular endothelial growth factor (VEGF),
        157, 180
Vascular flow, **51**, 52, 154
Vascularized bone marrow (VBM), 6
Vascularized composite allotransplantation
        (VCA)
    allogeneic immune response, 5
    alloimmune response, 5
    biomaterials, *see* Biomaterials
    CR, *see* Chronic rejection (CR)
    drug delivery, *see* Drug delivery
    goal, 27
    history, *172*, 172–173
    immune system, 5

    immunomodulation, 30–32
    immunotherapy and limitations,
        173–174
    localized therapy and topical creams, 174
    mixed chimerism, 6
    pioneers, *173*
    protocol and for-cause skin biopsies, **49**
    survival, 47
    tolerance induction, 6–7
    Tregs, 28
Vascularized composite tissue allografts, 62–63
Vascularized grafts, 199
Vascular sprouting, 157
Vasculopathy, 56, 62, 63
VCA, *see* Vascularized composite
        allotransplantation (VCA)
VEGF, *see* Vascular endothelial growth factor
        (VEGF)
Viral vectors, 196–197

W

Wallerian degeneration (WD), 102–103
Windkessel effect, 51

X

Xenotransplantation, 201

Z

Zinc finger nucleases (ZFNs), 197

·